THE ECOLOGY OF EARLY DEAFNESS
Guides to Fashioning Environments and
Psychological Assessments

THE ECOLOGY OF EARLY DEAFNESS

Guides to Fashioning Environments and Psychological Assessments

EDNA SIMON LEVINE

COLUMBIA UNIVERSITY PRESS
New York

Library of Congress Cataloging in Publication Data
Levine, Edna Simon
  The ecology of early deafness.

  Includes bibliographies and index.
    1. Deafness—Psychological aspects.   2. Man—
Influence of environment.   3. Human ecology.
I. Title.   [DNLM: 1. Deafness—Psychology.
2. Environment.   WV 270 L665e]
HV2395.L39   362.4'2'019   80-27138
ISBN 0-231-03886-0

Columbia University Press
New York   Guildford, Surrey

10 9 8 7 6 5 4 3 2

To
Jean Leigh
and
Mary Switzer
Of cherished memory

CONTENTS

Appendixes

AN INTRODUCTORY
COMMENT

THE QUESTION is reasonably asked, why a book concerned with deaf persons begins as this one does, with a section on environment. As a rule, the principal focus of such publications is on "problems of the deaf": problems of behavior, of rehabilitation and habilitation, of communication, research, and more. We freely admit the importance of these topics, and in fact have included them in this volume. But at the same time, we submit that there is more to people than problems, and more to behavior than appears on the surface. We submit further that this "more" is to be found in the influences that shape the human condition, whether it be deaf or nondeaf, and that are subsumed in the concept of "environment."

Environment is an elusive concept that cannot be divided into neat little informational packets for ready consumption. That it exerts influences upon behavior has long been conceded by the behavioral disciplines. But it is only in recent times that environment has emerged as a power to be reckoned with. The revelations of ecology and of disadvantaged minorities have had much to do with this development. We still do not know the dynamics that tie individual to environment, but both society and the sciences are coming to recognize the authority of the environmental imperative. The evidence is unassailable.

As a result, a remarkably steady shift is taking place from focus on the person to focus on environment. Not only is the shift gaining increasing adherents among behavioral scientists, it also has inspired the founding of specialized branches of study. Even psychology, long addicted to focusing on "the individual," is joining the move toward a clearer understanding of the person through a deeper understanding of his shaping environment.

For those of us grappling with the complexities of behavior fashioned in a soundless environment, it is likely that present understandings will be broadened by a similar move. Toward this end, the behavior-environment linkage is examined in the beginning chapters of this book, including the behavioral impact of acoustically impaired environments.

The focus of discussion then moves to the target populations of the volume—the deaf population; and to the issues, deficits, options and conflicts commonly found in "deaf" environments. What emerges from the review is the startling match between deficits usual to such environments and deficits common to many of the occupants.

The implications of this phenomenon are carried over into the second major part of the book, which deals with psychological examination and assessment. To prepare the ground, brief orientative sections provide a historical scan of psychology and the deaf, the competencies required of psychologists to the deaf, and the nature and rationale of the four basic techniques of psychological examining—the case history, testing, observation, and interview.

Guides are then offered to help psychological examiners through some of the difficulties of applying these techniques to a deaf clientele. Separate chapters deal with their use at three age levels—infancy, school-age and youth, and adult. For each level, strengths and weaknesses of the techniques are summarized, special strategies suggested, instruments listed, and problems noted. To flesh out and humanize the guides, illustrations and anecdotes from life are included here and there in the discussion.

In fact, throughout the book, I have reached out to those directly involved in the deaf experience—to deaf persons and to parents of deaf children—for anecdotal material, for quoted or directly expressed views, for their experiences and reactions, and finally for the Epilogue to this book in order to bring its contents as well as the reader closer to the realities of being deaf. An effort has also been made to present both sides of debated issues insofar as space and available materials permit, with the special aim of challenging the reader's independent deliberations and decision-reaching.

Efforts have also been made to disclose the backgrounds of some of the current "innovations" in habilitation and education, whose roots often reach far back in history. It is this sort of knowledge that distinguishes scholar from technician and stimulates researchers to move forward instead of blindly rediscovering the past or statically focusing on the known or the obvious.

A strong implication emerging from this book is that the psychological examination is, as often as not, an assessment of a deaf individual's shaping environment as much as of the individual per se. The guiding thought is that an environmentally expanded frame of reference will give greater scope to those who serve deaf persons to follow unexplored paths of inquiry, acquire the sensitivities to perceive new relationships, clear up mysteries that have hitherto gone unsolved, and, above all, to recognize their own unique position as "environmental influences" in the lives of deaf individuals and as powerful advocates for improvement and reform in the environments that fashion deaf persons.

Part One
THE ENVIRONMENTAL IMPERATIVE: A PROLOGUE

1 An Ecological Perspective

We come into the world as a bundle of possibilities bequeathed to us by our parents and other ancestors. Our nurture comes from the world about us.

Dunn and Dobzhansky, *Heredity, Race, and Society*

MOUNTING ALARM over the fate of humans in ravaged environments has generated an unprecedented burst of inquiry into the relationship between man and milieu. The focus of the biological sciences is on the forces that maintain the human animal in a state of balanced give-and-take with the natural environment and its other occupants. Of major concern to the behavioral and the social sciences is adaptation to the distinctive human environments that house mankind. What are the cohesive forces that link human environments and human beings? What are the dynamics of interplay?

The multidisciplinary meeting ground for such issues is the evolving discipline of human ecology (Ehrlich, Ehrlich, and Holdren, 1972; Hawley, 1950; Meadows et al., 1972). Although diverse views still require synthesis into integrated theory, there are numbers of premises on which the disciplines see eye to eye. The one of central importance to this volume is behaviorally oriented. It involves the cycle of deficits in which impaired human environments lead to impaired psychological environments; impaired psychological environments to disturbed human behavior; and disturbed human behavior back again to the cycle of deficits but with magnified impact. The problem of survival in ravaged natural environments is matched by the problem of survival in impaired psychological environments.

Most disciplines in the sciences and humanities are taking ecology's warnings to heart. Even psychology, long a lip-service advocate of "the influences of environment," is coming to acknowledge the power of the environmental imperative (Maloney and Ward, 1973; T. Miller, 1974; Schaar, 1976). In turning to ecology for leads, the disciplines are experiencing an entirely novel view of humankind's place in nature's scheme of things.

The intricate details of ecological theory are documented in the literature (e.g., Odum, 1971; Winton, 1972). Simply expressed, ecology views *Home sapiens* as simply another life-form, subject to the same laws of survival that hold for all life-forms and that involve such tight reciprocal ties to environmental inputs and ecological checks and balances that "man, like all other living creatures, is both part and product of his own environment" (Caldwell, 1971, p. 25).

The shift in perspective from the person as a more or less independent unit to the person as a part of environment is not easy to grasp. It is even more difficult to apply, particularly for specialists in human service and above all for those who work with the physically disabled. In the latter case, the observed environment of the disabled appears precisely the same as of the nondisabled. It takes a deliberate effort of the imagination to visualize the environmental havoc a physical disability can create: the featureless world of the blind; the soundless world of the deaf; the distorted world of the crippled, shrunk to the limitations of physical deformity. The only visible analogues of these environmental distortions are the behavior deficits the disabled individual may display. In consequence, these seemingly independent human units convey the impression of being responsible for their own problems. "Blaming the victim" is the way Ryan puts it (1971). The disabled environment that houses the "victim," shapes his behavior, and spawns its deficits remains unseen.

The shift in perspective from individual to environment introduces other issues in human service. Now that environment has become known as a force to be reckoned with, bothersome questions begin to arise for service specialists in all disciplines. For example: How feasible is it to treat maladjusted individuals while ignoring their sick environment? Wherein lies the greater promise for sweeping human adjustment, with rehabilitating clients or with rehabilitating society? Is taking action to eradicate the social conditions that breed disablement appropriate to the goals and functions of rehabilitation? Gellman (1973) calls particular attention to this last question as a growing issue in rehabilitation. The question leads to another: Is taking action to eliminate educational conditions that breed scholastic failure appropriate to the goals and functions of habilitation?

Difficulties in applying new concepts to old problems can be enormous. As Caldwell remarks, "To look at familiar things from an unfamiliar point of view is always a difficult and troublesome experience" (1971, p. 2). It is particularly so when the new knowledge needed for new answers is still in short supply. But, using the field of the deaf as an example, the difficulties can be no greater than the frustrations of looking at the same familiar problems decade after decade, from the same point of view, and finding nothing ahead but the same familiar obstacles to their solution. With this in mind, the concept, "environment" is examined here as an introduction to the environments that shape the behaviors and problems of deaf persons.

Background

The concept of mankind as a product of environment is not new. Dubos (1968) reminds us that it goes back some 2,500 years to the Greek physician-philosopher Hippocrates, who vigorously endorsed the view. The belief was carried over the centuries in the writings of various visionary philosophers and theorists, and acquired prominence when its advocates clashed head on with the social Darwinists of the nineteenth century over the relative importance of heredity and environment as shapers of human behavior.

The ensuing nature–nurture controversy (Hogben, 1933; Pastore, 1949) ushered in a period of intense activity on the part of psychologists of the 1920s and 1930s. The focus was on mental ability; the key issue was whether heredity or environment determined level of intelligence; and the instruments of investigation were chiefly mental tests (Schieffelin and Schwesinger, 1930). Evidence on the issues was gathered mainly from two types of studies: one focusing on genetically related children (twins and siblings) reared in different environments; the other, on unrelated children reared together in common environments. Studies were also conducted with children whose parents came from different occupational and economic levels, and with subjects of different racial and national origins.

The investigations led to no definitive conclusion. Except for a few diehards, psychologists generally acknowledged that heredity and environment operate together as determinants of mental ability. Emphasizing the importance of environmental influences were Freeman and his associates (Freeman, 1934); stressing the importance of heredity were Burks and her co-workers (Burks, 1928). Shuttleworth (1935) tried to break the seeming stalemate by establishing what percentage of a person's mental ability is hereditarily determined, and what percentage environmentally determined. The effort yielded no valid results, hence no determination.

Time, ecological devastation, and the socioeconomically disadvantaged accomplished what Shuttleworth's statistical approach failed to do; that is, to provide clear evidence of the power (if not the exact proportion) of environmental influence in shaping the human condition, as demonstrated in life and in research (Bloom, Davis, and Hess, 1965; Margolin and Goldin, 1969). Victims of environmental deprivation became dramatic advocates for psychological environmentalists, and inspired a new surge of inquiry into human adaptation and environment–behavior interplay.

This development did not end the nature–nurture controversy—debate continues to this day (Gage, 1972; Jensen, 1969, 1972; D. Miller, 1978;

Shockley, 1972). Nor did it still the voices of genetically oriented behavior investigators. Their arguments against the growing trend toward a purely environmental psychology found a forum in a relatively new specialty, behavior genetics (Fuller and Thompson, 1960). As the name implies, the broad aim of behavior genetics is to track down the genetic roots of behavior traits and variations. However, some consider it a loosely organized field of study that has not yet firmed up its goals or investigative approaches. As Vale remarks, it is rather in the position of a "genetical gadfly about the head of a recalcitrant environmental psychology" (1973, p. 880). Nevertheless, it is a gadfly to be reckoned with.

In the course of this new surge of inquiry into environment–behavior dynamics, the question inevitably arose: What is environment? Research attempted an answer by way of experimental studies of various environmental isolates such as light, heat, sound, and other physical components (Environmental Abstracts, 1965), and of single responding behavior variables (Sells, 1963). The studies supplied interesting information about the isolates, but little about environment. As far as behavioral scientists were concerned, environment remained a dim, amorphous influence that eluded conceptualization and evaded management. Psychologists seized, therefore, upon the more tangible object in the environment–behavior dyad, namely, the individual, with psychological tests rather than environmental influences serving as the major guide to behavioral insights, predictions, and change—and this despite the weaknesses of the practice (Bersoff, 1973; Cronbach, 1975). In this context, the individual amounts to little more than a receptacle for behavior traits and personality patterns. As for environment, it was accorded passing recognition as a contributor to the human condition, but for all practical purposes, it remained—and still remains—the "neglected child of psychological assessment" (T. Miller, 1974).

The impotence of the individual/test formula was borne in upon psychology when the increasing numbers of humans in need, in poverty and disability, in degraded environments, and in mutiny and despair overflowed the boundaries of its traditional percepts and procedures. Obviously, for psychology to carry out its professional role in the midst of a techno-cultural revolution demanded new perspectives; old boundaries had to be stretched to accommodate new problems; outmoded rituals, scrapped. Propelled in part by this realization and in part by mounting ecological evidence that degraded physical environments mean degraded psychological environments, psychology at last began its move into the mysteries of environment (Craik, 1973; Wohwill, 1970).

Here it finds itself in the company of many other disciplines, all equally concerned with mankind's fate in a world in chaos and all engaged in examining the dynamics of interplay between human behavior and human environment. Although differing in approach and perspective, they stand in basic agreement that people "cannot achieve and maintain physical and mental health if conditions are not suitable for environmental health" (Dubos, 1968, p. 165), and are joined by a common hope of contributing to a determination of what environmental health is and how to achieve it (Caldwell, 1971).

That hope is only in the early stages of realization. For one thing, most if not all the disciplines involved are still struggling to conceptualize and assess environment. For another, there is as yet no significant amount of interdisciplinary coupling for a joint approach to key issues. Each specialty tends to pursue an independent line of inquiry, guided by its own concerns, percepts, and procedures. But as findings emerge, there is a striking convergence of evidence concerning the power of the human environment to influence human behavior.

Illustrative Evidence and Theory

The path of inquiry into what is commonly thought of as "the" environment leads into a maze of complex, dynamically interrelated "co-environments." Roughly grouped, these co-environments may be conceptualized as: (1) the natural environment, including geography, topography, climate, atmospheric conditions, and weather patterns; (2) the man-made physical environment of architecture, technology, heating, lighting, ventilation, interior decoration, special settings, etc.; and (3) the sociocultural environment, including cultural patterns and mores, controlling societal institutions, and personal, interpersonal, group, and societal behavior and interactions. Sketchy though these groupings are, they nevertheless hint at the vast dimensions of environmental research.

The effects on human behavior of selected variables in each of these categories provide the focus for numerous investigations (Insel and Moos, 1974; Moos, 1973). The cumulative findings confirm that behavior is sensitive to a wide assortment of environmental influences. For example, among the components of the natural environment, meteorological influences (Muescher and Ungeheuer, 1961), atmospheric conditions (Sells, Findikyan, and Duke, 1966), and climate have been associated with variations in behavior. In the man-made physical environment, numbers of variables including architecture, physical design, interior decoration, and types of settings have been found to influence behavior (Wohwill and Carson, 1972; Proshansky, 1976). With the broadened realization among environmental researchers that the human members of a setting are also contributors to its characteristics, this research is moving into the social and psychological ecology of human environments (Gibbs, 1979; Rogers-Warren and Warren, 1977; Wicker, 1979), despite many methodological difficulties (Bronfenbrenner, 1976).

Ecological Psychology Theory

A unique example of eco-psychological research is the work of Barker (1968) and his associates. They focused on the texture of the human environment, theorizing that human environmental settings possess behavioral as well as physical properties, the former derived from the behavior of the occupying groups. The concept is in line with ecological theory which, as noted, regards the human organism, its behavior, and its setting as composing an ecological unit. Accordingly Barker calls this school of psychology "ecological psychology."

Among the questions of concern to ecological psychology are: "What are environments like? How does man's habitat differ, for example, in developed and developing countries, in large and small schools, in glass-walled and windowless office buildings, in integrated and segregated classes? How do environments select and shape the people who inhabit them? What are the structural and dynamic properties of the environments to which people must adapt?" (Barker, 1968, pp. 3–4).

Answers to such questions obviously require access to real-life rather than laboratory settings, and such were the units selected for study. Termed "behavior settings" by the investigators, they consisted of a standing pattern of group behavior bounded by a nonbehavioral physico-temporal configuration termed the "milieu." The milieus used in the investigation were ordinary community locales such as drugstores, barbershops, various kinds of professional offices, recreation centers, and many other community sites common to a small town in Kansas, which served as the research "laboratory." In order for these milieus to qualify as behavior settings, they had to meet a number of structural and dynamic criteria laid down by the investigators, involving not only the milieu but also the patterns of behavior encompassed.

In all, several hundred categories of behavior setting were assessed and classified for both nonbehavioral properties and the related behavior patterns of the occupying groups. Of these, 220 were selected as the researched units. From the findings obtained, the investigators made the startling discovery that it was possible to "predict some aspects of children's behavior more adequately from knowledge of the behavior characteristics of the drugstores, arithmetic classes, and basket-ball games they inhabited than from knowledge of the behavior tendencies of the particular children" (Barker, 1968, p. 4). Similar trends have been reported by other investigators, as cited by Insel and Moos (1974).

Based on findings such as these, evolving eco-behavioral theory postulates that behavior and environment are not independent entities. Rather, organism and environment are reciprocally influencing systems, both of which, in the words of Brunswik, are "hewn basically from the same block" (1957, p. 5). The concept can be summed up as follows:

> The individual and his environment, equally physical (or "geographical") and social, although treated as two separate realities for discussion in fact are one. A person and his context and actions as well as a people and its environment, had best be seen as indivisible. . . . The holistic viewpoint envisions each individual acting in perpetual coordination with his fellows, and all of them in like manner interacting with their surroundings. (Wagner, 1972, p. 100)

Cultural Patterning Theory

Support for Wagner's statement comes from a variety of disciplinary investigations of behavior–environment interplay, even studies radically different from the eco-psychological approach. An example is the cultural patterning approach in which data are compiled from studies of mankind through time as obtained from anthropology, archeology, ethnology and ethnography, linguistics, cross-cultural studies, and to a lesser extent from the behavioral sciences. From these perspectives, it becomes possible to trace the unfolding story of the creation of man-made environments, and of the individual's inextricable relationship to them.

Simeons scans the making of one such environment in the following sweep of technological accomplishment achieved by puny humans in their determination to outwit the forces of nature as well as their own physical limitations:

> First [man's "presumptuous brain"] replaced body hair by the warmth of fire and later skins, clothing, and shelter. It extended the range and strength of man's arms with spears, clubs, and stones which in due course of time led to the blow-pipe, the dart, the boomerang, the bow and arrow, and finally to firearms. Muscular strength was increased by the invention of the lever, the wheel, the pulley, and then by engines driven by water, wind, and later steam, electricity, oil, and nuclear fission and by such appliances as cranes, pile drivers, steamrollers, and bulldozers. . . . Timid man must always have envied the horse for its speed. Having no hope of ever being able to compete with it on a biological level, he brilliantly did the next best thing, which was to catch the horse, tame it and climb on its back. When mere horse-muscles became too slow and inconveniently in need of rest and food, man, ever impatient and on the run, invented mechanical transport. . . . Being a strictly ground-bound creature, he mastered water with ships, submarines, and diving equipment. He took to the air first in balloon, then in aircraft, and is now reaching into space . . . trying to get closer to the infinity he will never reach. (1961, pp. 73–74)

With the invention of technological paraphernalia, the natural environment gradually gave way to a technological environment. As this happened, adaptive demands shifted from those laid down by nature to those imposed by humans.

Another of the man-made environments to impose its particular adaptive demands is the societal environment. In the climb toward civilization, *Homo sapiens* progressed over the millennia from life as a nomadic hunter and food-gatherer subject to the whims and hazards of nature to life as a food cultivator living in a settled community along with the farm animals he had succeeded in domesticating. As can readily be inferred, life in settled groups necessitated reciprocal obligations among the members, division of work, and cooperative activities. These were facilitated through continuing developments in man's most brilliant invention of all time—a mutually understood verbal language for interpersonal communication and for establishing accepted practices of group living. The climax of this long process is referred to by anthropologists as the Neolithic Revolution. It opened the door to societal concepts in human thinking, relations, and adaptations.

Finally, the pattern of communal living fostered the development of yet another distinctively human environment: the psychosocial environment. In order to conform to the dictates of the communal order, people had to learn to live with one another on a broader and more intimate scale than they had yet experienced. When this requirement entered the picture, so did an environment derived from the processes, reactions, confrontations, and defenses of interacting humans and groups of humans. The psyche flowered, and man became a psychological creature subject to the pressures and demands of a psychological environment.

In the course of creating these various environments, humankind had gathered unto itself a wealth of wisdom in the form of information, experience, know-how; communicative codes and modes; technological aids; patterns of societal organization; principles, ideals, religions; attitudes, habits, standards; in short a whole panorama of tested experiences, beliefs, and practices which had served for survival and advance. This was the rich cultural heritage transmitted to succeeding generations through teaching/learning processes for lack of genetic programming. Of this circumstance, it has been said that every one of us has "inherited" the wisdom of people whom we have never met in the flesh. Or in the words of an unknown Chinese sage: "I am one, but I am made up of many."

Looking back in time, the natural environment so much feared by our ancestors of prehistory fades into insignificance before the awesome complexity of the cultural environment in which we do our living, from which we derive developmental, cognitive, and affective sustenance, and which, in advanced societies, is woven from intricate culture patterns, involved societal practices, incredible technologies, and the press and pull of a wide assortment of behavior-influencing humans.

According to cultural patterning theory, people are doubly bound to this environment. They have poured much of themselves into its making. They are therefore part of it. But insofar as their own making is derived from its input, they are also its products. And as its product, the human personality is a complex "in which the emotional responses and cognitive capacities [are] programmed in accordance with the overall design or configuration of [the] culture" (LeVine, 1973, p. 53). Goodman expands on the theory: "Biology sets the basic processes of *how* man learns, but culture as the transmitted experience of preceding generations, very largely determines *what* man learns" (1967, p. 61); and it is the biogenetically and psychically mediated internalization of what man learns that is reflected in his "modes of thought, his perceptual and conceptual habits, his motor skills, gestures, and his emotional responses" (1967, p. 177). In short, the individual is a microcosm of the fashioning cultural and immediate environments.

No matter how diverse the investigative approaches to the puzzle of man and milieu, all seem to be heading toward the same conclusion: the environments so ingeniously fashioned by the human occupants are in the end the manipulators of their own fashioning.

Man–Milieu: Communicative Language-Links

The link that makes reciprocal interaction at all possible between the individual and the milieu is subsumed in the concept of "communication." By reason of this linkage-role, communication acquires the status of a life-support system. Without communication, there would be no man–milieu interplay; and without such interplay, no life.

This key role of communication is not usually recognized, buried as the concept is under an avalanche of multiple meanings, theories, and countless fragmenting investigations into its parts and processes. In the welter of issues, the behavior of humans as communicating organisms has hardly been touched by theorists. Ruesch, for example, complains that "in developing an overall theory of communication, the greatest need at present revolves around the inclusion of communicating persons" (1964, p. 255). In a similar vein, George Miller voices the impression that "some communication theorists regard the human link in communication systems in much the same way they regard random noise. Both are unfortunate disturbances in an otherwise well-behaved system and both should be reduced until they do as little harm as possible" (1967, p. 45).

The track along which communication moves in joining individual to milieu is subsumed in the concept of "language," the most ingenious of which, the verbal form, was invented by the same "human link" that seems such an annoyance to theorists. Little did humans of prehistory suspect, when they invented the word, that they were at the same time sowing seeds of query and debate that are flourishing to this day. Over the centuries, scholars have pondered such questions as: How were words created? Why is it that all people everywhere do not speak the same language? Why are certain things called by one name and not another? Out of these questions came others. One of the most provocative is still: What is language? From this we plunge into such issues as: What are the roads from thought to words? Which were first, the language patterns or the cultural patterns? Does the structure of a given language affect the thoughts, the memory, the perception, the learning ability of those who speak that language? And crisscrossing these and many other unresolved questions are numerous lines of inquiry into the structure and universals of language, its morphology, syntax, phonology, and semantics.

Putting aside these distractingly provocative issues makes it possible to perceive the basic reason why all life forms have communicative mechanisms: communication is essential for life and survival. Toward these ends, every living species possesses its own species-specific bio-communicative structures and "languages" for effecting information exchange with its habitual life environment.

For example at the low end of the phylogenetic scale we find the single-celled amoeba. Tiny and undifferentiated though this protoplasmic mass is, it is nevertheless programmed for survival through communication. Put a poisonous element in its surrounding fluid, and the amoeba responds by thrusting out pseudopods and running for life. But if the element is food, the amoeba responds by approach. Survival messages in these species are transmitted through simple chemical lines of communication. They suffice for the limited information needs of such elementary life forms.

As we progress up the evolutionary scale, communicative linkages joining organism and environment become increasingly complex with the increased needs of the more elaborate biological species for greater amounts and varieties of environmental signals, more diverse and effective response mechanisms, and more rapid information processing systems. When we reach the level of *Homo sapiens,* we reach the apex of bio-communicative engineering. Here the need is for a communication system of sufficient versatility and flexibility to enable humans to adapt to the many natural environments they inhabit throughout the earth as well as to the man-made environments of their own creation.

Preparation for managing this heavy load of communicative traffic begins with the individual's first environment—the intrauterine milieu. Evidence that communicative activity takes place before birth is amply documented in the literature, particularly in Gesell's classic studies which demonstrated that "behavior development is already underway at a post-conception age of eight weeks, when the fetus is a scant inch in length'' (Gesell and Ama-truda, 1947, p. 299).

Greene (1958) suggests that fetal environment includes not only the physical enclosure of the womb but also the intrauterine ''languages'' of the mother's body in the form of signals emanating from sounds, pressures, and vibrations coming from the mother's vascular pulses. Messages from these sources are received by the fetus, and the bits of behavior noted by Gesell and Amatruda are, in Greene's view, among the adaptive responses the fetus makes to its environment.

A provocative hypothesis is proposed by Moore and Shiek (1971) concerning fetuses with inherited high potential for intellectual superiority. The investigators believe that such fetuses are developmentally ready for a broader range of communicative input than is afforded by the sensorially limited environment of the uterus. They ask: ''Given a fetus with a brain in an advanced state of developmental readiness for stimulation, but residing within a restricted uterine environment, what should be the possible results?'' (1971, p. 454). They see the results as early infantile autism resulting from intrauterine environmental deprivation. Their hypothesis is reinforced by compelling comparisons between the intrauterine and postnatal behaviors of such infants. The investigators regard intrauterine influence as constituting a ''prenatal *psychological* environment'' (1971, p. 453) in which environmental influence on the fashioning of behavior is strikingly demonstrated.

Montagu views the infant's earliest communicative experience with the mother's body as constituting ''his first language'' (1971, p. 110). The use of ''language'' in this sense will undoubtedly raise the eyebrows of linguistic purists. The classic linguistic concept of language is a system of arbitrary conventional symbols which are primarily vocal and produced by the organs of speech (Hartmann and Stork, 1972; Pei, 1966; Pei and Gaynor, 1954).

This concept makes language essentially a verbal system, which would rule out such nonverbal forms of human communication as the whistle-talk of the Mazateco (Cowan, 1948), the drum language of primitive peoples (Frobenius, 1960), the body language of everyday communication (Fast, 1970), and the sign language of the deaf (Stokoe, 1960). However, concepts vary even among linguists. A dissenting view is expressed by the same Pei who contributed to the classic concept cited above. He states, ''In their anxiety to restrict language to a pattern of sounds, too many linguists have forgotten that the sound-symbols of the spoken tongue are neither more nor less symbolical of human thought and human meaning than the various forms of activity (gestural, pictorial, ideographic, even artistic) by which men have conveyed significant messages to one another since the dawn of history'' (Pei, 1949, p. 10).

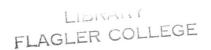

In my view, language is linked to *lingua,* the tongue, only in the etymological sense. The real seat of language is the mind. Further, the phylogenetic function of language is not in the service of human discourse; it is in the service of species' survival. In this frame, language includes all modes of expression used by humankind in effecting reciprocal communicative relations with their various life environments. It is in this sense that the term "language" is used here.

From a first communicative experience by way of the "languages" of the mother's body, the individual gradually advances in the course of time and maturation into a complex of human interaction settings, each with its characteristic patterns of language usage. The settings, as described by Ruesch and Kees (1956), include the intrapersonal, the interpersonal, the group, and the societal. The intrapersonal (or intrapsychic) setting is one in which individuals do their private thinking and ruminating. The interpersonal setting is generated by two interacting humans and the ways in which their distinctive traits mesh. In the next-broader setting the individual functions as a member of a group made up of several or many persons known to one another, each of whom occupies a specialized place in the group network. Finally there is the societal setting, created by the edicts of a society's controlling institutions and cultural mores, in which individual identity is lost and communication is an interaction of large bodies of persons.

To add to the communicative complexity, individuals in real life do not ordinarily function in just one setting at a time, but usually in several settings at the same time. A simple illustration is two people chatting at a party. The persons involved are thinking their own private thoughts (intrapersonal system) while at the same time conversing on other matters (interpersonal system), in the context of party distractions (group system), which in turn are imbedded in a sociocultural matrix (societal system). In such coexisting settings, communicative shifts are in constant operation, as are the languages of communication. Argyle (1967) reviews some of the languages of social encounter. In addition to spoken language, they include a wide variety of *nonverbal* forms: physical proximity and position (proxemics); bodily contacts; gestures; body movements and orientations (kinesics); facial expression; eye movements and glance; nonlinguistic aspects of speech such as intonation, rate, hesitation. Argyle also notes another important message conveyor in the language of behavior—its style, technique, strategies—all of which convey a particular message about the performing human.

How do such nonverbal forms acquire their distinctive meanings in a given society? Most are *learned* in much the same way as the meanings of linguistic forms, through exposure and experience. When they cannot be learned in this natural way, they must be taught in planned ways; because fitting comfortably into human interaction environments demands knowing all language-links of human encounter, the nonverbal equally with the verbal.

Scientific interest in the impact of nonverbal communication is rising at an extraordinary rate. Among the foremost contributors to the growing body of data are Ekman, Friesen, and their co-workers at the Laboratory of Human Interaction and Conflict at the University of California (Ekman, 1965; Ekman and Friesen, 1969). Studies of nonverbal behavior in psychopathological conditions are also receiving increased attention, thanks in part to the work of Ekman and Friesen (1974), Ostwald (1963, 1977), and the exceptional contributions of Ruesch (1957).

Goodman offers a cultural frame for studies on nonverbal communication. She observes:

> The survival of a human society and its way of life is heavily dependent upon interpersonal and intergenerational communication. . . . While the spoken and/or written language is perhaps the most obvious example of a system of expressive symbolism, there is in any culture a wealth of symbols of quite different sorts. Consider the "language" of gesture, facial expression, or posture, and how much can be communicated by a smile, a glance, a handclasp. Or think of the significance of such ubiquitous symbols as the flag, the national anthem, or national rituals. . . . Religious rituals have more explicit symbolic value, as do some of the more conventionalized art forms. The individual's clothing, house and other personal possessions speak more or less loudly to the initiated observer about the status of the owner. So too do his culturally patterned activities. (1967, pp. 44–45)

Goodman's phrase "the initiated observer" warrants particular attention since it introduces a crucial aspect of communication that is not generally noted in linguistic studies. Effective communication depends not only on a shared knowledge of the expressive symbolism of a given society but more particularly on shared familiarity with the habits, values, and mores of that culture. Without such familiarity, individuals from different cultures may speak the same linguistic idiom, but they do not necessarily speak the same language (Rudofsky, 1966). Linton calls cross-cultural consonance the ability to "think native," as applied to anthropologists living in a "primitive" society (1945, p. 101); Sussman calls it the ability to "think deaf," as applied to psychological workers with deaf persons (Levine, 1977).

Finally, Funk offers the following overview of everyday nonverbal symbols of human communication:

> We have so many ways of expressing ourselves without words. School bells and church bells call us to exercises, whistles remind us of factory hours or warn us of the danger from trains. Human whistles can command a dog or express surprise or invite a girl. Red lights and green lights say stop and go. There's a

white flag for surrender, a yellow flag for disease, a red one for danger. The nod or shake of a head is eloquent of yes and no. A raised hand asks attention, or in baseball, the spread and lowered hands of the umpire say safe. There are the applauding hands of approval and the stamping feet of impatience. A crossed finger can be a wish for luck. A wink almost anything you wish. And a thumb could be a request for a ride, or, properly applied to the nose, a dramatic gesture of derision. (1950, p. 5)

To sum up, the nonverbal and nonvocal languages of human communication are as essential as the linguistic components in linking mankind to environment. They perform a communicative function in their own right and supplement linguistic expression by extending its semantic range and giving its distinctive tone.

Semantics of Communicative Sounds

Largely overshadowed by the linguistics of communication are the meanings of communicating sounds. Many are contained in the music of the voice. In the absence of hearing, they and their generally unrecognized psychological impacts and values are powerless to perform their intended communicative functions. This section highlights some of these functions and, by inference, the voids created by their absence. This is more than an academic exercise. It touches the very heart of rehabilitation for the deaf. In rehabilitation theory, where an impaired function exists, compensations must be provided that are as closely equivalent as possible in purpose and service to those of the unimpaired function. But when we apply this concept to the habilitation of deaf children, we find ourselves faced with a knotty question: What *is* the function of hearing in human development and adjustment?

Thoughtful deliberation on the question leads to the realization that to provide full compensation for deafness requires knowing more than its manifest problems. It requires knowing what psychological benefits children who hear gain from the sounds around them that a child who cannot hear loses. *The psychological benefits bestowed by hearing are the corresponding needs imposed by deafness.* To provide a deaf child with these same benefits obviously requires knowing what they are. This is the logical point of departure. The problem is that departure is a very difficult operation. In respect to hearing, much has been written on the exquisite mechanism that makes hearing possible, but little if anything has been said on what hearing itself makes possible. In a similar vein, the literature is rich in studies of the acoustic properties of sound, but its psychological properties are hardly noticed. Yet unless they are brought to the surface and examined, their habilitative significance goes unrecognized.

It would be a Herculean task to fill the gaps in knowledge of the psychology of hearing. Here, on a more modest scale, we examine the psychological correlates of a small sample of sound-families, to illustrate something of what is missing from a human environment when they cannot be heard. For easier discussion, the sound-families are arbitrarily divided into factual-informative, affective, and self-perceptive groupings.

Factual-Informative Sounds

These are the sounds whose major semantic function is to convey fact. They are illustrated under three headings: verbal-informative, vocal informative, and nonvocal informative.

Verbal-informative. To convey fact through the spoken word is probably the most obvious and familiar function of sound. For small children, verbal sounds provide the first foothold into their cultural heritage and into the large bodies of knowledge they will need for maturation and adaptation. First through the spoken tongue, later supplemented by its written derivative, children learn facts on countless subjects ranging from things, places, peoples, and events to social customs, institutions, attitudes, prohibitions. They can go back in time to the great events of the past, and forward in imagination to the even greater possibilities of the future. They exchange views with their fellows and learn how others think and feel. They learn to understand behaviors and interpret happenings. They gain insights and form judgments, and all through the sounds of the spoken word. In short, the factual-informative inputs conveyed through sound represent key links in the chain of information that unites a child with the cultural milieu and an adult with the societal environment.

Vocal-informative. Conveying factual information is not limited to sounds encoded in words. Often it is not the word that informs but rather the tones in which it is uttered. Vocal intonations, inflections, stress, modulation, phrasing, timing—the musical elements of the voice—are all informers in their own right. The intonational features of spoken language have commanded the attention of numbers of linguists (Bolinger, 1964; Lieberman, 1967; Pike, 1945; Rommetveit, 1968; Schubiger, n.d.). The challenge can be inferred from Pike's statement:

> An extraordinary characteristic of intonations is the tremendous connotative power of their elusive meanings. One might hastily and erroneously assume that forms which change so rapidly and automatically could not be semantically potent. Actually, we often react more violently to the intonational meanings than to the lexical ones; if a man's tone of voice belies his words, we immediately assume that the intonation more faithfully reflects his true linguistic intentions. (1945, p. 22)

In addition to straightforward fact, inferential messages are also conveyed through vocal tones, as amusingly described by Connor:

The invitation or command, "Come in and sit down" seems simple and straightforward. But any husband can tell you that the speaker may mean, "I've called you twice and you haven't even answered me and supper is getting cold and we will be late again because you have to shave yet and you always make us late wherever we go and tonight of all nights I wish you would be on time because this is the first invitation I've ever got from Mrs. Morris and if we're late she'll never invite us again and so on and so on and so on." (1961, p. 52)

Sound also opens up wide avenues of factual information by way of the voice alone, quite divorced from verbal content. "We express not only fear, desire, and approval but many other states too when we click the tongue against the roof of the mouth (mild disapproval or reproach), hiss (strong disapproval), cut short a yawn (boredom of sleepiness corrected by regard for other people's feelings), expel the breath with a whistling sound (surprise), inhale with a somewhat osculatory effect (the last is self-explanatory)" (Schlauch, 1955, p. 7). The list of factual information conveyed by the voice-without-words could be extended indefinitely. To one who hears, each informative vocal sound conveys a factual message, and what is more, a message whose meaning is fairly well standardized within the culture and, in many instances, can even surmount foreign-language barriers.

Nonvocal-informative. Sound also conveys important factual messages from nonvocal sources. Among the most important are sounds that inform for the purpose of protection, such as traffic whistles, the fire alarm, the burgler alarm, the automobile horn, a siren, and, in the case of job protection, the alarm clock. Schlauch notes the variety of informative sounds conveyed by bells alone: "A bell which rings a certain number of times will announce to students a change of classes, to workers, a shift in jobs, to persons on a party wire of a telephone, summons to conversation with a friend. The bells on shipboard are highly conventionalized signals marking the passage of a day of maritime work. . . . The dirge of a funeral and the chimes of a wedding bell tell a whole story without words" (1955, p. 7).

Finally, a steady stream of information is continually relayed to us through sounds-at-large that come from our surroundings. Sounds from the street, from other parts of the house, sounds in our own room, all blend into an informative pattern that gives us a feeling of unity with our immediate world and of psychological security in it. Even when alone, we are neither isolated nor estranged, for we are never farther away than the sounds around us. We can rest secure in the knowledge that changes in sound will automatically alert us to changes in events. We can count on the sounds we hear not only to keep us in touch, but to keep us informed.

Affective Sounds

Emotional development is stimulated and emotional tonicity sustained through affective sounds. Their semantic appeal begins in early infancy with the cooing of a mother to her baby, and continues throughout life. The range of emotionally stirring messages transmitted through affective sounds is easily as broad as that conveying fact, and perhaps broader. Included are sounds of all kinds, both vocal and nonvocal, and in all varieties of emotional appeal from the pathetic whimper of a puppy to the stirring cadences of a symphony. Verbal elements are generally of minor importance in such sound. When present, their role is secondary to their tonal qualities.

Research on the communication of emotional meaning through vocal sounds, while still limited, has yielded some provocative findings. A chief problem of such research is to isolate the tones of the voice from verbal anchorage. Davitz (1964) cites a number of studies that bypass the problem, some by using neutral verbal elements such as the alphabet, and others by using filtered speech. "Regardless of the techniques used, all studies of adults thus far reported in the literature agree that emotional meanings can be communicated accurately by vocal expression" (Davitz, 1964, p. 23).

Several attempts have been made to judge various personal characteristics of a speaker through nonverbal vocal expression. In one of the earliest, according to Ostwald (1963), Pear (1931) investigated the responses of several thousand radio listeners of the BBC in England and Cantril and Allport (1935) repeated the work in the United States; it was found "that a speaker's nonverbal sound-making reveals reliable information about age, occupation, and appearance, [and] is occasionally helpful for evaluating personality attributes like extraversion and dominance" (Ostwald, 1963, p. 51). Starkweather (1961) reports an investigation along somewhat similar lines using nonverbal vocal sounds as cues in making judgments of personality and sensitivity to human feeling. He found that nonverbal vocal sounds appear valuable in predicting sound-makers' responses on projective tests and as indicators of strong, momentary emotional states (1961, p. 72). In the psychiatric area, Ostwald studied the vocal patterns of patients with psychopathological disorders, and urgently recommended a more active "search for correlation between acoustical and behavioral variables" (1963, p. 157) as an important aid in psychiatric diagnosis and treatment.

Hoggart concisely assesses the evidence on the role of the voice in communicating feeling: "It is easy to see that tone is more important than the dictionary-meaning of the words we use" (1972, p. 14). In a more poetic vein, Robson elaborates, "The mind's ear perpetually detects, discriminates, and perceives patterns of intensity or tone whenever the air moves in winds and whispers, in speech or music, in cries, chimes, storms, in the waves of the seas, or in the murmurs and pulse of cities" (1959, p. 85).

The various affective sounds noted in the preceding discussion are just a few of the kinds of affective sounds that stir persons to feeling. Pierce and David declare in wonder, "That our auditory senses can interpret all this is more marvelous still" (1958, p. 19). Some further examples of affective input through sound are grouped below into empathetic, persuasive, and esthetic sound families.

Empathetic sounds. These are the sounds whose emotional appeal tends to induce in a hearer a state of affective unity with another living creature by arousing in him the same emotion experienced by the sound-maker, or else an appropriately responsive emotion, as, for example, the sound of sobs reducing a hearer to tears, a cry of terror inducing a wave of panic in the one who hears it, the mew of a starving kitten producing an "empathetic" saucer of milk.

Persuasive sounds. This sound family includes sounds directed toward influencing attitudes, opinion, action. The individual who is the source of the sound can remain quite untouched by its affective appeal; the listener is the target. Foremost in the category of persuasive sound-makers are authority figures in all walks of life, from a cajoling parent to a raging demagogue. Persuasive sounds can be heard in such diverse messages as parental injunction and inducement, religious sermons, party manifestos, declamatory propaganda, political declamations, and advertising exhortations of all kinds. But whatever the message, it is the vocal rather than the verbal impact that is counted on to get to the heart of the listener.

Esthetic sounds. Esthetic sounds are those that stir feeling primarily through their appealing cadences. In the verbal area, examples are the sounds and sound images of great literature, of poetry. Before the words are muted in print, they are sounded out in the mind's ear of the author. Robson comments that "Poe proved that the esthetic power of language depended to a considerable degree on the *sounds* of the words" (1959, p. 11), and that "Hart Crane learned how the *sounds* of words could bombard his mind and evoke feelings out of associations dormant in his subconscious" (1959, p. 12). He tells further that "a word technician is concerned with how *auditory qualities* can express his thoughts, feelings, and emotions with more precise shades of meaning, greater accuracy in description, and a more decisive power of statement" (1959, p. 30; italics added in all three quotations).

In the nonverbal area, music is a prime example of esthetic sound. A number of studies of its psychological effects can be found in the literature (e.g., Farnsworth, 1969; Lundin, 1967), including its effects on behavior in such settings as factories, correctional institutions, hospitals, and psychiatric facilities (Soibelman, 1948).

Self-Perceptive Sounds

The ability to hear the sounds one makes plays a major role in self-perception and self-expression. An occasional look in the mirror during the day affords transitory visible proof of identity; but the sounds that issue forth from an individual provide continuing assurance. The sounds of the voice talking, humming, mumbling, interjecting; the sounds of the body, its footsteps, coughs, sneezes, the rumblings of an empty stomach, the rustling of clothes, all these and many more provide continuing assurance of existence, presence, of identity.

Another important function of the ability to hear one's own voice is emotional release. "Bursting with joy," for example, is largely the voice bursting forth in jubilation. And at the other end of the emotional spectrum, feelings of anger, frustration, and the like can be considerably relieved through vocal discharge. The ability to hear oneself assault vocally lessens the urge to assault physically. Another aspect of self-expression is the entertainment that hearing one's voice provides, as in singing, mimicry, performing, reciting, and the like, and in sharing the pleasure with others. Not to hear one's own voice is to be cut off from a vital part of the self and from a major expressive outlet.

Summary Comment

Current disclosures from research as well as from life provide mounting evidence of the power of environment in the fashioning of human behavior. Authorities from a wide variety of disciplines agree that whatever people know as human beings comes to them from environment; whatever mankind has achieved in the climb up the ladder of civilization was made possible through communication with environment and its human occupants. Human personality is fashioned largely by environmental influences; human achievement, by communication with the external milieu.

Particular attention is called to the powerful influences on human development and adjustment contained in the emotional, cognitive, and psychosocial meanings of nonlinguistic sounds. The psychological voids created by the absence of such sounds from deaf environments have seldom been noted. They demand recognition, investigation, and above all compensation.

Where, then, does environment end and the individual begin? This is the classic question asked by today's eco-behavioral investigators. Is there a dividing line between the two, or are both, as Brunswik suggests (1957), hewn basically from the same block? In terms of human service, the question becomes: Wherein lies the greater promise for human adjustment, with rehabilitating individuals or with rehabilitating their defective environments?

Such questions have yet to be answered. But the major theme emerging from studies of individual–environment interplay is simply stated and generally accepted: To better understand people, we must look to and understand the environments that fashioned them.

References

Argyle, M. 1967. *The Psychology of Interpersonal Behavior.* Baltimore: Penguin Books.

Barker, R. G. 1968. *Ecological Psychology.* Stanford, Calif.: Stanford University Press.

Bersoff, D. N. 1973. Silk purses into sow's ears: The decline of psychological testing and a suggestion for its redemption. *American Psychologist,* 28: 892–900.

Bloom, S. B., Davis, A., and Hess, R. 1965. *Compensatory Education for Cultural Deprivation.* New York: Holt, Rinehart and Winston.

Bolinger, D. L. 1964. Around the edge of language: Intonation. *Harvard Educational Review,* 34: 282–96.

Bronfenbrenner, U. 1976. *Reality and Research in the Ecology of Human Development.* American Psychological Association Master Lectures on Developmental Psychology Document. Washington, D.C.

Brunswik, E. 1957. Scope and aspect of the cognitive problem. In H. Gruber, R. Jessor, and K. Hammone, eds., *Cognition: The Colorado Symposium.* Cambridge, Mass.: Harvard University Press.

Burks, B. S. 1928. The relative influence of nature and nurture upon mental development. *27th Yearbook, N.S.S.E.,* Part I: 219–316.

Caldwell, L. K. 1971. *Environment: A Challenge to Modern Society.* Garden City, N.Y.: Anchor Books, Doubleday & Co.

Cantril, H., and Allport, G. 1935. *The Psychology of Radio.* New York: Harper.

Connor, J. 1961. Is it true or is it so? In C. Watkins and B. Pasamanick, eds., *Problems in Communication.* Psychiatric Research Reports 14. Washington, D.C.: American Psychiatric Association.

Cowan, G. M. 1948. Mazateco whistle speech. *Language,* 24: 280–86.

Craik, K. H. 1973. Environmental psychology. In P. H. Mussen and M. R. Rosenzweig, eds., *Annual Review of Psychology,* Vol. 24. Palo Alto, Calif.: Annual Reviews.

Cronbach, L. J. 1975. Five decades of public controversy over mental testing. *American Psychologist,* 30: 1–15.

Davitz, J. R., ed. 1964. *The Communication of Emotional Meaning.* New York: McGraw-Hill.

Dubos, R. 1968. *So Human an Animal.* New York: Charles Scribner's Sons.

Dunn, L. C., and Dobzhansky, T. 1952. *Heredity, Race, and Society.* Rev. and enlarged ed. New York: New American Library, Mentor Books.

Ehrlich, P. R., Ehrlich, A. H., and Holdren, J. P. 1972. *Human Ecology.* San Francisco: W. H. Freeman.

Ekman, P. 1965. Communication through nonverbal behavior: A source of information about interpersonal relationship. In S. S. Tomkins and C. E. Izard, eds., *Affect, Cognition and Personality.* New York: Springer.

Ekman, P., and Friesen, W. V. 1969. The repertoire of nonverbal behavior: Categories, origins, usage, and coding. *Semiotica,* 1: 49–98.

Ekman, P., and Friesen, W. V. 1974. Nonverbal behavior and psychopathology. In R. J. Friedman and M. M. Katz, eds., *The Psychology of Depression: Contemporary Theory and Research.* Washington, D.C.: Winston & Sons.

Environmental Abstracts SER 1. 1965. A Publication of the Architectual Research Laboratory, College of Architecture and Design, University of Michigan.

Farnsworth, P. R. 1969. *The Social Psychology of Music.* Ames, Iowa: Iowa State University Press.

Fast, J. 1970. *Body Language.* New York: M. Evans and Co.

Freeman, F. N. 1934. *Individual Differences.* New York: Holt.

Freud, S. 1947. *The Ego and the Id.* London: Hogarth Press.

Frobenius, L. 1960. *The Childhood of Man.* New York: Meridian Books.

Fuller, J. L., and Thompson, W. R. 1960. *Behavior Genetics.* New York: John Wiley & Sons.

Funk, W. 1950. *Word Origins.* New York: Grosset & Dunlap.

Gage, N. L. 1972. Replies to Shockley, Page, and Jenson: The causes of race differences in I.Q. *Phi Delta Kappan,* March 1972: 422–27.

Gellman, W. 1973. Fundamentals of rehabilitation. In J. F. Garrett and E. S. Levine, eds., *Rehabilitation Practices with the Physically Disabled.* New York: Columbia University Press.

Gesell, A., and Amatruda, C. S. 1947. *Developmental Diagnosis.* 2d ed. New York: Paul B. Hoeber.

Gibbs, J. C. 1979. The meaning of ecologically oriented inquiry in contemporary psychology. *American Psychologist,* 34: 127–40.

Goodman, M. E. 1967. *The Individual and Culture.* Homewood, Ill.: Dorsey Press.

Greene, W. J., Jr. 1958. Early object relations, somatic, affective, and personal. *Journal of Nervous and Mental Diseases,* 126: 225–53.

Hartmann, R. R. K., and Stork, F. C. 1972. *Dictionary of Language and Linguistics.* New York: John Wiley & Sons.

Hawley, A. H. 1950. *Human Ecology.* New York: Ronald Press.

Hogben, L. 1933 *Nature and Nurture.* New York: W. W. Norton.

Hoggart, R. 1972. *On Culture in Communication.* New York: Oxford University Press.

Insel, P. M., and Moos, R. H. 1974. Psychological environments: Expanding the scope of human ecology. *American Psychologist,* 29: 179–88.

Jensen, A. R. 1969. How much can we boost the I.Q. and scholastic achievement? *Harvard Educational Review,* 39: 1–22.

Jensen, A. R. 1972. *Genetics and Education.* London: Methuen.

Knapp, P. H. 1953. The ear, listening and hearing. *Journal of the American Psychoanalytic Association,* 1: 672–89.

Langer, S. K. 1967. *Mind: An Essay on Human Feeling.* Vol. I. Baltimore: Johns Hopkins University Press.

Levine, E. S., Ed. 1977. *The Preparation of Psychological Service Providers to the Deaf.* PRWAD Monograph No. 4. *Journal of Rehabilitation of the Deaf.*

LeVine, R. A. 1973. *Culture, Behavior, and Personality.* Chicago: Aldine Publishing Co.

Lieberman, P. 1967. *Intonation, Perception, and Language.* Cambridge, Mass.: M.I.T. Press.

Linton, R. 1945. *The Cultural Background of Personality.* New York: Appleton-Century-Crofts.

Lundin, R. W. 1967. *An Objective Psychology of Music.* New York: Ronald Press.

Maloney, M. P., and Ward, M. P. 1973. Ecology: Let's hear from the people. *American Psychologist,* 28: 583–86.

Margolin, R. J. and Goldin, G. J., eds. 1969. *Research Utilization Conference on Rehabilitation in Poverty Settings.* Monograph No. 7. Boston: Northeastern University.

Meadows, D. H., Meadows, D. L., Randers, J., and Behrens, W. W., III. 1972. *The Limits to Growth.* New York: Universe Books.

Miller, D. R. 1978. Nature/nurture and intelligence in current introductory educational psychology textbooks. *Educational Psychologist,* 13: 87–91.

Miller, G. A. 1967. *The Psychology of Communication.* Baltimore: Penguin Books.

Miller, T. L. 1974. Environmental effects: Neglected child of psychological assessment. *The School Psychology Newsletter* 28. American Psychological Association.

Montagu, A. 1969. *Man: His First Two Million Years.* New York: Dell Publishing Co., Delta Books.

Montagu, A. 1971. *Touching: The Human Significance of the Skin.* New York: Columbia University Press.

Moore, D. J., and Shiek, D. A. 1971. Toward a theory of early infantile autism. *Psychological Review,* 78: 451–56.

Moos, R. H. 1973. Conceptualizations of human environments. *American Psychologist,* 28: 652–65.

Moos, R. H., and Insel, P., eds. 1974. *Issues in Social Ecology: Human Milieu.* Palo Alto, Calif.: National Press Books.

Muescher, H., and Ungeheuer, H. 1961. Meteorological influences on reaction time, flicker fusion frequency, job accidents, and use of medical treatment. *Perceptual and Motor Skills,* 12: 163–68.

Odum, E. P. 1971. *Fundamentals of Ecology.* 3d. ed. Philadelphia: W. B. Saunders Co.

Ostwald, P. 1963. *Soundmaking: The Acoustic Communication of Emotion.* Springfield, Ill.: Charles C. Thomas.

Ostwald, P., ed. 1977. *Communication and Social Interaction: Clinical and Therapeutic Aspects of Human Behavior.* New York: Grune & Stratton.

Pastore, N. 1949. *The Nature–Nurture Controversy.* New York: King's Crown Press, Columbia University Press.

Pear, T. H. 1931. *Voice and Personality as Applied to Radio Broadcasting.* New York: John Wiley & Sons.

Pei, M. 1949. *The Story of Language.* New York: J. B. Lippincott Co.

Pei, M. 1966. *Glossary of Linguistic Terminology.* New York: Columbia University Press.

Pei, M. A., and Gaynor, F. 1954. *A Dictionary of Linguistics.* New York: Philosophical Library.

Pierce, J. R., and David, E. E. 1958. *Man's World of Sound.* Garden City, N.Y.: Doubleday and Co.

Pike, K. L. 1945. *The Intonation of American English.* Ann Arbor: University of Michigan Press.

Proshansky, H. M. 1976. Environmental psychology and the real world. *American Psychologist,* 31:303–10.

Robson, E. M. 1959. *The Orchestra of the Language*. New York: Thomas Yoseloff.

Rogers-Warren, A., and Warren, S. F. 1977. *Ecological Perspectives in Behavior Analysis*. Baltimore: University Park Press.

Rommetveit, R. 1968. *Words, Meanings, and Messages*. New York: Academic Press.

Rudofsky, B. 1966. *The Kimono Mind*. London: Victor Gollancz.

Ruesch, J., and Kees, W. 1956. *Nonverbal Communication*. Berkeley and Los Angeles: University of California Press.

Ruesch, J., and Bateson, G. 1951. *Communication: The Social Matrix of Psychiatry*. New York: W. W. Norton & Co.

Ruesch, J. 1957. *Disturbed Communication*. New York: W. W. Norton.

Ruesch, J. 1964. Clinical science and communication theory. In D. McK. Rioch and Winstein, E. A., eds., *Disorders of Communication*. Association for Research in Nervous and Mental Disease, Research Publications, Vol. 42. Baltimore: Williams & Wilkins Co.

Ryan, W. 1971. *Blaming the Victim*. New York: Random House.

Schaar, K. 1976. Environment and behavior. *APA Monitor,* 7: 4–5, 18–19.

Schieffelin, B., and Schwesinger, G. C. 1930. *Mental Tests and Heredity*. New York: Galton Publishing Co.

Schlauch, M. 1955. *The Gift of Language*. New York: Dover Publications.

Schubiger, M. n.d. *The Role of Intonation in Spoken English*. Boston: Expression Co. (c. 1933.)

Sells, S. B., ed. 1963. *Stimulus Determinants of Behavior*. New York: Ronald Press.

Sells, S., Findikyan, N., and Duke, M. 1966. *Stress Reviews: Atmosphere*. Technical Report No. 10, Institute of Behavioral Research, Texas Christian University. Fort Worth.

Shapiro, H. L., ed. 1956. *Man, Culture, and Society*. Reprinted 1970. New York: Oxford University Press.

Shockley, W. 1972. A debate challenge: Geneticity is 80% for white twins I.Q.'s. *Phi Delta Kappan,* March 1972: 415–19.

Shuttleworth, F. K. 1935. The nature versus nurture problem: II. *Journal of Educational Psychology,* 26: 655–81.

Simeons, A. T. W. 1961. *Man's Presumptuous Brain*. New York: E. P. Dutton & Co.

Soibelman, D. 1948. *Therapeutic and Industrial Uses of Music: A Review of the Literature*. New York: Columbia University Press.

Starkweather, J. A. 1961. Vocal communication of personality and human feelings. *Journal of Communication,* 11: 63–72.

Stokoe, W. C., Jr. 1960. *Sign Language Structure*. Buffalo, N.Y.: Studies in Linguistics, University of Buffalo.

Vale, J. R. 1973. Role of behavior genetics in psychology. *American Psychologist,* 28: 871–83.

Wagner, P. L. 1972. *Environments and People*. Englewood Cliffs, N.J.: Prentice-Hall.

Whatmough, J. 1956. *Language: A Modern Synthesis*. New York: St. Martin's Press.

Wicker, A. W. 1979. Ecological psychology: Some recent and prospective developments. *American Psychologist,* 34: 755–65.

Winton, H. N. M., comp. and ed. 1972. *Man and the Environment.* Bibliography 1946–1971. New York and London: Unipub, Inc./R. T. Bowker Company.

Wohwill, J. F. 1970. The emerging discipline of environmental psychology. *American Psychologist,* 25: 303–12.

Wohwill, J. F., and Carson, D. H., eds. *Environment and the Social Sciences: Perspectives and Applications.* Washington, D.C.: American Psychological Association, Inc.

2 Acoustically Impaired Environments: Psychological Correlates

. . . . everybody who acquires deafness goes through hell.
Peck, Samuelson, Lehman, *Ears and the Man*

JUST AS our physical being depends for life upon the air we breathe, so does our psychological being depend for life upon the sounds we hear. When sound is blotted out of an environment, various psychological voids are created that need to be filled. Yet adaptive pressures are not lessened because of the narrowed milieu. It makes no difference whether an individual can or cannot hear, or whether a person does or does not have the resources for coping; the environmental imperative prevails in accordance with its own immutable demands.

This is the situation facing the largest group of physically impaired persons in the United States, conservatively estimated to number some 13 million hearing-impaired individuals (Schein and Delk, 1974). This vast body includes hearing losses ranging in a steady continuum from the minor to the profound; impairments that appear at any time from birth to old age; and hearing difficulties that develop slowly and unobtrusively or strike suddenly and severely. The numerous variables represented in this population have spawned a host of classification systems and terminologies for hearing impairments as well as varying census figures, as will be discussed later. The aim here is to discuss the cycle of deficits in which impaired acoustic environments lead to impaired psychological environments, and impaired psychological environments to disturbed human behavior. To illustrate, we turn to three distinctly different types of impaired acoustic environments as represented by: (1) progressive deafness, traditionally termed "hard of hearing"; (2) sudden profound deafness, sometimes called "deafened"; and (3) profound congenital deafness, included in the category commonly termed "the deaf." By far the largest segment of the hearing-impaired population is made up of the hard-of-hearing and the deafened; the smallest, of the deaf.

Progressive Deafness

The situation in which persons with progressive deafness find themselves reflects the insidious environmental distortions commonly brought on by the condition. So unobtrusive may be the onset of hearing loss, and so gradual the increase, that often its presence goes unnoticed for years even by the victim. However, behavioral signs that something is wrong are manifest long before this time. They are simply attributed to other causes. The victim thinks the world has taken to speaking in a mumble. The world thinks the sufferer's personality is taking a turn for the worse. As described by Berry, "The father thinks that Tom is inattentive; the mother calls it preoccupation; the teacher suspects stupidity; his comrades think he does not care or that he is queer or self-centered" (1933, pp. 2–3). The human environment treats the child in as many different ways as there are misinterpretations of his behavior. With so many different images of himself reflected in the eyes of society, the child does not rightly know who he is.

A short-lived spurt of interest in this undramatic disability took place in the 1930s and 1940s, sparked mainly by Rudolf Pintner in the area of psychological research (Pintner, Eisenson, and Stanton, 1941), by a number of hard-of-hearing persons in hearing rehabilitation (Peck, Samuelson, and Lehman, 1926; Washington, 1958), and by several prominent otologists and psychiatrists whose patients included hard-of-hearing persons. Although most of the psychological studies of the period (Levine, 1956) were criticized by contemporary purists for inadequacies in research design, exercise of controls, and instruments used, the general results taken in conjunction with personal reports from persons with progressive deafness as well as from the observations of involved physicians pointed to serious problem areas in personality and adjustments.

It might be expected that the psychological disturbances reported in these early accounts would be notably lessened in the course of the decades as a result of the remarkable advances made in aural rehabilitation. However, this does not appear to be the case, as suggested by Rosenthal (1975). What has taken place since the 1930s and 1940s is a drastic lessening of interest in the hard-of-hearing and in related psychological research and publications. As a result, we find ourselves turning to the vivid narrative of the early reports to describe representative human responses to a progressively muted environment.

Hunt relates his experiences with an adult patient:

> Looking at this man, the otologist can readily visualize the boy he used to be. The boy who had the bad case of measles at the age of eight, perhaps. The one who was picked on in school for inattention, jeered at for making mistakes; who had to be forced to take part in group activities; who wasn't interested in girls. Making his painful way through childhood and adolescence, unguided, unaware of why he was always at a disadvantage, the young man chose his career . . . Now the man is grown. In spite of his unacknowledged handicap, he has forced from life the things he most wanted—a good job, marriage, family. He has arrived at the otologist's office—Why? Because he has everything the normal man wants out of life and he is in mortal fear of losing every bit of it.
>
> The otologist who examines this patient and writes on his record card, "Progressive deafness," has made only superficial diagnosis. The record might more accurately read: "Diagnosis: fear."
>
> Fear of failure, fear of ridicule, fear of people, fear of new situations, chance encounters, sudden noises, imagined sounds; fear of being slighted, avoided, made conspicuous—these are but a handful of the fears that haunt the waking and even the sleeping hours of the sufferer from progressive deafness. Small wonder that, at best, he tends to live in an atmosphere of despondency and suspicion. Small wonder that, at worst, he may not particularly want to live at all. (1944, pp. 4, 5)

Menninger sums up his experiences with progressively deafened persons in the statement, "It is as if something vital to one's existence had been torn from him" (1924, p. 146). Van Horn relates that for the teacher of lipreading, "threats of suicide, rage, depression, isolation, self-hate, shame, and suspicion are part of her daily contacts with her pupils as they go through the period of intense emotional struggle due to sudden loss of hearing or sudden realization that the handicap is permanent and progressive" (1929, p. 413).

Along the road the progressively deafened travel are young people who live in daily anxiety at the prospect of being caught in the joshing camaraderie of a hearing group; of being singled out in games; of being called on in class; and, worst of all, of missing the sweet nothings whispered into their impaired ears on dates. There are young brides filled with guilt at having burdened another with their deafness and deeply disturbed at the possibility of passing it on to those not yet born; anguished parents who cannot hear the baby's cry in the night or make anything of the excited prattle of their children; anxious wives who cringe at the thought of every social obligation that must be met; husbands and fathers faced with the prospect of becoming vocational students again in occupations where impaired hearing is no handicap.

The psychiatric term "isolation" is commonly used to describe the sensation of being cut off from the world which comes with lessened hearing ability. But the isolation thus experienced is not the same as that resulting from psychic disorder. In the latter case, "isolation" represents a defense employed by the individual to escape from an anxiety-provoking environment. But where isolation results from impaired hearing, it is not the individual who is seeking escape. On the contrary, it is the environment that is escaping from the perceptive grasp of the individual. By its very nature, decreased hearing ability simulates the sensation of increasing distance between the person and the source of sound. As hearing fades, sound seems to be coming from farther and farther away. Ultimately some sounds disappear altogether; others are distorted; patterns of sound are no longer recognizable. The resultant feeling of isolation, of detachment from the world, is forced upon all whose hearing no longer keeps them in touch with life.

Along with the feeling of detachment, a confusing distortion in audiovisual Gestalt arises from the sensorially illogical differences between the auditory estimates of the distance and source of sound and the actual visible evidence. It is as if sound were *heard* as coming from great distances and particular directions but *seen* to be quite near at hand and from a different direction entirely. Adding to this confusion are the distortions in the sounds that are heard:

> The deafened hear a great deal; they hear especially the louder strident sounds; street and mechanical noises fall heavily upon their hypersensitive ears. In certain types of deafness all sounds are distorted, and the sudden shriek of brakes or the wail of motor horns is agonizing. The cheerful phonograph discoursing harmless jazz for the dance is misery. Worst of all are the pathologically created sounds which have no external existence, and which we call tinnitus, or headnoises. He who has them, rarely, if ever, knows a moment of silence, and the torture they inflict can never be estimated by anyone who has never experienced them. Head noises alone would provide excuse for most of the mental aberrations of acquired deafness. (Peck, Samuelson, and Lehman, 1926, p. 37)

These authors also wish "to slaughter, if we can, a popular delusion, the classic association of deafness with silence. . . . Silence would fall upon the deafened like the gentle pall of sleep upon the weary" (pp. 36–37).

While the sufferers are engulfed in the struggle to bring this incredibly distorted influx of sound into a semblance of perceptive order, they are threatened by still another type of auditory problem—a decreased ability to gauge and monitor the sounds of their own voices. To persons with obstructive deafness, their voices may sound disproportionately loud, and to avoid what they perceive as shouting, they tend to speak lower and lower until they can hardly be heard at all. On the other hand, persons with severe nerve involvement have difficulty in hearing the sound of their own voices, and to overcome this, they speak with unnecessary loudness. As time goes on and hearing lessens, defective articulations commonly appear, together with other poor speech habits. Gifford and Bowler observe that "many of these hard-of-hearing people live in fear of their own voices. They are constantly on the alert to detect the unfavorable reaction of those with whom they talk, trying to regulate by this reaction the volume of their voice" (1942, p. 23). To the continuing strain of trying to understand is added the strain of trying not to be misunderstood.

From the tensions thus imposed on interpersonal communication, a rift develops between hearing-impaired individuals and the human environment. Society contributes in no small measure to the rift, albeit unintentionally. Nothing of the auditory turmoil experienced by the sufferer is visible except possible changes in behavior; and since these annoy, society retreats.

The ways in which progressively deafened persons react to a beginning awareness of the hearing problem led Peck, Samuelson, and Lehman to classify them as: "the 'Truth-at-any-price' type; the 'Hermits'; the 'Wont's'; and lastly, the 'Panaseekers' " (1926, p. 10). The "Truth" group has the stamina to accept the situation and take the necessary measures to meet the related problems. The "Hermits" withdraw. The "Wont's" defy every effort at rehabilitation, in the belief that it is society's duty to cater to their misfortune. The "Panaseekers" will not believe there is no cure, and "dash from scientist to charlatan in search of the 'sure-cure' " (1926, p. 10).

An important inference to be drawn from these categories is that a person's manner of reacting to deafness is an expression of basic personality. Where isolation and regression are the individual's established modes of dealing with emotional crises, the feeling of detachement that comes with impaired hearing may, under adverse conditions, easily slip into true psychic detachment. Inability to hear offers such persons a ready-made escape from tensions and responsibilities; they meet these with apathy, withdrawal, or regression to psychic infantilism. In other cases, inability to solve the conflicts activated by hearing loss leads to a hostile projection of the problems onto society, a "chip on the shoulder" attitude, a suspicious, defensive set commonly referred to in the field literature as the paranoid attitude of the hard of hearing. However, interpretative caution must be exercised before a diagnosis of psychopathology is made. On the basis of broad psychiatric experience with hearing-impaired persons, both Knapp (1948) and Zeckel (1950) agree that suspicion is frequently present but that, as often as not it is justified, for "people do avoid them, exploit them, and talk about them" (Knapp, 1948, p. 210).

Some individuals deny the reality of the facts that would otherwise generate deep anxiety. Fowler (1951, p. 2) observes that the "tendency to ignore or deny the first indications of deafness, aversion to consulting an otologist, and even to resent suggestions that hearing is not 'perfectly all right,' [and] persistent objections to using a hearing aid or studying lipreading, until long after these are clearly indicated" are common reactions in otosclerotic progressive deafness.

An interesting look into the emotional concomitants of objections to using a hearing aid is offered by Warfield from her personal experiences:

> It seemed to me that the life experience of a person such as myself divided into three periods, each with its own emotional factors: Needing a hearing aid. Getting a hearing aid. Forgetting your hearing aid.
>
> However long the first period lasts it is characterized by one outstanding emotion: anger. The person who does not hear well lives, as I have said, in an angry world of raised voices and exasperated faces. Moreover, he himself is angry. Angry with himself for being at a disadvantage. Angry with the rest of the world for keeping him at a disadvantage.
>
> The anger does not always show. Sometimes it takes the form of aggressiveness. Then you have the person who fights it out with the world, insisting that he can hear but that everyone else is mumbling. Sometimes the hidden anger emerges as indifference. Then you have the person who convinces himself and often succeeds in convincing the rest of the world that he doesn't care to hear—that noise is unpleasant and conversation is boring and deafness is fine. And sometimes the hidden anger reverses itself completely and emerges wearing a masquerade of sweetness and light.
>
> Next comes the period of getting a hearing aid. . . . On the emotional level, it means admitting to yourself and to the rest of the world that you lack something. . . . By getting a hearing aid you admit that you are crippled. And when you do that you run into the emotion that every crippled person knows: fear.
>
> Now comes the third emotional problem. One has overcome anger at being handicapped, lived through fear that a hearing aid will mean the loss of whatever is most valuable in life. The third problem is putting it on and forgetting it. . . . In this third period there still is a highly charged emotional factor. It is insecurity.
>
> . . . some hard-of-hearing people seem to come by inner security naturally and without too much effort. Some achieve it voluntarily, by associating themselves with hearing organizations or with friends who share their handicap. But a great many need help in finding their inner security. They need special understanding, special patience, and even a certain amount of special protection as they make their way slowly and sometimes painfully toward rehabilitation (1957, pp. 102, 103).

In short, it is personality and circumstances rather than hearing loss that determine individual reaction to the indignities of what Warfield calls the "crippled" state. As summed up by Zeckel, the defenses employed by deafened individuals are "not unique. . . . In a great number of cases we have seen that a neurosis existed before the patient lost his hearing. . . . In a great number of cases definite illness becomes manifest because of the additional handicap of deafness. . . . The less neurotic the patient is, the better he will adapt to his deafness" (1950, pp. 338, 340). In this connection, Rosenthal warns rehabilitation clients to beware of attempts by unqualified professional personnel to shift the locus of the problem "from your ears to your psyche" (1975, p. 76). The less expertise that specialists possess in their own disciplinary domain, the more apt they are to "shift the blame" to another discipline.

Where adjustment to hearing loss is ultimately achieved, the types of satisfactory compensation are summarized by Menninger (1924) as: (a) perceptual compensation, in which there is a deliberate as well as a more or less unconscious sharpening of sense perception so that latent sensory faculties are developed to fill the gaps left by impaired hearing (lipreading represents a visual perceptual compensation); (b) intellectual compensation, in which a philosophical attitude and a purposeful broadening of creative interests and outlets are employed to maintain psychic balance and vigor; (c) emotional compensation, through which individuals succeed in sublimating their disturbance and come to peace with themselves through healthy psychic devices, aided by the saving grace of a sense of humor; and (d) volitional compensation, through which the individual is impelled to achieve not only in spite of but because of disability.

Although Menninger's compensations were formulated more than a half century ago, they are still the recommended compensations today, as expressed in Rosenthal's (1975) positive cycle of steps for adjustment to hearing loss. The number of new psychological studies of hard-of-hearing persons has diminished considerably since the 1930s and 1940s, but the general findings are still the same; the earlier personal accounts of the psychological impact of progressive deafness are echoed in the present; society still recoils from what it cannot understand; a substantial prevalence of undetected hearing loss still exists among children despite the increase of auditory screening programs in the schools (Roberts and Federico, 1972); and pressing needs are still unmet.

In the belief that it requires the national voice of millions of hearing-impaired people and the authority of a national organization to recognize the problems and needs of the hard-of-hearing, the Consumers Organization for the Hearing Impaired, Inc. (COHI) was established in the late 1970s. Designated by its founders as "an organization committed to furthering the interests of hard of hearing persons" (*COHI Reporter*, March 1980, vol. 2, no. 1) a number of its purposes are:

- To create a unified national voice for all hard-of-hearing persons.
- To educate the public on the unique problems and potentials of hard-of-hearing persons.
- To clarify the difference between those who are hard of hearing and those who are deaf.

- To eliminate misunderstanding and discrimination against hard-of-hearing workers and job-seekers.
- To offer technical assistance and information on the needs and experiences of hard-of-hearing persons to organizations of consumers, professionals, manufacturers, and to government agencies.
- To form alliances and seek active cooperation with other organizations of consumers and professionals. (Excerpted from COHI membership application 1979–1980)

It may well be that the sparks generated by COHI will rekindle interest in progressive deafness and in the psychologically disruptive potentials of its bizarre acoustic environment.

Sudden Profound Deafness

Whereas many progressively deafened persons visualize silence as a blessed release from the piercing agonies of head noises and the raucous distortions of external sounds, for individuals experiencing sudden profound deafness, the silence is one of life's most terrifying experiences (Lehmann, 1954). It represents an abrupt plunge from the vigorous, energizing acoustics of a bustling world to the deadness of a tomb.

Hearing persons often experience the sensation on stepping into a completely sound-isolated room such as is used in the testing of hearing. The silence is suffocating. Ears seem to stretch out to catch whatever small sounds may be around. When none are heard, the individual nervously utters vocal sounds on his own; anything to dispel the almost physical discomfort that the absence of sounds produce. Not infrequently, feelings of panic set in, and the individual is forced to flee the cubicle, sometimes embarrassed but always relieved. Lucky the ones who can escape when anxiety becomes intolerable. The deafened are not among them.

In Childhood

Possibly the most confused victims of sudden profound deafness are young children. When, for example, small three-year-olds experience abrupt soundlessness, they have no way of knowing what has happened. Nor is there any way of explaining. Introspective reports from very young children are naturally impossible, and retrospective accounts are rare. But observation of behavior supplies clues to the children's feelings. One three-year-old, in my clinical practice, thought people stopped talking aloud simply to tease. Her bitterness with this cruel joke led her to lash out at them physically whenever they spoke to her. She carried her bitterness into habilitation, where she lashed out emotionally with indifference and negativism. The child never overcame her hostility toward the hearing world even in adulthood. Another three-year-old, realizing that people had suddenly become soundless, sought out other kinds of noises, and went about the house banging pots and pans, hitting furniture, slamming drawers, doing anything that previous experience had told her produced noise. Her face would light up whenever any of the noises penetrated the wall of silence. This child took to the hearing aid with joy. The former child with customary negativism.

Another example of sudden deafness in childhood concerns a seven-year-old who came down with spinal meningitis and had to be hospitalized. The ensuing events are as alive in the mind of the now adult narrator as if they happened yesterday:

When I woke up I was in a strange small white room all by myself. My first sensory impression was music in my head. It went on endlessly and I was positive it was coming from next door. It became so annoying that I began to bang on the wall to get it to stop. Eventually it did.

A day or two later, my parents appeared for the first time. My mother stood in the doorway and did not come in. She was overcome with emotion. However, my father walked over to me and began to talk with deliberately exaggerated mouth movements. I understood him perfectly well. I thought I was hearing him, and that because of my prior experiences with the strange noiseless yet noisy environment, I suspected that I would also have to mouth to my father in order to be understood. And that is how we communicated.

A day or two later, I asked my father why I could not hear his voice. He said that because we were on the 10th floor of the hospital where the air is very thin, nobody could hear, and everybody had to watch the mouth. He told me this was called lipreading, and that that was the way everyone was communicating here on the 10th floor. At that point I asked about my sister who had been hospitalized at the same time, also with meningitis. Does she have the same problem? No, he replied, because she is on the 8th floor, and that hearing problems began only on the 10th floor. Then why couldn't I join her on the 8th floor, I wanted to know. He replied that the 8th floor was only for babies, and since I was a big boy of seven, I would be very unhappy there.

After about a week, I was moved into a ward where the beds were separated by glass partitions. Much to my joy, my sister was wheeled into the compartment next to mine, still on the 10th floor. I assumed that her move upstairs would now result in her being unable to hear, and that I had a head start over her in lipreading.

However, I was due for a rude shock when my parents came on their next visit. They continued to ''talk'' to me in that old laborious mouthy movement; but when they spoke to Norma, communication seemed very natural and unforced. I noticed the difference immediately and became very perplexed. I wanted to know how come my sister was able to hear even though she was on the 10th floor where the air was thin. My father answered that my sister had a natural aptitude for lipreading, and that I had better practice harder. As the big brother, I felt very put out, and resolved to become the best lipreader on the 10th floor.

A month passed and we were on our way home. One of my most vivid recollections was when we emerged into the bright sunny street looking for a taxi to take us home. I strained for the hearing I fully expected to return now that I was on street level. But no such thing happened. Again came the questioning, and again my father was prepared with an answer. This time I was told that because I had been up on the 10th floor for so long, it would take time for my hearing to return. I had to be patient.

I continued to observe my sister and her remarkable lipreading ability; and then one day I came to the conclusion that she was able to hear after all. I became angry and jealous, and for the first time began to question my father's honesty with me.

I began to ask more and more frequently when my hearing would return, until finally my father could find no more evasions. He summarized the matter by saying that people recover from these problems at different rates, and I must be patient; and above all continue gaining lipreading proficiency.

My return to my old school was a joyous occasion for me; but problems quickly arose, with the teacher continually running in exasperation to the principal saying that I was holding back the class. They knew that I was now deaf, and they couldn't cope with it. Soon thereafter I entered my first school for the deaf, a day school. The move was filled with trauma for me, since for the first time the fact of deafness began to settle in on me as a permanent condition. I would not accept it and refused to identify with deafness. In fact I would not even use the word "deaf." I preferred "can't hear." I remained at this school a month, and was then transferred to a residential school for the deaf on the advice of the family physician. He probably thought such a setting would reconcile me to deafness. It did not. I felt as if I were in a prison, and that my heretofore loving parents had rejected me and put me away. To make matters worse, my lack of identification with deafness had somehow created the impression among the staff that I was either emotionally disturbed or mentally retarded. From the third grade in hearing school I was now placed in the kindergarten. It was only after I picked up a piece of chalk and wrote my name and address on the blackboard that the teacher began to suspect I had been improperly placed.

My unhappiness in the residential school took its toll on my health and emotions. I began to lose weight and to bed-wet. Although I came home on weekends, I still felt rejected. Finally after a month of endless frustration and misery, my parents convinced me that a return to the day school would be a much happier move because I could come home every day. Things began to improve after that. I settled down somehow, began to make my peace with deafness, and progressed so well scholastically that thanks to my lipreading proficiency among other things I was able to enter a hearing high school on graduation and complete my education in the regular schools and universities. Most of my friends were hearing persons.

As I said, I made my peace with deafness, but it took a great many years before I could fully accept the deaf world and participate in the deaf community. I still feel the emotional scars of my early experiences. (Personal communication to author.)

The narrator of these experiences is now a distinguished member of the deaf professional community. He contributes these painful reminiscences so that professional personnel and bewildered parents alike will be alert to the consternation and anger that sudden deafness arouses in a child whose hunger to hear is still active and alive and has not been stilled by deafness.

In Adulthood

For hearing adults to be suddenly plunged into silence can be an even more shattering experience than for children. Terror, panic, and disorientation are common first reactions: terror at being cast out of a lifelong environment; panic at being out of touch with reality; disorientation at being trapped in a place with neither acoustic substance nor auditory input. The victim feels as if blinded by silence.

After the initial shock has somewhat abated, a variety of ego-blows begin to inflict their depressing messages on the deafened. The alarm clock no longer arouses them to their importance in the world's work. There is no familiar household bustle to welcome them when they come home; no outside sounds to keep them informed of the passing scene.

Former diversions cannot ease their grief and mourning. Radio, television, music, the theater, carefree get-togethers with friends—none of these old reliables can comfort them with their magic. Even their bodies have joined the rank of soundless things. They talk and cannot hear the sounds of their voices. They cough, and again there is no sound. They walk and there is no accompanying footfall. They feel like creatures detached even from themselves. The only magic they now have to look forward to takes the form of communication aids and therapies, and these are viewed as crutches for a cripple.

A rare opportunity for the systematic study of a sizable group of deafened persons was offered by the deafened veterans of World War II, and was collaboratively conducted by the Psychiatric and the Hearing Services divisions of Deshon General Hospital (Knapp, 1948). The subjects were soldiers with varying amounts of hearing loss, but in most cases reportedly "sudden." The most significant feeling-tone reported was loneliness; the most common fear, that of being thought stupid; and the most keenly felt anxiety, insecurity in social situations. Somatic complaints were also reported, particularly tension headaches. A universally felt lack was the loss of daily background sounds, with associated anxieties felt in regard to traffic, crowds, inability to hear an alarm clock or an order. Also missed were the sounds of nature—the rain, the wind, birds, and the like. The tension of silence, as of holding one's breath until sound breaks through, was a common source of distress.

The relationship between amount of hearing loss and the effect upon the social organism is summarized by Knapp as follows:

> At the threshold of incapacitation, patients were not greatly dependent; frequently their sole complaint was that the world did not talk loudly enough.

More often they spoke of how great a strain it was to hear, especially in groups. Still it was possible to "get by" socially. In the 50–70 decibel range, more marked impairment appeared. It often led to a more grossly abnormal facial expression and mannerisms, as well as to more severe emotional reactions, especially of withdrawal. The effort necessary to maintain social bonds sometimes hardly seemed worthwhile. The totally deaf patients felt that these bonds were definitely ruptured. Lipreading, though useful, could not substitute for the quickness and warmth of words that were heard. The men had to adjust as best they could to partial isolation and helplessness. (1948, p. 207)

Knapp also noted differences between cases of true sudden deafness and those with histories of chronic auditory impairment. The study suggests that although patients with true sudden deafness are more apt to be "tinged with depression," they are psychologically more flexible than the chronic cases who have over time "reached equilibrium"; that although the latter experience a less drastic sense of loss, it is a more warping one. The trauma of true sudden loss tends to generate more intense struggles than the gradual pace of progressive impairment, and it is thus more accessible to treatment.

Individual reactions of the subjects supported the finding, in studies of other types of deafness, that the ultimate determinant of adjustment lies with the premorbid personality structure. Where the structure is unhealthy, mild loss can cause profound disturbance; where the structure is sound, the problems of even severe loss can be managed.

The compensatory strategies employed in successful adjustment are essentially the same as those summarized earlier from Menninger for progressive deafness. The neurotic defenses are also the same. These are roughly classified by Knapp as follows: (1) "overcompensated," outgoing, striving, an exaggerated display of jovial behavior with great emphasis on talking rather than listening; (2) denial of hearing loss; (3) retreat from society; (4) neurotic displacement of anxiety into the sphere of somatic preoccupations and complaints; and (5) neurotic exploitation of hearing loss, with the hearing aid used as a "badge of invalidism."

Quite likely the full impact of sudden hearing loss on most of Knapp's subjects was lessened as a result of the rehabilitation services they were receiving. It is particularly interesting, therefore, to note the reactions of hearing subjects who were experimentally deafened for twenty-four hours, as reported by Meyerson (1948). His subjects, a number of children and college students, had the advantage of knowing that their handicap was temporary; but even so the investigator notes the appearance of "bored, stupid, or inappropriate behavior," evidences of fatigue and irritability, change in quality and intensity of voice, and a tendency to "preoccupation." The college students further reported feelings of frustration and aggression resulting from their inability to fully understand oral communication, and a tendency to give up and withdraw from further frustrations. Among the children's reactions were increased tension and restlessness, increased alertness to nonverbal clues, decreased initiative in seeking social contacts, and either delayed reaction to oral communication or no reaction. As summarized by Cornell, who subjected himself to a similar experiment for seven days, "They (the deafened) are living in a partial auditory vacuum—a world of silence mixed with distorted and unfamiliar sounds" (1950, p. 14), a fair summation of dissonant input from an acoustically shattered environment.

Congenital Deafness

Of the three acoustically damaged environments reviewed in this chapter, that created by profound congenital deafness is the least traumatic emotionally but imposes the most severe and most sweeping deprivations developmentally. The victim experiences no emotional shock through lost hearing because there never was any meaningful hearing to lose. But developmentally, the absence of meaningful sound since birth means the absence of sounds that bring language and information, that stir feelings, influence actions and attitudes, confirm identity, allow expressive release, impart esthetic pleasure, and unite the individual to the company of humankind. And this, in turn, means the absence of sounds necessary for normal processes of enculturation, maturation, and adaptation. Such is the environment of those traditionally termed "the deaf." The unique human problems so created, and their wide ramifications, are reviewed in the chapters that follow. We pause here to lay the groundwork by discussing the historic difficulties in conceptualizing the human products of a soundless environment. Who are the deaf?

From ancient times until well into the Middle Ages, the deaf were considered uneducable, hence fools, idiots, scarcely human (Hodgson, 1954). They were treated accordingly. It was not until the sixteenth century that doubt was cast on this stereotype by the first tutors to the deaf, who had been entrusted with the education of the deaf scions of noble houses. Their miraculous success inspired others to try their hand at teaching the deaf. Gradually the concept gained ground that the deaf were not only humans but educable humans. The scope of education broadened.

During the following centuries, schools were established for all the deaf, not only the favored few, and specialists from other disciplines became involved in this education. Eventually the need to identify and define "the deaf" for census and educational purposes became a practical necessity.

In the United States, examples of the difficulties of definition reach back to the beginning efforts of the Federal Census Bureau. In the early nineteenth century, before the teaching of speech to the deaf had become common, deaf persons were simply designated as "deaf and dumb." But when

speech teaching became accepted procedure, ''dumb'' was no longer appropriate, and the deaf were defined as persons who had lost their hearing
before the age of 16 years and were unable to talk because they could not
hear. In 1890, the speech criterion acquired even stronger emphasis, and the
deaf were defined as only those who were also ''dumb''; deaf persons who
could speak were not included in the category. The concept was soon abandoned, and the next census defined as deaf all who could not understand
loudly shouted conversation. This raised a furor among hard-of-hearing persons whose hearing losses had become profound. They were appalled at
being classed with the ''deaf and dumb'' stereotype. At this point, the
Bureau of the Census decided to settle the issue by casting all definitions
into one hamper. The classification ''deaf'' now included children under 8
years of age who were totally deaf, older persons who could not understand
loudly shouted conversation even with the help of a hearing aid, and adults
who were born deaf or had been totally deaf from childhood. Understandably this strategy too was doomed to failure, and in 1930 the Bureau of
the Census conceded defeat, washed its hands of the deaf, and left the job of
defining and enumerating them to whatever other agencies were courageous
enough to undertake the task.

The problem of definition was not dropped with the failure of the Bureau
of the Census. Educators of the deaf, in particular, needed to know how
many children and how wide a range of hearing losses they were expected to
serve so that adequate instructional provisions could be made. The struggle
therefore continued, with the deaf being shifted about from one definition to
another.

The next major efforts were made by the White House Conference on
Child Health and Protection (1931) and by the Conference of Executives of
American Schools for the Deaf (1938). In the former effort, the main criterion for definition and for differentiating ''deaf'' from ''hard of hearing'' involved the usability of hearing for the acquisition of speech and language (p.
277); and in the latter, the functional use of hearing ''for the ordinary purposes of life'' (pp. 2–3). Neither definition inspired field consensus.

In the meantime, rehabilitation of the deaf was gaining a sure place in the
field, accompanied by a variety of rehabilitation specialties, each with its
own concept of ''deaf'' and its own classification of hearing impairments.
The result was a definition explosion.

At the first national conference held in this country to develop uniform
statistics and definitions of deafness (*Proceedings, Conference on the Collection of Statistics of Severe Hearing Impairments and Deafness,* 1964), it
was reported that ''there are at least six [different definitions of ''deaf'']
from as many different professional areas, such as the definition of the
audiologist, the rehabilitation worker, the social worker, the psychologist,

the otologist, and the educator of the deaf" (p. 2). The estimate of six definitions advanced to seven in 1974 with the term "pre-vocationally deaf,"
coined by Schein and Delk for enumerating the deaf population of the
United States; the term includes "those persons who could not hear and understand speech and who had lost (or never had) that ability prior to 19 years
of age" (1974, p. 2). The prevalence of such persons is estimated by the investigators as 200 per 100,000 population. And seven definitions advanced
to eight in 1975 with that used in Public Law 94-142, namely "a hearing
impairment which is so severe that the child's hearing is non-functional for
the purposes of educational performance."

At about the same time, a number of definitions proposed by an Ad Hoc
Committee to Define Deaf and Hard of Hearing were accepted by the Con-
ference of Executives of American Schools for the Deaf (Report of the Ad
Hoc Committee, 1975). Included among them are "General Definitions,"
"Definitions," "Definitions for Educational and Research Considerations,"
"Definitions Related to Age of Onset," and "Associated Descriptions of
Educational Deafness." The general definitions are as follows:

> *Hearing impairment.* A generic term indicating a hearing disability which
> may range in severity from mild to profound: it includes the subsets of deaf and
> hard of hearing.
> A *deaf* person is one whose hearing disability precludes successful processing
> of linguistic information through audition, with or without a hearing aid.
> A *hard of hearing* person is one who, generally with the use of a hearing aid,
> has residual hearing sufficient to enable successful processing of linguistic infor-
> mation through audition. (1975, p. 509)

Since none of the foregoing definitions sufficiently describes the target population of this book, definitions are bypassed here in favor of the following
descriptive summary of "deaf":

The *deaf* constitute a minority population of persons with potentially normal mental and psychological endowments,

1. Whose *physical impairment* lies in severe, irreversible damage to the
sensori-neural and/or cortical structures necessary for normal hearing, a condition which is present since birth or from the formative years of childhood
and is not amenable to current medical or surgical treatment;

2. Whose *disability* is a loss of functional hearing of such severity that
the ability to understand conversational speech through hearing is severely
impaired even with the help of a hearing aid;

3. Whose major *handicaps* stem from the resultant break in the lines of
auditory contact with environment, a condition which possesses the potential
to:

    a. Limit the intake of messages mainly to visual channels;
    b. Prevent the normal acquisition of all forms of verbal language;
    c. Reduce or eliminate input of the emotional correlates of sound;
    d. Impair the establishment of normal communicative exchange with society;
    e. Hamper the processes of enculturation and adaptation.

Included in the deaf minority are numbers of hearing-impaired persons who are "deaf" by preference rather than definition, who find life more fulfilling and comfortable in the deaf world than as "crippled" members of hearing society.

The singular environment in which the deaf are reared is potentially as narrowed psychologically as it is deadened acoustically. Although it is often referred to as a "soundless world," certain acoustic forces do break through in many instances; but these are experienced mainly as noises. What does not come through is the flow of the voice, and herein lies the devastating deprivation of a soundless world. When the voice is not heard in its natural form and flow, neither are words. When words are not heard from birth onward, they cannot be learned in the natural way. If they remain unlearned, normal encounters with the world suffer stark disruption. Something of what this means is expressed in the following analogy:

> If I had the power to forbid you to communicate, forbid you to listen, to speak, to read or to write, I could reduce you in one stroke to intellectual slavery. I could reduce your environment and social structure to that of an animal. I could completely stop the teaching-learning process. I could lock your intellect. (Welling, 1954, pp. 1–2)

The degree to which congenital deafness can inflict its handicaps depends largely on the habilitative strategies used to fill the environmental voids. The human outcomes reflect habilitation's successes or failures, as discussed in later chapters. In the meantime, we ponder the question whether it is better to have heard and lost, or never to have heard at all.

The Environment of Societal Attitudes

To society at large, impaired hearing is an irritating block to quick, easy communication. If there is to be contact with the person behind the block, a barrier needs to be negotiated. But this takes understanding and patience—a patience to which modern living is not geared, an understanding that society has not yet attained.

In addition, society commonly reacts with aversion to physical deviations, especially to such incomprehensible ones as impaired hearing, which does not show, hence provides no clues to its impact or effects. As Hardy once described the situation, the victim " 'limps' only socially, 'fumbles' only psychologically, 'stumbles' only vocationally" (1952, p. 1). The acoustically impaired environments responsible for such cripplings remain invisible.

At the other extreme of misunderstanding is society's naive faith in the magic of lipreading and the hearing aid to effect complete restoration of function, and the confusion that ensues when the magic fails to produce the expected result. "There must be something else wrong with him" is the public verdict. But possibly the cruelest practice of all is the "comic figure" stereotype so frequently attached to hearing-impaired individuals.

Peck, Samuelson, and Lehman tell of their personal experiences with attitudes in connection with progressive deafness:

> Every deafened person knows, and knows well, the sting of contempt. It is shown so quietly and unobtrusively: . . . in the office, the church, the circle of friends, the family group, and even in the home. . . . We have observed the husband whose contempt for his deafened wife extends to all deafened women of middle age; the wife whose husband is bravely realizing deafness and who accentuates his deficiency on all occasions. We have observed the victims of such contempt; the slightly hard of hearing young woman, well-bred, well-educated and not unpleasing in appearance, dropping out of society because she is so resolutely cold-shouldered that self-respect will not permit her to continue. We have seen a young girl who is struggling with developing deafness criticized by her mother for lack of social success, while her sister, with normal hearing, makes it a practice never to introduce her to the members of any group. We have known a businessman who won his way to conspicuous success through the gathering mists of deafness, hard-headed and heavy-fisted, determined and dour. His family enjoys every luxury that his wealth can supply, yet he sits at his table, silent and lonely. And who has not seen a deafened person wait with a resigned or bitter smile for the end of a colloquy carried on in an undertone, regardless of his presence, by the members of a hearing group who would be genuinely shocked if they could realize the full cruelty of their casual rudeness! . . . Is it not natural, then, that deafened people should seek their own kind? (1926, pp. 117–18)

Rosenthal sums up in the statement, "Suspicion of the hearing-impaired is deeply rooted in our culture and has been more fierce and durable than stigmas affixed to people with other handicaps" (1975, p. 95). Rosenthal, too, speaks from personal experience.

As to the deaf, Sussman (himself a congenitally deaf person) tells of the effects of adverse public attitudes upon the self-concept of deaf persons. He relates that attitudes of the hearing toward the deaf are a "burning issue" in deaf society, "particularly where attitudes are devaluative, depreciative and discriminatory" (1976, p. 9). They can be an annoyance, a "thorn in the side,'' and even an obsession. He goes on to say that the deaf do not consider deafness per se to be their chief handicap, but rather the negative attitudes of hearing society.

In his study of 129 deaf adults, Sussman found significant relationships between their self-concepts and their perceptions of attitudes of others toward deafness, with self-concepts contaminated by devaluating attitudes. He explains:

> One may raise the question as to whether attitudes as perceived by deaf people are in tune with reality. The possibility of misperception or misinterpretation undoubtedly does exist. Nonetheless, we ourselves have also to be in tune with reality. Deaf people *are* discriminated against in more ways than one. They do experience discrimination and devaluative attitudes even within the field of deafness itself. Prejudice against deaf people is still rampant in our society despite increasing enlightenment. Deaf people have been hurt and treated badly by society especially when it comes to employment opportunity and job mobility. It is a rare deaf person who has not as a child been ostracized, ridiculed, and denigrated by nondisabled children. Such memories are painfully poignant. (1976, p. 10)

Perhaps the most deeply resented attitude is the pervasive paternalism that enmeshes deaf people, with the chief offenders being parents, educators, and other professional persons who persist in regarding the deaf as ''children,'' regardless of age.

The harm inflicted upon hearing-handicapped persons by a denigrating society extends even into rehabilitation. Time and gain, the energies, expertise, and successes of conscientious rehabilitation personnel are completely undone by a society or employer who will not open the door to a deaf rehabilitant. This same situation characterizes other disability areas as well, despite the many earnest efforts to ''educate the public'' (Garrett and Levine, 1962, 1973). But the public, it turns out, is neither ready nor eager for direct confrontation with the facts of disability.

In the field of the deaf, projects to inform the public are ongoing operations of all national and local organizations and concerned individuals. One example is the National Theatre of the Deaf. The original proposal to establish a national theater of the deaf was first submitted to the Office of Vocational Rehabilitation by this writer in the early 1960s. The inspiration was a brilliant performance of Othello by the Gallaudet College Dramatic Group. With the encouragement and help of Anne Bancroft, the noted actress, and of Mary Switzer, then Director of the Office of Vocational Rehabilitation, planning grant RD-974-5 was awarded the American National Theatre and Academy (ANTA) in 1961 to set up a plan of operation. Although the plan was approved in principle, it could not be funded at the time, and the project waited for several years until the Eugene O'Neill Memorial Theatre Foundation, of which David Hays was an Administrative Vice-President, decided to reactivate the original proposal, with my permission and encouragement. Under the direction of David Hays, the National Theatre of the Deaf has given a brilliant account of itself and of the talents of its deaf performers. In so doing, it has not only made theatrical history, but more importantly has served a major advocacy function for the deaf in the ranks of the public at large.

Another of my advocacy efforts focused on a different kind of population—non-deaf children. This focus was prompted by the problems encountered by many mainstreamed deaf children when exposed to regular-school pupils and personnel who were completely unfamiliar with the facts of prelinguistic deafness. This particular "public-education" strategy took the form of an award-winning, illustrated book written for young hearing children to explain the meaning and ramifications of deafness in simple terms and with simple analogies (Levine, 1974). The hope was that inculcating understanding and attitudes of acceptance among the hearing at the child level would not only help mainstreamed deaf children but would also create lifelong attitudes of acceptance toward the deaf.

These are only two of the many public-education strategies used in the field of the deaf. Inroads are indeed being made in "rehabilitating" the attitudes of society toward its hearing-impaired members, but much remains to be done.

Summary Comment

The discussion in this chapter has two main purposes: first to disclose something of the grotesqueries of acoustically damaged environments; and second, to illustrate the behavioral repercussions that can ensue when human need is met by distorted environmental input. In this instance, both need and input involve damaged auditory links to environment, but the same pattern obtains for other needs and other links. In all instances, ravaged human environments lead to impaired psychological environments; and impaired psychological environments to disturbed human behavior.

References

Berry, G. 1933. The psychology of progressive deafness. Reprint. *Journal of the American Medical Association,* 101: 2–3.

Conference of Executives of American Schools for the Deaf. 1938. Report of the Conference Committee on Nomenclature. *American Annals of the Deaf,* 83: 1–3.

Cornell, C. B. 1950. Hard of hearing for seven days. *Hearing News,* 18(3–4): 14.

Fowler, E. P. 1951. Emotional factors in otosclerois. Reprint. *Laryngoscope,* 61: 2.

Garrett, J. F., and Levine, E. S. 1962. *Psychological Practices with the Physically Disabled.* New York: Columbia University Press.

Garrett, J. F. and Levine, E. S. 1973. *Rehabilitation Practices with the Physically Disabled.* New York: Columbia University Press.

Gifford, M. F. and Bowler, M. L. 1942. Quoted in C. G. Bluett, comp. *Handbook of Information for the Hard of Hearing Adult.* Sacramento, Calif.: California State Department of Education.

Hardy, W. G. 1952. *Children with Impaired Hearing: An Audiologic Perspective.* Children's Bureau Publication No. 326.

Hodgson, K. W. 1954. *The Deaf and Their Problems.* New York: Philosophical Library.

Hunt, W. W. 1944. Progressive deafness rehabilitation. *Laryngoscope,* May, pp. 4–5. Reprint.

Knapp, P. H. 1948. Emotional aspects of hearing loss. *Psychosomatic Medicine,* 10: 203–22.

Lehmann, R. R. 1954. Bilateral sudden deafness. *New York State Journal of Medicine,* May 15, pp. 1481–88.

Levine, E. S.. 1956. *Youth in a Soundless World.* New York: New York University Press.

Levine, E. S. 1974. *Lisa and Her Soundless World.* New York: Human Sciences Press.

Menninger, K. A. 1924. The mental effects of deafness. *Psychoanalytic Review,* 11: 146.

Meyerson, L. 1948. Experimental injury: An approach to the dynamics of physical disability. *Journal of Social Issues,* 4: 68–71.

Peck, A. W., Samuelson, E. E., and Lehman, A. 1926. *Ears and the Man: Studies in Social Work for the Deafened.* Philadelphia: F. A. Davis Co.

Pintner, R., Eisenson, J., and Stanton, M. 1941. *The Psychology of the Physically Handicapped.* New York: F. S. Crofts & Co.

Proceedings, Conference on the Collection of Statistics of Severe Hearing Impairments and Deafness in the United States. 1964. Bethesda, Md.: Public Health Services, National Institute of Neurological Diseases and Blindness, National Institutes of Health, HEW.

Report of the Ad Hoc Committee to Define Deaf and Hard of Hearing. 1975. *American Annals of the Deaf,* 120: 509–12.

Roberts, J., and Federico, J. V. 1972. Hearing sensitivity and related medical findings among children. *Vital and Health Statistics,* Series 11, No. 114.

Rosenthal, R. 1975. *The Hearing Loss Handbook.* New York: St. Martin's Press.

Schein, J. D., and Delk, M. T. 1974. *The Deaf Population of the United States.* Silver Spring, Md.: National Association of the Deaf.

Sussman, A. E. 1976. Attitudes toward deafness: A dimension of personality. *Hearing Rehabilitation Quarterly,* 2: 9–10.

Van Horn, M. 1929. In a discussion of: The mental effects of deafness, by R. Brickner. *Volta Review,* 31: 413.

Warfield, F. 1957. *Keep Listening.* New York: Viking Press.

Washington, M. L. 1942. Quoted in Federal Security Agency, *Rehabilitation of the Deaf and the Hard of Hearing: A Manual for Case Workers.* Vocational Rehabilitation Series Bulletin No. 26. Washington, D.C.: Office of Education.

Washington, M. L., ed. 1958. *Hearing Loss . . . A Community Loss.* Washington, D.C.: American Hearing Society.

Welling, D. M. 1954. Communicate! *Utah Eagle,* 65 (March): 1–2.

White House Conference on Child Health and Protection, 1931. *Section III, The Deaf and the Hard of Hearing.* New York: Century Co.

Zeckel, A. 1950. Psychopathological aspects of deafness. *Journal of Nervous and Mental Diseases,* 112: 337–40. Reprint.

Part Two
PRELINGUISTIC DEAFNESS: KEY FASHIONING ENVIRONMENTS

3 Early Environmental Influences

Everything he knows as a human being, man has had to learn from other human beings.

Montagu, *Man: His First Two Million Years*

FOR CHILDREN who cannot hear, adaptive demand stems from a mesh of generally confusing, frequently confused, and often discordant environments. There is the immediate environment created by deafness—the soundless world—into which congenitally deaf children are born. There is the sociocultural environment created by the hearing and for the hearing, but to which deaf children are expected to adapt. There is the human environment composed of parents, family, and an assortment of other authority figures including professional personnel, who too often have as little understanding of deaf children as the children have of them. There is a variety of special education environments created by the hearing for the deaf which represent a deaf child's principal formative milieu. There is the child's intrapersonal environment, the inner self, that strives to come to adaptive terms with the demands of the other environments, and failing this, to fend off psychic insult through a variety of behavioral and psychopathological strategies. Finally, there is an environment of labels, stereotypes, and definitions that await a deaf child even before it is born.

A frequent question is whether the deaf inhabitants of this environmental mesh have a "different" psychology from the hearing. In answer, it can only be said that the psychological development of deaf individuals is subject to the same principles as for the rest of mankind. It is not the deaf person's psychology that is innately different—it is the deaf person's environment that is unique. People who are deaf are psychologically normal human beings striving to adjust to a hearing society in the face of subnormal environmental input and abnormal environmental pressures.

The Infant Environment

Children who are born deaf are closest to their hearing peers in environmental input and behavior during early infancy. At this threshold stage of life, all infants are protected from excessive environmental stimulation and assault because of their incompletely developed sensory systems. Environment is sensed rather than perceived. As described by Gesell and Ilg:

> the young baby senses the visible world at first in fugitive and fluctuating blotches against a neutral background. Sounds likewise may be heard as shreds of wavering distinctness against a neutral background of silence or of continuous undertone. Doubtless he feels the pressure of his seven pound weight as he lies on his back. Perhaps this island of pressure sensation is at the very core of his vague and intermittent sense of self. He also feels from time to time the vigorous movements which he makes with his mouth, arms, and legs. Doubtless he has delightful moments of subjectivity at the end of a repleting meal and he has episodes of distress from hunger and cold. Such experiences in association with strivings impart vividness to the early mental life of the baby even though the outer world is still almost without form and void. (1943, p. 22)

At this time, the infant has no notion of where he ends and environment begins. So far as he is concerned, all is one; and the one is largely a mass of sensory impressions. The groundwork for awareness of self is laid when developmental changes in the sensory and neuromuscular systems act to propel the infant into physiologically compatible explorations of environment. It is out of these explorations that the self gradually emerges as distinct from surroundings.

The implication of these early events is that input from the sensorially dimmed outer environment of hearing infants in the first weeks of life is much the same as from the sensorially impaired outer environment of deaf infants of the same age. In both cases, behavior is regulated by similarly patterned inner environments composed of innate factors, reflexes, instincts, sensory impressions, feelings of comfort/discomfort, and the like. Therefore, observed behaviors are so similar that it is well-nigh impossible to tell the deaf baby from the hearing one. Nor is it likely that any suspicion of deafness will flash a warning to an enchanted observer of a behaving deaf infant.

It is also unlikely that behavioral differences will be observed when, in the course of maturation, organism and outer environment begin to form their mutually interacting pact for the differentiation and internalization of experiences. This is so because it is vision that plays the leading role in an infant's first efforts at independent environmental exploration. As expressed by Gesell and Amatruda, "infants are born with visual hunger" and "in the early months looking is half of living" (1947, p. 257). There is logic to this developmental sequence. In order for infants to motorically explore their new world, they must first have some idea of its "geography." Vision provides such clues. At this stage, deaf and hearing infants are both visual creatures.

At the same time that this new world is coming into sharper visual focus, the infant's developing neuromuscular system is sparking a push toward motor exploration. "As once he showed visual hunger, now he shows touch hunger" (Gesell and Amatruda, 1947, p. 101). The infant reaches out to touch, feel, taste, probe, accompanying all these actions by automatic vocalizations. Again, the pattern of behavior is the same for deaf as for hearing infants.

Although the events involved in this very early organism/environment interplay are instigated by complex physiological processes, an infant is not a robot. Psychological elements are present even as the infant's "self" begins to emerge from the initial mass of sensory impressions. The self can be felt as a successful self, a distressed self, a frustrated self, or a non-self, depending upon how well environmental input meets bio-maturational need.

The infant feels himself a successful self when he needs to look, and there are satisfying things for him to see; when he needs to touch, and there are gratifying things for him to feel; when he needs to be relieved of discomforts, and there is succor. He is a distressed, frustrated, or non-self when his developmental needs are neglected or are not met at the right time, in the right way, or in the right amount, as Ruesch (1957) would say. These latter babies are already victims of environmental deprivation, and they register the results in personality and behavior, as shown by institution-syndrome infants (Dennis, 1960; Spitz, 1945). The successful self, on the other hand, reaches out to environmental unknowns with healthy curiosity and with feelings of security acquired in the course of previously satisfying excursions into the environment.

The time soon comes when visual and motor inputs are not enough to satisfy the push toward broader environmental interplay. The infant is already acquiring a grasp of the geography and "feel" of his small, immediate world. The "wisdom" of development now decrees input from sources outside the range of sight and touch in preparation for enculturation. This need is met by the sense of hearing. At the same time that visual and motor needs are being met, the sense of hearing is occupied with refining and decoding the blur of sounds in its perceptive environment. As auditory discrimination sharpens, the sense of hearing begins to take on heightened and purposeful listening. A cardinal purpose is to pave the way for linguistic interplay with the human environment.

Observable differences between deaf and hearing babies appear when the results of sound-awareness begin to be manifested in behavior. As hearing babies become increasingly aware of the sounds in their environment, the visual and touch hungers that guided their earlier explorations are gradually matched if not exceeded by auditory hunger. At first, sound was just another diffuse element in the baby's undifferentiated state, and infant vocalizations were a motor-automatic manifestation. But as babies begin to attend to this particular sensation and as discrimination sharpens, they gradually come to perceive differences in the sounds around them and to discover that they themselves are a source of some of these sounds, a discovery that stimulates increasing vocalizations. Bit by bit, the differences take on meanings. One kind of sound informs the baby that someone is hurrying to him; another brings to mind a rattle; still another means that food is on the way; and soon babies discover that they can control and interact with the human elements in the environment through variations in the sounds they themselves produce. Long before a baby is aware of words, it is alert to the fact that sounds embody concepts, and that concepts embody meanings. What is more, the infant reacts to familiar sound-concepts mentally, emotionally, and socially; and to unfamiliar ones with curiosity bent on mastery.

As maturation proceeds, the sounds of speech come within the babies' range of auditory discrimination. The stream of spoken language that flows into their ears begins to take on verbal form. And now their earlier practice in associating gross sounds with conceptual equivalents stands them in good stead. They merely apply the same principle in associating word-sounds with their conceptual equivalents. But always, the word that is heard gains its meaning from the concept or experience with which the baby is already familiar. Without this frame of reference, words remain just sounds and nothing more.

The whole cycle of language acquisition soon becomes a wonderful game. The baby listens, imitates, practices, experiments. More and more word-sounds find their way into the experiential frame; more and more are reproduced. Language begins to fill an expressive as well as a receptive need, and in due course comes to be used for thinking as well as for communicating with others. Eventually language and concept fuse, and the child is well on the way to becoming a verbal being and full heir to the developmental benefits bestowed by hearing.

But long before this happens, the baby has been responding to concepts even though they were contained in gross sounds alone. Babies are conceptual beings long before they become verbalized ones, just as was their ancestor of prehistory who invented verbal language even before possessing the words in which to embody his thoughts.

In contrast, without the stimulus of sound, a deaf baby's vocalizations gradually diminish and in time cease. There is no beginning speech, no speech at all. There is usually some response to various noises and other loud sounds or to their felt vibrations. But all this does is to convey the false impression that this is a hearing baby.

This does not mean that deaf babies do not put two and two together and come up with a concept. Whereas hearing babies listen, deaf babies watch. They watch for clues from facial expressions, gestures, objects, activities. They try to abstract meaning from the unfamiliar by watching a course of events and observing the outcome. However, the impaired, unaided, and untrained auditory mechanism does not supply the kinds of information the babies need as a foundation for interpersonal exchange and enculturation. Thus, while the baby who hears is forging ahead developmentally by virtue of lines of auditory communication, the one who does not hear is left behind in a soundless world.

The Soundless Environment: Pre-detection Phase

Deaf babies are blissfully unaware that their hearing peers are profiting from auditory experiences that will never be theirs. There are still many exciting visual attractions in the soundless world to spark curiosity and compel investigation. The alert deaf baby makes associations, performs abstractions, coordinates experiences into elementary operations of intelligence, and otherwise conceals deafness by achieving remarkable mental feats guided mainly by visual input and propelled by curiosity and exploratory hungers.

As these babies grow to early childhood, their deafness still undetected, they see a whole new world unfolding about them. The visual and motor hungers that propelled their earlier excursions into environment are now exceeded by an intense mental hunger. The children want to know the whys and wherefores of what they see. Surging through their minds are many questions that seeing alone cannot answer. "Who is that?" they would like to know. "Why do they do that? What does this mean? Where are we going? What will happen to me? Why? Why? Why?" But they cannot ask, for they have no words; no words to ask, no words to understand. Never having heard any, they do not even know such things as words exist. So the world remains a silent motion picture, and their questions remain unanswered. The children can only feel the strain and tensions of their wish to know, of the need to satisfy the psychological imperatives of development.

Alert children continue to "hide" their deafness by responding actively and intelligently to many of the challenges in their small life sphere. They play, they explore, they think things out for themselves. They even effect communicative links with the hearing environment. They receive messages by reasoning from facial expression and body movements in relation to a given situation. They transmit messages through privately invented systems of gestures and pantomime. But as time goes on, these are not enough. Gestures cannot keep pace with a child's growing mind. They convey only rudimentary messages. The need to know extends far beyond these.

As for receiving messages, this too becomes increasingly difficult. The children see people about them working lips and faces at one another with intent and purpose and are aware that something important is taking place; but they cannot fathom what it is. They watch silent people responding soundlessly to one another and cannot grasp the magic that conveys messages between them, initiates their responses, and directs their behavior. The members of their own hearing families try to bring them within their circle through these same strange means; but even they cannot break through the walls of silence that separates the deaf child not only from them but from all others as well. As for the families, they are uneasily aware that the child is somehow "different," but they quiet anxiety by telling themselves that all will be well; it is just a matter of time.

Thus many small deaf children find themselves trapped in communicative bondage. They may withdraw in apathy and dependence. But whatever the response, so long as deafness remains undetected, the walls remain.

By way of contrast, for the child who hears, the air throbs with sounds that bring information, explanation, preparation; with sounds that stimulate emotional development and sustain emotional tonicity; that arouse curiosity, direct attention, influence action; that confirm identity and offer emotional release; above all, with sounds that bring language and effect enculturation. There are sounds that "impress, cajole, threaten, influence, inform, shape, deceive, conceal, alert, warn, question, query, explain, demonstrate, argue, and perhaps a few hundred more" (Chapanis, 1971, p. 937). Simply by walking down the street with open ears, the hearing child is exposed to a cross-section of cultural input from a wide range of sources. The child hears the neighbors, playmates, passersby; discussions, quarrels, gossip, threats, jokes, accusation, cries, laughter, shouts; the sounds of the street —automobiles, the fire engine, the ambulance siren, airplanes overhead. Above all, such children hear themselves. All that they hear is grist to enculturation. Caught up as they are in the hubbub of living, hearing children feel the beat of life.

Deaf children hear nothing of all this. Their "public," when they are very young, generally consists of the one or two persons in their immediate world who are closest to them, who are aware that these children are "different" without yet knowing why, and who try to effect some degree of meaningful communication with them. These persons are the deaf child's society; they interpret the meanings of its visual events.

The kinds of information thus relayed depend on the particular event, on the skill and patience of the "interpreters," and on a child's own flair for piecing together isolated clues into meaningful wholes. Often the wholes thus painfully pieced together end up as misinterpretations. But even at best, no matter how skillful the human mediator and how intelligent the child, small deaf children still make only superficial contact with their cultural milieu and with a society that tends to recoil from those who are different. In contrast to their hearing peers, a deaf child's status is that of an onlooker hoping to get the point of what is happening, and longing to be taken into the flow of activities.

Some deaf children are driven to fight for attention, or they may stand on the sidelines feeling that they are somehow different; they know not how. Feeling that they do not belong; they know not why. They only know that they are unable to participate like other children in the give and take of community happenings, that something is wrong; they know not what.

Whether a deaf child becomes part of the give and take depends largely on the human mediator. All else being equal, it is this person's management that determines whether or not the child will slip away into the apathy of indifference, the helplessness of overdependence, the hostility of frustration; or whether the child will have the stamina and security to meet life head on. It is this person's attitudes and practices that determine whether or not a community will open the door to a small, different child. And, as a rule, it is this person's perceptions that first detect the possibility that the child's difference is due to deafness.

In the usual course of events, the role of human mediator is first filled by parents, generally the mother. How great the handicaps are that may accrue from undetected deafness and from the forced dependence of small deaf children on mother-mediators is closely linked to parent reactions to deafness and maternal management of the child.

Parent–Child Relations

In applying principles of parent-child relations to deaf children, it is necessary to realize that in the majority of cases, deaf children are born to hearing parents and that most of these parents have had little if any previous experience with deafness. Their ideas about the disability are vague in the extreme, and their feelings are colored by the common misconceptions of society.

It is also important to bear in mind that children often have a deep symbolic meaning to parents. For example, they may symbolize virility, an extension of the ego, the means of attaining status, the ideal self, an outlet for "the things I couldn't do or have when I was a child." These values are derived from the parents' own early experiences and are therefore deeply rooted. When a deaf child is born to nondeaf parents, the emotional reaction is apt to derive its charge as much from the symbolic meaning of an impaired child as from the implications of deafness.

These are some of the problems encountered on the parents' side of the wall of silence. As time goes by, others arise. Yet the principles of parent–child relations are not altered because of these circumstances. They remain an integral part of the developmental master plan in which early sensory input is intended to familiarize infants with the physical aspects of the world into which they were born; and early parent input, to lay the foundations for becoming a part of this world. How well a child succeeds depends on the soundness of the foundations; and this in turn depends on the nature of the child's early relationships with the first human "teachers"—the parents —and on the manner in which developmental imperatives are met.

In the case of a deaf child, the need for healthy parent–child relations is doubly important, because of the psychological hazards involved in the close and confining dependence on parents that deafness forces on very young deaf children.

Theories and patterns of parent–child relations are amply documented in the literature of psychology and psychiatry. The focus here is on common reactions of parents to a first deaf child, and the spillover into the child's developmental environment.

Hearing Parents

When a healthy, seemingly nondisabled baby begins to behave in an atypical manner, parents are naturally concerned (Becker, 1976). At first it is hard to tell exactly what is wrong, and parents' expressions of anxiety are usually dismissed as overconcern. "Just wait," they are advised. "He'll outgrow it."

They wait. The baby does not outgrow it. Concern mounts.

As a rule, it is to the physician that parents first turn in their anxiety. But, as Fellendorf and Harrow (1970) report in a comprehensive survey of parent counseling-experiences, too many medical specialists lack expertise in diagnosing infant deafness, or are reluctant to be the bearers of sad tidings, or lack knowledge of referral resources for hearing-impaired babies and their parents. To add to the confusion, the child, in many instances, does react to certain sounds, giving the impression of being a hearing child. Again parents are offered the "he'll outgrow it" placebo. And again they wait.

Often the deafness is discovered only after prolonged periods of waiting in vain for speech to appear. In the meanwhile, concern heightens, bewilderment increases, suspicions about the child's mental abilities make their appearance, and doctor-shopping begins. The child, well aware of being the center of anxiety, begins to absorb the tensions that contaminate the developmental environment.

A correct diagnosis, when it is finally made, does little to ease the situation. For hearing parents who know next to nothing about deafness, to have a child of their own "stigmatized" by this mysterious "deaf and dumb" affliction can be a shattering experience, particularly when, as so often happens, "cause is unknown." McAree (1970) and Spradley and Spradley (1978) give sensitive personal accounts of the feelings experienced. Common first reactions are panic, guilt, blame, and despair. There is the mortification of having to inform relatives, friends, neighbors, a community. There is sometimes marital disruption.

The waves of disturbance experienced by many hearing parents of a first deaf child commonly find release in various types of psychological defenses: overprotection, denial, rejection in different guises, open rejection, cure-seeking, doctor-shopping, and outright consternation. To make matters even more bewildering for the child, the type of parent behavior can change from day to day, depending on a parent's fluctuating moods, and reactions to the child can differ widely from one professional authority figure to another. The wonder is that a deaf child's psychological structure can withstand the buffeting of such erratic input.

As for the parents, before they have had time to fully absorb the first shock, they find themselves facing a new problem: the matter of schooling. This is another agonizing period. Knowing that a child is deaf does not automatically mean knowing the ramifications of the disability, let alone the child's instructional needs, the various methods used, and the philosophies behind the methods. Yet educational decisions must be made, and soon; too much time has already been wasted through undetected deafness. But where to turn for help?

Parents now turn to the team experts in hearing rehabilitation. And here they encounter the full force of dissension concerning terminology, school placement, communication methods, and more (Panel on Parent Education, 1974). They are told the child is "deaf," "severely hard of hearing," "hearing impaired"; they are variously advised to send the child to a residential school, a day school, a day class, a regular class in a "hearing" school; they are lectured by proponents and opponents of oralism, total communication, acoupedics; they are given conflicting professional opinions on the subjects of hearing aids, lipreading, speech instruction, home teaching, home management.

It is a strong parent who can emerge unshaken from such well-intentioned but discordant convictions. And still unanswered is the question: Which educational philosophy best meets the needs and abilities of this particular child? Educational predictions for very young deaf children are as yet more a matter of clinical judgment based on the advisor's experience and expertise than of the questionable predictive ability of objective measures. What assurances are there, then, that the choice made is the right choice?

These are no new questions. They have tormented every parent of a first deaf child since education of the deaf began. During the nineteenth century, parents started to band together to help one another find answers. Under the leadership of determined members, they began to form parent associations. Among the first was the Boston Parents' Education Association for Deaf Children, founded in 1894 (Best, 1943, p. 362). Others followed, along with increasing numbers of articles on the advantages of early instruction, tips for parents, methods advocacies, and more (Fellendorf, 1977). Today parent associations and parent programs are a common resource in educational facilities for deaf children as well as at regional, national, and international levels; and parent involvement in educational decision-making has received unprecedented federal support through PL 94-142, the Education of All Handicapped Children Act (U.S., Congress, 1975), to be discussed in chapter 5.

However, the experiences of professional workers involved in parent guidance (e.g., Bennett, 1955; Harris, 1960), taken in conjunction with the findings of exceptional amounts of emotional disturbance among deaf pupils (Schlesinger and Meadow, 1972), suggest that parent education programs can go only so far in reducing the traumatic effects of a hearing parent's confrontation with child-deafness. Bennett (1955) observes that emotional disturbance can persist in some parents to an incapacitating degree and can affect every area of parent–child relations, including educational decision-making. Herein lies a serious potential danger of PL 94-142: although granted the authority, so few parents are ready either emotionally or informationally for objective educational decision-making at the time when first decisions must be made.

Parent disturbances are expressed in many ways. When they are manifested as rejection of the child, the school is often forced to assume a parent role out of sheer concern for the rejected child. If a significant other figure enters the child's life, whether in the school or elsewhere, and provides the love, recognition, and motivation the child needs to forge ahead, then not too much harm has been done. The parents have simply lost a child. But if no other significant figure appears, the child himself may well be lost, and go through life forever seeking from others the care and attention that should have come from the parents.

Where parent disturbance shows itself in overcontrol, one pattern is a need to wipe out the "stigma" of deafness as rapidly as possible by pressuring the child to quickly acquire the accouterments of "normalcy," particularly in terms of speech. Often, parents as well as professional workers are completely oblivious to the fact that there are limits of tolerance to input. When these limits are exceeded, the results show up in various pathological ways. One of the most common can be found under the umbrella "learning disability," which hides not only *"teaching* disability" but also many deaf children who are seeking escape from the disruptive effects of being pushed beyond their limits.

In his masterful treatment of the behavioral aspects of human communication, Ruesch observes (in regard to nondeaf children) that the rather characteristic disturbances resulting from excessive pressures include rigidity in perception and action at the expense of flexibility, and adherence to rules and principles of behavior are apt to occur when "parents become impatient with the child's nonverbal forms of communication. . . . Premature verbalization and apparent skill with numbers take the place of much-needed experience in the process of interaction" (1957, p. 96). These comments have remarkable relevance to the situation in which many young deaf children find themselves.

Another form of child control is seen in parents whose need is to dramatize themselves as the major figures in the confrontation with deafness, as martyrs, protectors of a helpless child. In such instances, the parent takes on a dominating role that far exceeds the limits of practical necessity, robbing the child of identity, limiting the exercise of independent action to a minimum, retarding development, and otherwise laying the foundation for an infantile and ineffective adult.

There are many other variations of unhealthy child management by parents who cannot accept the reality of deafness. Whatever the variation, it is determined by the psychological needs of the parent at the expense of the developmental needs of the child. But no matter how self-deceived parents may be regarding their feelings for the child, the child "knows." No amount of surface display of love and concern can fool the penetrating perceptions of childhood. Children know when they have been measured and found wanting. They register their protests and unhappiness in the only way open to them—in behavior—at which point they are labeled "maladjusted" or "emotionally disturbed." But what else can they be? They are, after all, simply reflecting the pathologies of their maladjusted environment.

Fortunately, there are numbers of deaf children whose parents possess the stability and stamina to cope with the initial shock of diagnosis. After a reasonable period of mourning-for-loss, they buckle down to the job of becoming effective parents to a child who happens to be deaf and whose greatest need is for communicative interplay with the world around. The "curriculum" for such parent-preparation is generally put together by the parents themselves from a variety of sources that are available to them—the literature and lectures on deafness, child development, and on field resources and options; visits to facilities; discussions with experts in various disciplines and with other parents; membership in parent organizations; participation in adult deaf activities; and more. From information so obtained, screened by sound common sense, these parents draw out the special guides and techniques to provide their deaf child with the formative and informational inputs normally supplied through hearing. Increasing numbers of hearing parents are turning to the nonverbal language of signs (Sternberg, 1981) to provide their deaf babies with the communicative equivalents enjoyed by hearing babies of the same age (Stoloff and Dennis, 1978).

To put the guides into practice is no easy task. Often decision-making can tax the emotional control of even the most stable parents, as, for example, in weighing the advantages versus the dangers to a deaf child of such potentially hazardous but socially desirable activities as street play, bicycle riding, roughhouse games with the neighborhood children, and many other kinds of independent social interaction. It takes special skills and self-control to caution a deaf child to "be careful" without frightening or discouraging him.

Interestingly enough, many of these "adjusted" parents have found their own lives greatly enriched through the circumstance of having a deaf child. Dale quotes one of them: "It seems awful to say this, but I'm sure my husband and I have had a much more interesting life since we discovered Peter was deaf. We've met so many wonderful people, read more than we ever did, and somehow little things don't seem to worry us as they did" (1967, p. 28). I have heard many similar comments. Such parents have learned to see the normal child behind the façade of deafness. The relationship between them and their deaf children is a joy to both.

Deaf Parents

Deaf parents of deaf children escape the disruptive potential that the discovery of deafness has for hearing parents. The soundless world into which their child is born is their world. They have been reared in its subculture, use its unique manual communications, have experienced its problems, and generally feel equipped to guide the child over many of the obstacles. Furthermore, they are familiar with habilitative measures and educational procedures through personal experience, and seldom challenge professional educational responsibility. Most feel comfortable with their deaf children.

It is when a first hearing child is born to deaf parents that anxieties are apt to arise. Although most wish for hearing children (Rainer, Altshuler, and Kallman, 1963), when the wish is granted, doubts may arise. They wonder if they have the knowledge and ability to share the child's hearing world. Who will teach the child to talk? How will they function in the unfamiliar setting of a "hearing" school and hearing parent associations? Will their child's hearing friends look down upon his deaf parents? Will the child himself be ashamed of them? Such worries are obviated when a deaf child is born.

For the deaf infant, there are a number of potential advantages in having deaf parents. For one, the infant is spared the impact of disturbance common to hearing parents of a first deaf child. For another, the "visual hunger" with which babies are born is apt to be more readily and fully satisfied by visually oriented parents such as the deaf than by auditorially oriented hearing parents. As a result, the deaf baby of deaf parents is generally involved in stimulating parent–child gestural communication as early as the first months of life. Furthermore, to satisfy the baby's "mental hunger," the early gestural message forms are easily transposed into the structured manual communication forms used by deaf persons. These give the deaf child, while still in babyhood, a feel for the use of patterned language in interpersonal communication. Unlike deaf children of hearing parents, many deaf children of deaf parents are experienced communicators well before preschool age. By the time the deaf child enters school, interpersonal communication has become a way of life.

However, early parent–child communication does not necessarily ensure healthy parent–child communication. It only ensures an early intake of parental influences. These may be for better or for worse, depending on the parents. A "for better" picture comes with deaf parents who make sure that the child is provided with the input that fits developmental imperatives, emotional needs, and cultural adaptation. A "for worse" picture comes with a scattering of deaf parents who lack the maturity, knowledge, and intuitions necessary for child-rearing. Examples are cited by Schlesinger and Meadow:

> We have met immature deaf parents with their children who were unable to see their infant as a feeling baby. Their infants remained nameless for prolonged periods of time, they were "mascoted" and treated like dolls or objects. Some immature deaf parents have felt so incompetent in the task of child-rearing that their infants were cared for by maternal grandparents. (1972, 26–27)

With mature deaf parents as well, hearing grandmothers are frequently called upon for help especially with a first child. Initially, grandmothers serve as attentive ears for baby sounds and cries, and to lend a hand with household chores. But as time goes by, many become closely involved in child-rearing and decision-making. They, too, were the parents of deaf babies and have a wealth of experience to share with these "babies," now parents themselves. Although it is usually overlooked, the importance of the grandparent role in the rearing of deaf children was acknowledged by a special workshop for grandparents conducted by the Atlanta Speech School

(Rhoades, 1975). In addition to grandparents, another frequently overlooked group is composed of oral deaf parents of deaf infants. Special programs for such parents are conducted by the Lexington School for the Deaf (Held, 1975).

Research summarized in later chapters indicates significant advantages to a deaf child in having deaf parents. However, it would be interesting to know how many of these children owe their developmental foundations to hearing grandmothers or other hearing mediators. Unfortunately, such data were not included in the studies.

Although much remains to be learned about the actual child-rearing practices of deaf parents, common sense would lead to the conclusion that any advantages a deaf child derives from parental influences depend on the effectiveness of the parents as people rather than on their audiograms.

The Environment of Labels and Stereotypes

An environment of labels, terminology, and stereotypes awaits a deaf child from the moment of birth. Apart from their obvious connotations, more subtle and generally unrecognized influences are involved in each of the many labels that might be attached to a particular child.

For example, Wilson, Ross, and Calvert conducted an interesting study to determine which of eleven terms was preferred by a group of 69 hearing college students to describe individuals having some degree of hearing loss. The terms judged were: deaf, deaf-mute, deaf and dumb, hearing impaired, hard of hearing, hearing loss, partially hearing, partial hearing loss, limited hearing, hearing handicapped, and partially deaf. The preferred choice was "hearing impaired." It "evoked fewer negative semantic associations than any of the other common terms and phrases used to denote a hearing deficiency" (1974, p. 413).

Although the investigators point out the value of the generic use of the term "hearing impaired," they also hypothesize that the more favorable image evoked by this term as compared with "deaf" would produce higher scholastic expectations, hence better achievement, from children labeled "hearing impaired" than from the same children if they were labeled "deaf." Such is the subtle power of labels to influence outcomes.

Similarly with definitions: every definition of "deaf" evokes a different image of a deaf person in the user's mind; every term used to designate "deaf" creates a different feeling for what it implies. When there are as many different personifications of "deaf" as there are interpretations, there are bound to be just as many different opinions about management. In consequence, a deaf child runs a continuing risk of being forced into a setting that fits the label but not the child.

There is also a tendency to change a deaf child's label in recognition of outstanding achievement, a kind of promotion from "deaf" to "hard of hearing" or "hearing impaired." However, scholastic success does not alter the basic physiological picture of prelinguistic deafness nor of its fundamental implications. In my opinion, an exceptional child who happens to be deaf should be rewarded with recognition as an outstanding *deaf* child rather than with a change of label. All that label-change does is to create more confusion than now exists in what Wilson and associates (1974) call the "semantics of deafness." The historic burden the deaf have borne of being cast as labels and stereotypes rather than as people is not the least of the handicaps of deafness. As Schreiber remarked, "It is a tribute to the deaf that they survive at all under such conditions" (1969). It may be that to a certain extent deafness protects.

References

Becker, S. 1976. Initial concern and action in the detection and diagnosis of a hearing impairment in the child. *Volta Review,* 78: 105–15.

Bennett, D. N. 1955. Parents as teachers of the preschool deaf child. *Journal of Exceptional Children,* 22: 101–3, 122.

Best, H. 1943. *Deafness and the Deaf in the United States.* New York: Macmillan Co..

Chapanis, A. 1971. Prelude to 2001: Exploration in human communication. *American Psychologist,* 26: 949–61.

Dale, D. M. C. 1967. *Deaf Children at Home and in School.* London: University of London Press.

Dennis, W. 1960. Causes of retardation among institutional children. *Journal of Genetic Psychology,* 96: 47–59.

Fellendorf, G. W., ed. 1977. *Bibliography on Deafness.* Washington, D.C.: Alexander Graham Bell Association for the Deaf.

Fellendorf, G. W., and Harrow, I. 1970. Parent counseling 1961–1968. *Volta Review,* 72: 51–58.

Gesell, A., and Amatruda, C. S. 1947. *Developmental Diagnosis.* 2nd ed. New York: Paul B. Hoeber.

Gesell A., and Ilg, F. L. 1943. *Infant and Child in the Culture of Today.* New York: Harper & Brothers.

Harris, N. 1960. A pilot study of parental attitudes. *Volta Review,* 62: 355–61.

Held, M. 1975. Oral deaf parents communicate with their deaf infants. *Volta Review,* 77: 309–10.

McAree, R. 1970. What price parenthood? *Volta Review,* 72: 431–37.

Montagu, A. 1957. *Man: His First Two Million Years.* New York: World Publishing Co.

Murphy, A. T., ed. 1979. The families of hearing-impaired children. *Volta Review,* 81: 265–384.

Panel on Parent Education and Combating Misinformation. 1974. *Proceedings of the Forty-Sixth Meeting of the Conference of Executives of American Schools for the Deaf, Inc.,* Tucson, Arizona: Arizona School for the Deaf and the Blind. Pp. 8–18.

Rainer, J. D., Altshuler, K. Z., and Kallmann, F. J., eds. 1963. *Family and Mental Health Problems in a Deaf Population.* New York: New York State Psychiatric Institute.

Rhoades, E. A. 1975. A grandparents' workshop. *Volta Review,* 77: 557–60.

Ruesch, J. 1957. *Disturbed Communication.* New York: W. W. Norton & Co.

Schlesinger, H. S., and Meadow, K. P. 1972. *Sound and Sign.* Berkeley: University of California Press.

Schreiber, F. 1969. The deaf adult's point of view. Lecture presented at the Teacher Institute, Maryland School for the Deaf, October 1969.

Spitz, R. 1945. Hospitalism: An inquiry into the genesis of psychiatric conditions in early childhood. *Psychoanalytic Study of the Child,* 1: 53–74.

Spradley, T. S., and Spradley, J. S. 1978. *Deaf Like Me.* New York: Random House.

Sternberg, M. L. 1981. *American Sign Language: A Comprehensive Dictionary.* New York: Harper & Row.

Stoloff, L., and Dennis, Z. G. 1978. Matthew. *American Annals of the Deaf,* 123: 442–47.

U.S., Congress. 1975. Education of All Handicapped Children Act of 1975. Public Law 94–142. November 27, 1975.

Wilson, G. B., Ross, M., and Calvert, D. R. 1974. An experimental study of the semantics of deafness. *Volta Review,* 76: 408–15.

4 The Language Environment

> The bond between an individual and society is supplied by language.
> Whatmough, *Language: A Modern Synthesis*

COMMUNICATIVE RESTRAINTS of the kinds imposed by prelinguistic deafness would be expected to narrow a language environment and reduce the number of language forms used by its occupants. Such, however, is not the case with the deaf. In fact, considerably more "languages" are found among the deaf than among their hearing peers.

Represented in the deaf language environment are what Charlton Laird (1953) calls the "four vocabularies" of literate peoples—the speaking, writing, reading, and recognition vocabularies. In addition, there are language forms special to the deaf, such as lipreading, fingerspelling, the American Sign Language, and various systems of manually coded English.

One might suppose that with all these language forms at their disposal, the deaf would have easy communicative access to society. How they actually fare is the subject of this chapter. Discussion focuses on selected features of the principal "languages" in the deaf environment and on their mastery.

Verbal Language Forms

Linguistic Aspects

A few introductory comments on verbal language provide a context for the unusual situation facing deaf persons in mastering this language form.

In order for the communicative function of any language to be fulfilled, the members of a given community must share a common symbol system expressed and received in mutually used and understood patterns. It may come as a surprise to learn that this was not always the case with the English language in established societies. Bowen relates that the first English grammars were written out of the despair of scholars of the eighteenth century with the chaotic state of the language: "there was no agreement on spelling, style, or usage . . . and no authority one could appeal to in order to resolve questions of correctness" (1970, p. 36). He further remarks that these early grammars were designed primarily to prevent the deterioration of the English language by writers of the period.

The grammars may well have salvaged the English language, but an even more momentous contribution was to spark the scientific study of verbal language. The term "linguistics," by which this branch of study is known, was first used in the mid-nineteenth century, and until the early half of the twentieth century the main focus was on written language. Then, under the influence of Sapir (1921; Mandelbaum, 1956) and Bloomfield (1933), the focus shifted to the spoken form. As explained by Sapir, "the actual history of man and a wealth of anthropological evidence indicate with overwhelming certainty that phonetic language takes precedence over all other kinds of communicative symbolism" (Mandelbaum, 1956, p. 2).

An important outcome of the shift to the spoken tongue was to expose the astonishing ambiguities of even ordinary conversation, as expressed in the saying: "I know you believe you understand what you think I said, but I am not sure you realize that what you thought you heard is not what I meant." The linguistic unknowns underlying that doggerel intensified the search into the mysteries of verbal language acquisition and of the rules governing its grammar and use. Of the ensuing theory explosion, Johnson-Laird wryly remarks, "The literature continues to grow faster than knowledge" (1974, p. 135).

Dettering (1970) groups language-acquisition theories into two main "biases": the rationalistic, which emphasizes an innate ability for acquiring verbal language while minimizing the influences of environment: and the empirical, which views verbal language in terms of both speech and grammatical construction as being acquired mainly through input from the cultural milieu and as being as much a product of environmental determinism as is any other acquired human behavior.

The theory that has had the greatest recent impact on linguistic thinking is a type of generative grammar termed transformational, in particular the type developed by Noam Chomsky (1957, 1965, 1968). Since aspects of the theory have entered the field of the deaf through research and practice, a short discussion is in order. Fuller references to psycholinguistic theory formulations can be found in Lyons (1970) and in the comprehensive reviews of Fillenbaum (1971) and Johnson-Laird (1974) and in current linguistic literature.

Chomskyan transformational-generative grammar is affiliated with the rationalistic school in accordance with its postulate that children are born with an "innate idea" of the rules of grammar, and that this innate faculty accounts for the extraordinary rapidity with which very young children are able to master complex syntactic structures. The postulate represents a radical departure from long-held views of language acquisition as a product of outside influences imposed on the child by the linguistic environment through imitation, conditioning, or reinforcement. In the Chomskyan view, the acquisition of language is essentially a child-created phenomenon in which the child's deep innate cognitive structures transform perceptions into kernel sentences, consisting, it may be, of only one word. In the process of maturation, these are transformed into infantile grammatic structures, which in turn and with striking rapidity are transformed into the structures of the mother tongue. Involved in the process are various controlling factors, both within children, such as memory, and outside them, such as the immediate linguistic environment represented by parental speech against which children test their own emerging speech. In the course of expanding their language competencies, children unknowingly acquire for themselves the rules governing the grammar of the language. It is in this sense that children are considered language creators.

A major focus of Chomsky's work has been to search out and formalize the system of rules that constitute grammar. Included in the system are: (a) the *rules of syntax,* which govern the order and relationship of words in well-formed sentences; (b) the *rules of phonology,* which specify the phonetic character of the sentence generated by the syntactic rules; and (c) the *semantic rules,* which interpret the meaning of a sentence. The syntactic rules generate what Chomsky calls the *deep structure* of a sentence; the phonological rules, the *surface structure* in the form of actual sentences produced by the language-user; and the semantic rules of interpretation assign the meaning as derived from the deep structure.

Chomsky's greatest contribution is considered the inclusion of a *transformational* component into linguistic modeling. Through a series of steps, procedures, and rules too complex to be cited here, the transformational component converts the deep abstract structure of a sentence into its linguistic surface structure, and makes it theoretically possible to extend and expand the structural patterns of well-formed sentences to account for the infinite variations produced by language-users. Chomsky designates as *competence* the idealized, perfect grammatical use of a language, as distinguished from *performance,* which refers to the actual productions of the language-user. One of the tasks of generative linguists in describing the language of a particular speech community is to examine the consistency between competence and performance.

The remarkable impact of Chomskyan theory not only on linguistic science but also on language instruction in the schools (Markwardt and

Richey, 1970) does not imply universal acceptance. Certain linguists maintain with Bierwisch (1969) that a sentence derives its meaning as much or more from the other sentences with which it is associated in a frame of discourse as from its syntactic structure. Others hold that "competence" in the use of language is as much determined by the social situation in which it is used as by the ability to produce syntactically well-formed sentences (Bernstein, 1971). Possibly the most controversial difference exists between proponents of the Chomskyan belief in an innate syntactic faculty and those who maintain that whatever innate predispositions there may be are strongly influenced by environmental variables in language acquisition, particularly by parent-child dialogue (Campbell and Wales, 1970). The old nature-nurture controversy comes to mind, albeit with a different focus.

Simplistically summarized, the crucial question in Chomskyan-inspired deliberations seems to be: How are the raw data of mind and thought transposed into their linguistic equivalents? That the process is rooted in biological engineering is not surprising. In the service of survival, innate communicative engineering characterizes all living species, each with its own species-specific "language" for effecting adaptive organism–environment interplay, as for example the chemical "language" of the amoeba, the dance "language" of the honeybee (Von Frisch and Lindauer, 1965), the voice of the dolphin (Lilly, 1969), and the verbal language of *Homo sapiens*. In the case of the latter species, the need to cognitively internalize vast amounts of complex adaptive information, for lack of instinct programming, makes it essential that the young develop information input and exchange mechanisms as rapidly as possible to keep up with the adaptive demands of the cultural milieu. Again, biological engineering meets the need by activating what Marshall (1970) refers to as an early "critical period" in brain development, during which the brain is especially "tuned" to language acquisition. Hence the rapidity with which young children are able to acquire mastery of the mother tongue as well as of other languages.

Problems arise not in accepting these obvious facts, but in digging beneath the surface to get at the processing details. Lenneberg's (1967) efforts to track down the biological foundations of language have yielded abundant data, but "scholars are still unable to propose a biological *theory* of language—a formal model of a brain mechanism consistent with the physiology described by Lenneberg and with . . . psychological data" (Marshall, 1970, p. 241).

On the linguistic side, scholars are still theorizing about the structural properties that distinguish human language from all other animal languages, namely its syntax, phonology, and semantics; still deliberating on a human being's ability to produce and understand an infinite variety of sentences never before heard; still theorizing on the rapid acquisition of verbal language by the human young; and still searching for universals in the world's languages.

Overriding the unknowns and debates of linguistic inquiry is the driving concept that the structure of a language reflects the multiple functions of that language; that an understanding of the ways in which the words and sentences of a language relate to one another underlies an understanding of the ways in which words and sentences relate to reality.

On one point at least there is complete agreement, namely, that verbal language development is initiated through hearing. The grammar of a language flows into the ears of hearing children from babyhood onward throughout the whole of a waking day, in all its syntactic complexities, phonetic variations, semantic multiples and parallels, and intonational subtleties, and this comes about not only through the parent-child dialogue so favored by researchers, but through all the conversations that nondeaf children hear and overhear in their linguistic milieu. Little pitchers have big ears, the saying goes, and thanks to such copious, constant auditory input, by the time hearing children are ready for school, their common coin of communicative exchange includes verb forms, infinitives, relative pronouns, question formulations, passives and actives, conjunctions and prepositions, negatives, colloquialisms, and more. Further, not only are these children able to produce and understand sentences they have never before heard, they can also use and understand the semantics of intonation, pitch, stress, and all the other musical elements of a communicating voice. The biological foundations are there; hearing activates their operation; environment provides the input.

Verbal Language and the Deaf: Root Problems

When congenitally deaf children begin to learn verbal language, they find a ready-made body of voiceless, unknown words waiting to be mastered which they have never heard and never will hear in their natural-sounding form and flow. A hearing child *acquires* verbal language through audition, but a deaf child must memorize it piece by piece, mainly through visual input. And whereas a hearing child *creates* his language, deaf children find it imposed on them from the outside. They have played no part in its making, either semantically or syntactically. Mastery rests mainly on rote memory.

Memorizing Words and Meanings. The first verbal discoveries that prelinguistically deaf beginning learners make are that things have names, that activities have names, that they themselves have a name. They learn that these "names" are "words" and that words have meaning. They are shown how words look on the blackboard or spelled on the fingers. They learn that if they watch very closely, they can see how a particular word looks on the lips of a speaker, and how it differs in appearance from other words. Of course they cannot understand any words until they are taught the meanings. They must therefore memorize the various visible appearances and meanings of every word they add to their verbal vocabulary.

To help them in the task, illustrative pictures are used and specific word meanings are drilled and drilled until they are fixed in memory. But pictures are not the real thing; and many very young children, hearing as well as deaf, do not realize that the picture of an airplane, for example, stands for the actual plane as it soars through the sky. The connection between the picture and the object for which it stands must be made clear to them. If it is not, then the picture is the "airplane" and the thing in the sky has another name, as yet unknown. In programs in which teaching is conducted through speech, the children are spoken to constantly so they will see how whole thoughts and connected language as well as single words look on the lips. And before very long, children in these programs begin the most exacting task of all, and that is to use voice, breath, and articulatory organs in oral expression. This too they must fix in memory for every word they learn to say.

As time goes on, deaf children are taught that things have qualities as well as names. Things can be big, small, round, red, pretty, and so forth. It goes without saying that the children were aware of such differences in appearance all along; they simply lacked the words to cloak the observations. But as the word-meanings are given, linguistic perplexities begin to arise. From the children's point of view, if one can see a ball, or a pencil, or a boat, why not a big, or a small, or a red? And if blue distinguishes one dress from another, why not a "dress blue" instead of a "blue dress"? The words mean the same; what difference should word order make? Linguistic perplexities multiply as word-meanings must be learned that cannot be illustrated by pictures, such as "the," "a," "but," and "if," to say nothing of the semantic complications that arise from multiple word meanings, and the differences in meaning of such expressions as "to look at," "to look like," "to look out," "to look for," "to look out for," and eventually from having to memorize the word order that gives meaning to sentences. There are not enough hours in a school day to touch all linguistic bases when the meaning of a language must be learned bit by bit through vision, drill, and memory.

To learn verbal expression in this slow, piece-by-piece way is not only linguistically unnatural, it is psychologically incompatible with a small child's developmental imperatives and an older pupil's informational needs. A deaf child's chief defense against serious communicative deprivation is a master teacher who, to paraphrase Simmons (1968), knows *what* the pupil needs to know and *why*, before deciding on how best to teach it. But the problem here lies in the serious shortage of teachers who are qualified and adequately trained to teach deaf children (Connor, 1971; Council on Education of the Deaf, 1974; Delgado, 1973).

When the delicate yet crucial matter of teaching communication to a deaf beginning pupil is left to the inexperienced and poorly trained, the "what" and the "why" of teaching customarily focuses on words and vocabulary building; the "how" on the method of instruction espoused by the school. Progress is measured in terms of number of words mastered, and these generally bear a closer relationship to mode of communication than to the child's experiences and expressive needs. For example, words traditionally chosen for beginning lipreading are ones that are readily seen on the lips— fish, bow, airplane; while those chosen for speech are ones that present the least difficulties in articulation. Then there are other words for reading plus words coming through the hearing aid, to say nothing of fingerspelled words and words taught in various sign systems. The child sees unrelated words coming at him from all kinds of places: from the lips, the blackboard, the hearing aid, from books, and from the fingers, from everywhere seemingly but from the world of his interests and experiences. But unless the words a deaf child is taught relate to life, that child is being taught a dead language. In such vocabulary-oriented teaching, mental hungers are fed with an assortment of memorized word meanings instead of with the semantics of experiences and concepts; and communicative drive withers under drill, repetition, and correction.

To keep verbal language alive for small deaf children and the spirit of inquiry flourishing is a glowing competence of the true master teacher. Unless this is done, there is grave danger that the child's mental set will take on the same rigidities as practiced in teaching. In this connection, Mildred Groht (1958), the renowned proponent of natural language for deaf children, used to tell of a teacher in a "deep-south" school who was conscientiously intent on drilling the day's vocabulary when a sudden snowstorm appeared. The teacher religiously kept to the day's schedule. When the visiting supervisor asked why the teacher did not take advantage of this unique opportunity to tell about "snow," the teacher explained that the word was not on the day's vocabulary list. Another incident that I witnessed illustrates instructional rigidities reflected in pupil behavior. This young deaf child dug in his heels and refused to enter a particular room for his lipreading lesson on the ground that it was not his regular "lipreading" room. It was his speech-teaching room. Where the teaching of verbal language to deaf children lacks spark, relevance, and flexibility, so eventually will the ones being taught. The whole point of learning to communicate is lost. The pupils have simply learned to memorize; they have not "learned to learn" nor learned to think.

Numerous highly respected professional persons outside the field of the deaf entertain the idea that children who cannot hear the mother tongue can learn by reading. The fact of the matter is that reading places greater demands on linguistic competence than does talking; and when average deaf pupils open a book based on the interests of their particular age group, they see not a story but a conglomeration of unknown words, confusing idioms, and unfamiliar constructions. To hold on to the thread of a narrative while trying to decode the elements is enough to discourage all but the stoutest of hearts, the sharpest of minds, and the most persistent of spirits. Where these qualities are lacking, less hardy spirits handle the matter by spinning a narrative out of selected words and familiar phrases. Sometimes they hit the mark; often they do not, as illustrated by the following incident that occurred in a school for the deaf.

The personnel director of a large business concern employing deaf persons became greatly alarmed at the number of personal data forms in which the answer "yes" had been given by the deaf job applicants from this particular school to the questions "Have you ever been in a mental hospital?" and "Have you ever had fits?" She hurriedly phoned the school principal for explanation, and was promptly reassured. None of the applicants had ever been committed to a mental hospital. None had ever had fits. The problem lay in their reading of the language of the application form.

Regarding the first question, the words "mental" and "hospital" had never been taught as the unit expression "mental hospital" but simply as isolated words. Consequently the deaf applicants were unfamiliar with the expression. But they were completely familiar with the word "hospital." All had at one time or another been to the school hospital or had visited friends in other hospitals. "Hospital" was part of their experience, and the word stood out like an old friend. Accordingly, they geared their response to this familiar word, and in so doing obligingly answered "Yes" to the question "Have you ever been in a mental hospital?"

As to "Have you ever had fits?" all the young applicants had just completed a course in dressmaking. Great stress had been placed on the need for accuracy in the cut and fit of the garments they had made. What could be more reasonable than to assume the word "fits" in the question had the same meaning as in dressmaking? So here too the answer yes seemed entirely suitable. As George Miller remarks, "Words signify only what we have *learned* they signify" (1951, p. 5; italics added).

This anecdote provides a small sample of the difficulties of memorizing the semantics of a language word by word, without benefit of hearing. Complex though the problems are, there is a still greater one, and that is memorizing the syntax of the language and learning the contributions of syntax to meaning.

Memorizing Syntax. Teachers struggling to teach verbal language to con-

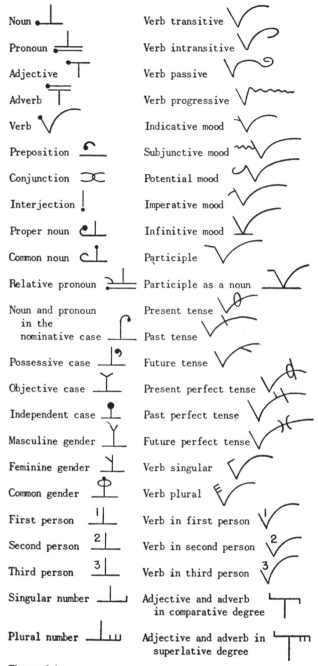

Figure 4.1.
A system of symbols used in the study of grammar.
From Nelson (1949).

Conjunction (co-ordinate) . . . . Ⅸ

Conjunction (subordinate) . . . . Ⱨ

Adverbial conjunction . . . . Ⱨ⁵

Relative pronoun

    Nominative . . . . Ⱨ S

    Possessive . . . . Ⱨ 2

    Objective . . . . Ⱨ O

Special Symbols

Noun or name word . . . . **N**

Auxiliary verb . . . . **+ or −**

Progressive form of verb . . . . **V̿**

Present tense . . . . **V̍**

Past tense . . . . **V̀**

Future tense . . . . **V́**

Object of participle or infinitive . . **O̅**

    Noun or pronoun . . . . **N̅C̅**

    Adjective . . . . **A̅C̅**

Nominative independent . . . . **[S]**

Nominative absolute . . . . **(S)**

Indirect object . . . . **− O**

Ellipsis . . . . **✳**

Interjection . . . . **!**

The Essentials

Subject . . . . S

Verb (general symbol) V

    Intransitive . . . . V͡ͻ

    Transitive, active . . . . V͡‾

    Transitive, passive . . . . ͡‾V

Object . . . . O

Complement (adjective) . . . . AC

Complement (noun and pronoun) . . . . . . NC

Modifying Forms Indicated by Numbers

Noun or pronoun in apposition I

Possessive 2

Adjective and article 3

Prepositional phrase 4

Adverb and adverbial phrase 5

Infinitive 6

Participle 7

Figure 4.2.
Another system of symbols used in the study of grammar.
From Nelson (1949).

genitally deaf pupils are hard pressed to see among them any evidence of the Chomskyan concept of an "innate idea" of syntactic structures. Equal difficulty is experienced in accepting Lenneberg's supportive statement for the innate idea theory, that although "congenital deafness has a devastating effect on the vocal facilitation for speech, yet presentation of written material enables the child to acquire language through a graphic medium *without undue difficulties*" (1964, p. 67; italics added). What Lenneberg's statement does illustrate is the enormous difficulty even exceptional persons have in conceiving the linguistic void created by congenital deafness, and the learning problems of children who do not know there are such things as words, who have never experienced such things as sentences, and have yet to encounter such things as rules of grammar.

The instructional way has not yet been found for arousing an innate idea of syntactic structures in the minds of children who have never heard the verbal tongue. This has not been for lack of trying. The excellent reviews by Nelson (1949) and Schmitt (1966) summarize over 30 instructional approaches and philosophies that have been used with deaf pupils in this country since the early nineteenth century. Fellendorf's bibliography (1977) of articles from *The Volta Review* and the *American Annals of the Deaf* gives a vivid picture of the instructional strategies used by ingenious teachers in their determination that their deaf pupils master verbal language.

A major difficulty in all approaches is the scarcity of pictorial aids for illustrating syntactic relationships and fixing them in the minds of the pupils. Schmitt expresses it well when he says, "Language development for the deaf might be said to entail building the English language into the child" (1966, p. 86). The building-in process is based on memorizing. With syntax as with vocabulary, mastery rests on memory.

To bolster memory, the earlier educators devised visible aids in the form of complicated symbol notations for the parts of speech, and elaborate sentence diagrams to indicate syntactic relations. Several are depicted in figures 4.1 and 4.2. Certain of these aids to memory appear to present a greater tax on memory than would syntax itself. Most have gradually fallen into disuse. The outstanding exception is the Fitzgerald Key (1926), which is a sentence pattern guide to help deaf children form and correct their own sentences. The key still enjoys considerable use in schools for the deaf (Hudson, 1979). Later devised but less generally used syntax- and vocabulary-teaching strategies are competently summarized by Schmitt (1966).

Other types of language-support strategies are more recent additions to the educational scene. These include such approaches as educational media, mainstreaming, total communication, and early fitting of hearing aids. A common underlying goal of all of these is improved language learning. Finally, from the ranks of Chomskyan linguists comes a recommendation by

McNeill (1966), proposing the use of "expansion-like" instruction in which a young deaf child's beginning exposure to verbal language would be in the form of "child speech," in accordance with the baby-talk patterns that characterize the beginning speech of hearing children, and would then "expand" from that point with the introduction of increasingly advanced structures. Determining whether these moves will result in a more productive teaching–learning environment for deaf pupils will require prolonged and carefully controlled longitudinal study.

As matters stand, an examination of the verbal language habits of the deaf as obtained from written samples over the decades shows no historic change despite the variety of instructional methods tried. For example, the most important "errors of construction" found by a teacher of the deaf in 1897 "from a perusal of examination papers" were:

Misuse of the verb,
Misuse of the adjective and adverb,
Misuse of the relative clause,
Confusion of direct and indirect quotations,
Careless use of pronouns, especially in lack of agreement with antecedent,
Misuse or omission of the articles,
Transposition of adjective and noun,
Transposition of letters in familiar words. (J. L. Smith, 1897, p. 205)

The errors noted by Smith bear striking resemblance to the defects reported in recent times. For example, Quigley, Power, and Steinkamp (1977) found that particularly difficult structures for the deaf subjects of their research include: the verb system, the use of pronouns, infinitives, and gerunds; and the use of relative pronouns, phrases, and clauses.

How such impaired linguistic structures appear in sentence form is illustrated by the following examples taken from a list recorded by Fusfeld (1958) and written by applicants for admission to Gallaudet College:

1) I began to love it as to be my favorite sport now.
2) To his disappointed, his wife disgusted of what he made.
3) He always patiented with his wife because she always boss over him.
4) Many deaf people play or act nicelessly to the people if they get mad with them.
5) I was happy to kiss my parents because they letted me playing foot ball. (pp. 261–62)

The following example shows how the impaired structures read in narrative form, as excerpted from Fusfeld (1955):

Some people must take with many deaf people. They like to help them became they were smart. They must to kind to them. Maybe many deaf people will like

them became a freind. Yes, they were sorry for them because they can't heard
and they don't understand what the people said. (p. 2)

The language used here is fairly good "deaf" language, as deaf language
goes. Readers can judge for themselves by comparing it with the following
direct transposition from the sign language of an intelligent but uneducated
deaf adult:

> Improve cold snow tonight. North coming cold now maybe. Many people pass-
> ing here fast shot cars 70 hour. Time now 12:46 A.M. Sleep now—Sunday, to-
> morrow plus now. (Personal communication)

Other examples of written productions, from superb to jargon, are given in
the course of later discussion to illustrate, among other things, the exceptional range of linguistic fluency in the deaf population.

A composite description of the freely written language of deaf research
subjects can be abstracted from various authoritative sources (Blanton, 1968;
Heider and Heider, 1940a,b; Kates, 1972; Myklebust, 1960; Quigley,
Power, and Steinkamp, 1977; Simmons, 1962). "Deaf language" has a
strong "rubber-stamp" quality, rigid in style and loaded with stereotypic
repetitions suggesting memorized units rather than generative productions.
The simple, short sentences resemble the patterns of much younger hearing
children, and the narrowed vocabulary (Cooper and Rosenstein, 1966) is
characterized by a large proportion of everyday nouns and verbs at the expense of many other parts of speech. Among the common errors are omission of essential words, use of wrong words, addition of excessive words,
and incorrect word order. The Kates study (1972) gives additional information obtained from a comparative analysis of the written productions of subjects exposed to three different instructional communicative environments:
oral, combined oral-manual, and fingerspelling, while the Blanton research
(1968) mentions a singular and extremely provocative aspect of "deaf
language"—the deficiency in affective language and evaluational responses.

A more recent research move has been to probe beneath the descriptive
findings obtained from freely written language samples, into syntactic patterns as obtained through the more controllable cloze procedure. Leaders in
the move are Russell, Quigley, and Power (1976), who, with their associates, addressed such issues as the order of difficulty of syntactic structures
for deaf children, the establishment of syntactic rules, developmental stages
of syntactic rules, acquisition of distinct syntactic structures, and syntactic
structures in reading materials. One of the most productive outcomes of this
6-year research is the Test of Syntactical Abilities (TSA), designed to serve
as a diagnostic and assessment instrument and as a guide for teachers in
programming syntactic instruction.

Questions arise concerning the relationship between reading ability and the syntactic deficiencies of the deaf. Quigley, Power, and Steinkamp (1977) express the opinion that "the gap between the deaf subjects' knowledge of specific syntactic structures and the appearance of those structures in the widely used *Reading for Meaning* series . . . was so great for almost every structure, even for the 18-year-old subjects, that we feel justified in concluding that most deaf students cannot read the books that they are supposed to be reading and from which they are supposed to be learning" (p. 81). This opinion is supported by national achievement test data for hearing-impaired students collected since 1968 by the Office of Demographic Studies of Gallaudet College. Reporting on the 1974 reading achievement test findings, Trybus and Karchmer (1977) state that the median reading score for students ages 20 or above "corresponds to a grade equivalent of about 4.5. In other words, half the students at age 20 (or any younger age) read at less than a mid-fourth grade level, that is, below or barely at a newspaper literacy level," and that "at best, only 10% of hearing-impaired 18-year olds nationally can read at or above an 8th grade level" (1977, p. 64). There are some in lay and professional circles who counter with the observation that similarly low reading levels are not uncommon among hearing students as well. They overlook the fact that the low-reading hearing pupil has abundant auditorially acquired language which is denied the deaf. The hearing pupil has a *reading* disability; the deaf pupil, a *language* disability. These are two very different things.

Traditionally under fire for this sorry state are the communicative methods used in instructing deaf pupils. Advocates of instruction through speech hold that the grammar of the American Sign Language interferes with the learning of English grammar, while advocates of manual methods of instruction contend that the slowness and difficulties of teaching deaf pupils mainly through spoken language retard the whole learning process.

Also subject to blame are the rigidities of the subject-verb-object pattern in teaching word order to deaf pupils. Here, the usual focus is on fitting expressive language into a fixed mold; sentences are drilled in isolation without showing how they relate to one another in a frame of discourse, and alternate sentence forms and transformations are generally left for "later." Wilbur (1977) in particular believes that this approach contributes heavily to the syntactic problems of the deaf.

To sum up, the semantic/syntactic deficiencies of the deaf have a long history and do not yield to usual instructional strategies. It may be that by the time deaf children are exposed to formal language instruction, they are past Marshall's "critical period" in which the brain is especially "tuned" to language acquisition. If this be so, then current moves for auditorially amplified and/or manual language-input beginning in babyhood, before this critical period is past, warrant special attention.

Mastering Verbal Methods of Interpersonal Communication

Research shows no lack of mental or cognitive abilities on the part of the deaf which might account for their deficiencies in reading and writing. This being so, we turn to the verbal forms used by deaf persons in interpersonal communication: spoken language, lipreading, and fingerspelling.

Spoken Language. Of all the language forms used by man, spoken language is the commonest and most useful coin of communicative exchange. It requires the smallest vocabulary for everyday use (Laird, 1953), yet for all its small size goes the farthest not only in interpersonal exchange but, perhaps more importantly, in providing people with impressions of one another as human beings, and with feelings about one another. Spoken language creates personal awareness.

Spoken language is as remarkable in its production as in its use. It is created by an exquisite coordination of the movements of various respiratory and articulatory muscles, ably and succinctly described by Eisenberg (1976). The lungs supply the energy source for speech in the form of a column of expired air; the vocal cords at the larynx convert the column into a series of puffs or bursts whose energy registers as sound; and sound, in turn, is "shaped" into speech by the resonating cavities of the upper respiratory tract, and patterned in accordance with the particular adjustments and positions of the articulatory organs.

The role of hearing in this process is to stimulate vocal sound-making, convey the patterns of spoken language, and provide a monitoring mechanism for the sound-maker. A major purpose and accomplishment of the prolonged practice in vocal sound-making by hearing babies is to automatize coordination between respiration and articulation.

For the unaided ears of congenitally deaf babies, there is neither the stimulus for vocal practice nor the joy of feedback. The deafness-imposed silence wipes out a whole program of "drill" through which a hearing baby gradually acquires the ability to "breathe" speech. By the time most deaf children are taught to speak, respiration and articulation are two things apart.

Details of various methods and devices used in teaching speech to the deaf can be found in the copious literature on the subject (Calvert and Silverman, 1975a,b; Fellendorf, 1977; Strong, 1975). Briefly, the two main approaches are termed multisensory and unisensory. In the multisensory approach, tactile, visual, and auditory senses are all used, aided by various teacher-made reinforcements (New, 1940, 1949, 1954; Vorce, 1974), and, in certain programs, by technological aids that supply visible and/or tactile transformations of speech patterns (Boothroyd, 1975; Boothroyd et al., 1975; Larkin, 1976; Peterson, 1962; Pickett, 1976; Pronovost, 1978; Strong,

1975). The pupils watch how a word looks as spoken by the teacher and as visually transformed or tactually represented by the technological aid being used; feel the vibrations the word makes in the teacher's nose, throat, and face; hear what they can of how the word sounds through amplified residual hearing; commit the inputs to visual, tactile, and auditory memory; synthesize the memories into imitative utterance, subject to correction; and then drill until the word they are learning to say acquires intelligibility in the judgment of the teacher and in the pattern of the technological aid. Emphasis is on articulation. Special training in coordinating articulation and respiration is rarely given. This system of instruction is known as the *oral/aural* approach (Simmons-Martin, 1972).

In approaches that are unisensory, the teaching process emphasizes the use of one sensory input. In the *Tadoma method* (Gruver, 1955), for example, the tacile-kinesthetic avenue is used. The child feels the vibrations and muscular movements made by the spoken word by placing his hands on the teacher's face, and then on his own face in order to imitate what he has felt of the teacher's utterance. In order for the child to get the full effect of vibration, a blindfold is used, or the child's eyes are shut so that vibration becomes the only speech-lead. The "blinding" operations are discarded once vibratory sensitivity is well established. Inspiration for the Tadoma approach came from the better speech various deaf-blind persons were observed to have as compared with deaf persons.

More recent unisensory procedures owe their inception to remarkable advances in hearing aid technology (Risberg, 1971; Israel, 1975), in audiological and other techniques for early detection and diagnosis of impaired hearing (Downs, 1968; Lloyd and Dahle, 1976; National Joint Committee on Infant Hearing Screening, 1971, 1973), and in the early use of hearing aids, in some programs during the first few weeks of life (Griffiths, 1975). Taken together, these advances have generated the possibility of creating a "hearing" environment for deaf children from infancy onward, thus activating the practice necessary for coordinating respiration and articulation, and giving the children enough of the sounds of spoken language to develop their own systems of encoding what they hear into meaningful language.

Prominent among the auditory-unisensory approaches are the *Acoupedic* system (Niemann, 1972; Pollack, 1964, 1970), which is based on early detection of hearing impairment, early fitting of hearing aids, a normal learning environment, and the development of language solely through audition, and the *Verbotonal* system (Craig, Craig, and DiJohnson, 1972; Eisenberg and Santore, 1976; Guberina, 1964), which follows the early intervention pattern of the acoupedic program and the use of special equipment for low-frequency amplification along with body movements and musical stimulation to give pupils a feel for the rhythms, stresses, and phrasings of speech.

There is also the *Auditory Global* approach (Calvert and Silverman, 1975a), which, while not exclusively auditory-unisensory, places the same emphasis on early auditory input of fluent connected speech as do programs that are. In conversations with numbers of severely, congenitally deaf young adult "successes" of auditory programs, I have been deeply impressed with the excellence of their spoken language in sound and fluency. In some cases, the difference from "hearing" speech was barely noticeable. The need to study these phenomena is a pressing one.

Concerning the deaf at large, intelligible speech appears the exception rather than the rule. Brannon concludes his review of research by saying that "it is very difficult for the average congenitally deaf person to achieve useful levels of speech intelligibility. It is low in most, perhaps 20–25%" (1966, p. 130). Brannon's estimate is not far from that obtained by Tato and Arcella in an investigation of the speech intelligibility of 20 educated young deaf adults as understood by a group of normally hearing listeners familiar with "deaf" speech: "The average percentage of these 20 cases shows less than 30% (27.424) as regards the intelligibility of the speech of deaf-mutes in conversation" (1955, p. 162).

Other studies of speech intelligibility also come close to these estimates. Markides (1970) found that about 31% of the words spoken by hearing-impaired day and residential school subjects were intelligible to their teachers, and 19% to those unfamiliar with deaf speech. Ling (1976) cites a doctoral study by Heidinger (1972), which found that less than 20% of the words in short sentences spoken by deaf pupils in a residential school were intelligible to three experienced teachers of the deaf, and another doctoral study by C. R. Smith (1972), which found a mean of 18.7% in word intelligibility as judged by 120 listeners unfamiliar with deaf speech. Ling cites numerous other studies that yield similarly poor findings. Of deaf persons with high speech intelligibility, Brannon astutely comments, "The crucial factor seems to be not non-verbal intelligence but *the ability to make use of residual hearing,* even among those with losses of 75 decibels or more" (1966, p. 130; italics added).

The sound of "typical" deaf speech is difficult to describe since it is a composite of a number of speech defects plus deficiencies in syntax and vocabulary. A sure give-away is voice quality. In a study conducted by Calvert (1962), teachers of the deaf variously described the quality as tense, breathy, harsh, and throaty. The deaf, it must be remembered, do not "breathe" speech. It seems forced from the throat. This defect in speech breathing is a major contributor to the deficiencies of deaf speech but is hardly ever subjected to training despite the alerts sounded in the pioneer research of Hudgins (1936, 1937, 1946).

Nickerson (1975) provides a comprehensive review of investigations of the speech characteristics of deaf persons in regard to timing and rhythm, pitch and intonation, velar control, articulation, and voice quality. He makes the special point that although the defects noted in these areas can be separated for purposes of analysis, they cannot be separated for purposes of remediation. "A problem-by-problem approach to training may be bound to yield only limited success" (1975, p. 358). Nickerson deplores the fact that no successful alternative approaches have yet been devised. Ross (1976) sums up the state of the art in teaching the deaf to speak with the question, "If a hearing impaired child can communicate effectively, using both oral expression and reception, only to his teachers and his immediate family, can this be considered successful oral communication?" (1976, pp. 324–25).

In Ross's view an important contributor to this unsatisfactory situation is the unsatisfactory state of speech instruction, notably the failure to use the expertise of audiologists and speech pathologists, who are better trained than are teachers of the deaf. The importance of the speech pathologist is also stressed by Bennett (1974), while Ross and Calvert (1977) offer an impressive guidelines-document for the establishment of audiology programs in educational facilities for hearing-impaired children. The premises on which the guides are based are "1) the normal primacy of the auditory channel for speech and language development, 2) the evidence relating to the extent of residual hearing among 'deaf' children, and 3) the currently inadequate exploitation of residual hearing" (1977, p. 153).

To sum up: the speech patterns of the deaf are typically impaired by deficiencies in timing and rhythm, pitch and intonation, velar control, articulation, and voice quality, plus deficiencies in syntax and vocabulary. Research indicates no lack of mental or vocal ability on the part of the deaf for learning speech. Therefore, the accusing finger points to ineffective instructional practices as the most likely cause of deficiency (*Newsounds, 1977*).

The expectation grows increasingly strong that creating an "auditory environment" for the deaf from infancy onward through expert amplification of residual hearing reinforced by expert auditory training will result in significant gains in spoken language.

Lipreading. Lipreading is the visual reception and comprehension of messages conveyed in spoken language. For persons with impaired hearing, it is a key communicative link to the speaking world.

Certain terminological purists do not take kindly to the term "lipreading." Some maintain that the hearing-impaired receiver of spoken language is not reading *lips* but rather the *speech* that issues forth from them. They prefer the term "speech reading," originally proposed in 1889 (E. A. Fay, 1889) and now given new life. Others contend that the lipreader is not reading *speech* but the "thoughts transmitted via the visual components of oral discourse" (O'Neil and Oyer, 1961, p. 2). An alternate term, "visual hearing," used by Mason (O'Neil and Oyer, 1961, p. 147) has won a few proponents. By and large, however, the old standby "lipreading" remains the most commonly used, with "speechreading" a close second.

One popular belief is that lipreading is a verbatim visual intake of every word uttered by a speaker; another is that the ability is automatically activated as compensation for impaired hearing. Both beliefs are wide of the mark. Lipreading is by no means the magic route to speech comprehension that it is often supposed to be. Numerous hearing-impaired persons cannot master the skill despite exceptional language levels and mental endowment. Even where lipreading is above average, the lipreader comes up against such visual obstacles as stiff lips, poker faces, facial expression concealed by sunglasses, protruding teeth, moustaches, mouthings and grimaces, all of which make it impossible to see clearly the fleeting mouth movements that provide the clues to what the speaker is saying. To add to the difficulties, there are countless words that require little if any lip movement for utterance and so cannot be seen at all. Finally, there are numerous words of completely unrelated meaning that look exactly alike on the lips, as, for example, abuse and amuse; bloom and plume; and smell and spell; clam, clamp and clap; bump, mum, pump, and pup.

What goes into the making of a good lipreader is still an open question. The search for an answer has led into a number of possible related areas, including *intelligence* (Lewis, 1972; O'Neill and Davidson, 1956; Pintner, 1929; Reid, 1947; Roche et al., 1971; Simmons, 1959); *audition* (Erber, 1971, 1972; Ewertsen Nielsen, and Nielsen, 1970; Siegenthaler and Gruber, 1969); *visual acuity* (Braly, 1938; Erber, 1971; Hardick, Oyer, and Irion, 1970; Stockwell, 1952); *visual memory* (Blair, 1957; Espeseth, 1969; Furth, 1961; Hiskey, 1950; Neyhus, 1969; Pintner, 1929; Sharp, 1972; Simmons, 1959); *visual synthesis* (Sanders and Coscarelli, 1970; Sharp, 1972; Simmons, 1959); *amount of facial exposure* (Berger, Garner, and Sudman, 1971; Lowell, 1959); *gestures* (Berger and Popelka, 1971; Popelka and Erber, 1971); *concept formation* (O'Neill and Davidson, 1956; Simmons, 1959; Tiffany and Kates, 1972); *rhythm* (Heider and Heider, 1940a,b; Sharp, 1972; Simmons, 1959), and more, such as attentiveness, attributes of the speaker-sender, and the investigative materials used (O'Neill and Oyer, 1961), the most popular of which are motion picture tests of lipreading ability (Heider and Heider, 1940b; Mason, 1943; Morkovin and Moore, 1948–1949; Utley, 1946). Erber (1977) cites other tests of lipreading ability and proposes some evaluative approaches of his own. However, as Clarke and Ling remark, "Publications on speech reading . . . have contributed very little new information to our corpus of knowledge concerning this skill" (1976, p. 23). In a similar vein, Farwell concludes her comprehensive review of research with the statement, "Speechreading, the hallmark of deaf education, remains an enigma'' (1976, p. 27). Open to question are the tests used in the various studies, the samples surveyed, and the methodological procedures employed. In my opinion, it is doubtful whether the isolates involved in lipreading will disclose the dynamic interplay and counterbalance of attributes, abilities, and special skills that go into the making of a good lipreader.

We turn therefore to the lipreaders themselves for some of the real-life facts concerning the art. How the process works in life is described by Rosenthal:

> lipreaders don't "read" so much as pick up clues from the mouth, face, and body expressions to fill in the spaces of sounds they don't hear. This isn't easy. For every English-language speech movement one can read, there are two or three that are all but impossible to read. Lipreading is more like filling in the blanks of a crossword puzzle than reading a mouth syllable-by-syllable or word-by-word. You lip-read by combining movements deciphered visually with knowledge of the conversation's context, just as with a crossword puzzle you combine the letters you already have with the clues provided about the word you are trying to figure out. (1975, p. 158)

Rosenthal's word picture summarizes the experiences of many lipreaders.

Further information comes from a study conducted by Fusfeld (1958), who analyzed the reports submitted by the members of two groups of deaf college graduates, both groups of above-average achievement but one composed of good lipreaders, the other of indifferent ones. According to a member of the latter group, successful lipreading depends on a favorable interplay of a number of related factors:

> 1. Factors inherent in the speaker, namely, his bearing, the character (positive or negative) of his lip-movements, the inherent nature of his vocabulary and subject matter, his pronunciation, his facial expression, his intelligence; 2. Factors peculiar to the lipreader, as, amount of hearing left, vocabulary, understanding, eyesight, intelligence; and 3. Factors external to both, such as distance between speaker and lipreader, amount of light, extraneous facial features, i.e., moustache, dentures, hearing aids, sex. (Fusfeld, 1958, p. 239)

In regard to sex, Rosenthal observes that "women tend to be better lipreaders than men . . . no one knows why" (1975, p. 158). He also notes another important factor in effective lipreading—the lipreader's ability to cope with the fatigue induced by having to concentrate perpetually on a speaker's face while at the same time performing the mental gymnastics necessary for comprehension.

On the basis of his experience as a teacher of the deaf, Scouten (1969) summarizes the essentials for lipreading as: vocabulary; syntax; synthesization, meaning the ability to grasp instantaneously whole units, whole words, whole phrases and whole sentences; intuition, the ability to "put two and two together"; and experience in the use of the English language. He adds, "If any one of these five essentials is diminished, speechreading skill is diminished" (pages unnumbered).

Various approaches are used to help lipreaders fill in what Rosenthal calls the empty "spaces" between perceived lip movements. The oldest approach is instruction, introduced in this country in 1864 by Harriet B. Rogers (Peck, Samuelson, and Lehman, 1926) and used primarily with the hard of hearing. Among the most prominent instructional methods are the Nitchie (1930), the Müller-Walle (Bruhn, 1930), and the Jena (Bunger, 1944). Copious references to instructional methods and practice materials for lipreaders can be found in Fellendorf's bibliography (1977). It has also been found that the hearing aid and auditory training can be of great help in cueing the lipreader (Heider, 1943; Prall, 1957; Siegenthaler and Gruber, 1969). Another aid is an ingenious device designed by Upton (1968), in the form of eyeglasses fitted with five tiny lamps which supplement lip clues by means of light-flash information about a speaker's articulations. Another form of visible cue is the Mouth–Hand System (Holm, 1972), developed early in this century by Georg Forschhammer, headmaster of a Danish school for the deaf. In this system, phonetic hand-position symbols accompany a speaker's utterances as visible aids to the lipreader for invisible or ambiguous articulations. In this country, the Cued Speech method developed by Cornett (Clarke and Ling, 1976; Cornett, 1967, 1975; Moores, 1969) employs the same principle of manual phonetic cues.

No matter what the approach, success in sustained conversational lipreading and especially in instructional classroom lipreading demands one competence above all others, and that is an understanding of the vocabulary and syntax of the language uttered by the speaker. Unknown words and unfamiliar syntactic patterns cannot be meaningfully lipread. Not that linguistic ability guarantees lipreading ability. There are numbers of linguistically gifted deaf persons who are poor lipreaders. However, good lipreaders are good linguistic performers. And here we encounter a major obstacle to lipreading on the part of deaf children and language-deficient deaf adults. Costello (1958) observes that the deaf child

> lives in a world of here and now, without words, without an orderly language pattern, and in many instances without the concepts which language symbols presuppose. Thus the achievement of speech-reading for the deaf child is not confined to training on the differentiation of the perceived visual signals. It involves perceptual growth, concept formation, development of vocabulary, and ability to deal with the meaning conveyed by myriads of language patterns.

Because of a deaf child's unformed linguistic state plus the ambiguities inherent in lipreading and the strains imposed on a lipreader, Vernon estimates that "the average deaf child understands about 5% of what is said in lipreading" (1972, p. 531).

However, many young deaf children respond appropriately to considerably more than 5% of the messages a speaker conveys and so give the impression they are lipreading. They are not lipreading in the classic sense, but are doing what I have come to call "concept-reading." They take in the total situation, focus on the particular aspect involving themselves and the speakers, put "two and two together," and respond to the concepts abstracted. The true test of lipreading ability comes when the child is exposed to sustained conversation and to spoken instructional language in the classroom. Here it is likely that the ability to understand lipread language will not rise much above Vernon's estimate for the young "average deaf child."

Similarly for language-deficient deaf adults, ordinary conversation contains more blank spaces than lipreadable clues. And again, some ingenious deaf adults are occasionally able to fill in the blanks through remarkable associative feats and mental agility. In so doing, they perform not as lipreaders but seemingly as mind readers. But the strains of such performance are enormous, and it cannot survive sustained conversation or substitute for lipreading ability.

Among the most important communicative lacks in lipread language are the messages conveyed by vocal intonation: the warmth, the subtleties, the rhythms and stresses, the whole "orchestra of the language" (Robson, 1959), as contained in the sounds of the voice. There are no substitutes for these in lipread language. To use facial expression and gestures as substitutes is risky. Exaggerated facial expressions tend to distort lip movements, and punctuating gestures tend to distract the lipreader. So for the profoundly deaf, lipread language can be a rather flat form of communication.

Yet despite all the difficulties, there are those among the profoundly deaf since birth who are phenomenal lipreaders; but such persons are exceptional in other respects as well. Among the deaf at large, in lipreading as in speaking, reading and writing, only a small percentage can be considered efficient achievers in the verbal arts.

Fingerspelling. Fingerspelling, sometimes called dactylology, is a manual form of verbal language based on the formation of the letters of the alphabet by designated positions of fingers and hands; in this country one hand is used (see Appendix C), and in the English system both hands are used. Words and sentences are spelled out in these manual alphabets in what Fusfeld calls "a sort of writing in the air" (1958b, p. 268).

Fingerspelling has long been used as a method of communication. Abernathy's absorbing historical sketch (1959) traces its use to the ancient Egyptians, Hebrews, Greeks, and Romans. He relates that pictures of dactylology can be found in Latin Bibles of the tenth century and that during the Middle

Ages it was used by monks in enforced silence and by others for secret or silent communication. However, fingerspelling does not appear to have been used with the deaf until the early seventeenth century, when a one-hand alphabet was introduced by Juan Pablo Bonet of Spain as an aid in teaching the deaf to speak.

In this country, Zenas F. Westervelt, Superintendent of the Western New York Institute for the Deaf at Rochester, envisioned a broader use for finger-spelling than as a speech aid. He was convinced that the Manual Alphabet offered the ideal means for teaching the deaf grammatically accurate verbal language. He also felt that the easy visibility of fingerspelling could help in lipreading as well as in speech instruction. In 1876, Westervelt introduced fingerspelling into his school as the chief instructional method, beginning with the earliest kindergarten level, to the complete exclusion of nonverbal manual methods both in and out of class (E. A. Fay, 1889, 1896). This created something of a furor among the doubting Thomases of the day, but many of their criticisms were stilled by G. O. Fay's glowing first-hand report (1889) of the success of Westervelt's daring innovation.

Westervelt's manual alphabet method, known today as the Rochester method (Galloway, 1964; Scouten, 1964), is still practiced at the school he headed, now named the Rochester School for the Deaf, and at a few other schools, though with some modifications. Basically, it remains dedicated to the verbal instruction of deaf pupils through the concurrent use of finger-spelling and lipreading, with a strong support program of reading and speech. However, in certain schools the pupils are free to use nonverbal manual communication outside the classroom. Also, not all schools follow the procedure of using fingerspelling with preschool children (Morkovin, 1960; Scouten, 1967); some do not begin its use until the intermediate level.

For researchers, these and other institutionally inherent variables raise confounding problems in investigating the reported benefits of fingerspelling in the education of the deaf. Quigley (1969) skillfully maneuvered around the problems without completely overcoming them in an investigation of three "Rochester method" schools, each of which had as comparison-control two residential "non-Rochester" schools similar in size and student make-up to their experimental mate. On the basis of an exceptionally thoughtful interpretation of results, Quigley concludes:

1. The use of fingerspelling in combination with speech as practiced in the *Rochester Method* can lead to improved achievement in deaf students, partic-ularly on those variables where meaningful language is involved.
2. When good oral techniques are used in conjunction with fingerspelling, there need be no detrimental effects to the acquisition of oral skills.
3. Fingerspelling is likely to produce greater benefits when used with younger rather than with older children. It was used successfully in the experimental study with children as young as three and a half years of age.

4. Fingerspelling is a useful tool for instructing deaf children but it is not a panacea. (1969, pp. 94, 95)

In another of the relatively few comparative studies of instructional methods of what might be termed the "pre–Total Communication era," Johnson (1948) conducted a study of pupils at the Illinois School for the Deaf from the oral, acoustic, and manual departments respectively in regard to reading, lipreading, speech-hearing, hearing plus lipreading, fingerspelling, and fingerspelling plus signs. Johnson's findings indicated that the only two methods that could be used with any degree of accuracy when communicating with pupils as a group were fingerspelling and reading. Johnson also advised that since lipreading comprehension by the oral pupils was so inferior to their ability to understand fingerspelling, it might be a wise move to replace lipreading with fingerspelling for all oral pupils who lacked usable hearing activity, a history of hearing experience, or high lipreading scores.

Hester (1964) reported on the merits of fingerspelling in instructional communication through various comparisons of pupils taught by fingerspelling for up to 5 years with pupils of the same age and condition who had not been exposed to fingerspelling. The results of testing showed that the pupils taught through the combined use of fingerspelling and speech achieved higher scores in reading and in lipreading than did the pupils not taught in this way. However, in view of the number of variables which could not be controlled in this study, Hester concludes, "Although the objective results achieved so far do not prove very much, we think that the evidence indicates that the simultaneous approach (i.e., fingerspelling and speech) should be continued over a longer period of time with more accurate approach to objective measurement" (1964, p. 221).

Viewers of good fingerspelled communication are generally impressed with its speed and question how it compares in speed with writing, and how it compares in accuracy of reception with reading. In a small study, Fusfeld (1958) found that it took the 12 men and women who served as subjects half the time to fingerspell a passage of 39 words totaling 178 letters as to write the passage. Another small study was conducted by Stuckless and Pollard (1977) to compare the amount of verbal information visually processed by 19 elementary and secondary-school deaf students through reading and through fingerspelling. They found that printed words were more readily processed than fingerspelled words, hence more facilitative of comprehension. Other studies involving fingerspelling generally include the method in relation to multimodal (total) communication. Several are cited in Table 5.1.

Like other verbal forms, fingerspelling depends for its grammatical fluency on language competence; for expressive speed, on manual and digital dexterity as well as stamina; and for reception, on the viewer's ability to synthesize the letters formed by the flying fingers into a flow of language.

Martin Sternberg, a consummate master of all manner of communications used by the deaf, has this to say of fingerspelling:

> To the uninitiated, this method might seem as distracting as reading a message as it is being typed out on a machine—and much more difficult. With perseverance comes expertise, as in so many other skills. The skier, for example, starts with the snow-plow, slowly acquires his ski legs, begins to use his body to maneuver around curves; his legs gradually relax, and he begins to enjoy skiing, rather than fighting it. So with fingerspelling. Staccato, letter-by-letter fingerspelling, often accompanied by vocally sounding out the letters, is helpful to no one. With practice, this should give way to a feeling for the rhythms of fingerspelled words or portions of words. We begin to render them in a series of smoothly flowing bundles of movements, each in turn flowing into succeeding ones. Good fingerspelling is easy to comprehend, and a truly skilled fingerspeller is a joy to watch. It is entirely possible to inject elements of manual alliteration (a deliberate downsweep on the repeated letter is one way). Assonance, too, can be rendered through rhythmic movement of the hand while fingerspelling the portions of the word in question. Onomatopoeic fingerspelling is particularly beautiful. Bernard Bragg's "Reflections" is a classic example of spelled-out words creating pictures. Here both hands, facing one another, spell out words simultaneously, conjuring the image of a mirror. The possibilities are endless. One can utter fingerspelled shouts, fingerspelled whispers, simulate a fingerspelled conversation between two persons, using both hands to represent the communicators and their interaction. Mary Beth Miller does a memorable vignette of a pair of lovers immersed in sweet nothings. You can see the coyness of the girl; the self-assurance of the boy. All this through the way her fingers move. The conversation is there, yes, but so is a great deal more. (private communication)

Bernard Bragg and Mary Beth Miller, mentioned above, are gifted deaf theatrical performers.

The "great deal more" with which Sternberg concludes his narrative conveys that beneath the stodgy designation "fingerspelling" is a lively form of communication that is capable of manually producing not only verbal language but also many equivalents of the orchestra of the language—its intonation, stress, modulation, timing, rhythm—thus giving surprising dimension to the vitality, impact, and versatility of this language form. The likelihood is that expert fingerspelled language imparts considerably more semantic scope and subtleties to communication than is possible with lipread language. Understandably, fluent fingerspelling is a technique that is beyond the syntactic and semantic disabilities of the deaf-at-large.

The American Sign Language

Although verbal language is the commonest form of human communication, gesture language is the earliest. Pei relates that "gestural language is commonly conceded to have preceded oral speech, some say by at least one million years'' (1949, p. 13). He continues:

> It is further estimated that some seven hundred thousand distinct elementary gestures can be produced by facial expression, postures, movements of the arms, wrists, fingers, etc., and their combinations. This imposing array of gestural symbols would be quite sufficient to provide the equivalent of a full-blown modern language. It is quite conceivable: first, that a gestural system of communication could have arisen prior to and independently of spoken language; second, that such a system, had historical precedents been favorable, might have altogether supplanted the spoken tongue; third, that it could today supply the world's needs for an international common system. (1949, pp. 13–14)

An especially provocative aspect of gestural language is its apparent closeness to the raw data of the thoughts of pre- or non-linguistic humans. In its primal state, gesture language would seem to be an almost direct rendition in ideo-kinesic form of mental concepts as they flow through the mind. Owing to millennia of contacts with cultural and linguistic influences, gestural language as used today has lost much of its primal character; but wherever and however it is used, it remains a language whose basic vocabulary consists of concepts rather than words. Such is the American Sign Language of the deaf.

Known also as Ameslan, the American Sign Language (Sternberg, 1981; Stokoe, 1978) is an ideo-kinesic form of communication commonly used by the American deaf. As practiced by these persons, Ameslan is more than the ''manual'' language it is usually called, since more is involved than the hands; nor is the language restricted to conventional signs, since more is involved than gestural symbols. The language is, rather, a meshing of many kinds of body movements and positions into a flow of picto-kinesic expression. Depending on the situation as well as the expertise of the ''speaker,'' the traditional sign language of the deaf is composed of varying quantities and qualities of natural gesture, conventional signs, fingerspelling, facial expression, body movements, postures and positions, and many other kinesic subtleties.

Not all deaf persons know the language of signs, some because they have been reared in purely verbal environments and adhere to the oral philosophy, and others because they have never learned any conventional method of communication. Among the latter can be found extraordinary pantomimic talents.

The individual signs from which the language derives its name depict concepts and ideas expressed through conventional positions and movements, mainly of the hands and arms, and come from a variety of sources. Some are natural gestures or combinations of gestures. For example, the sign for "eat" is simply the bunched fingers of one hand pecking at the mouth; for "gluttony," the same sign but more forcibly made using both hands as if cramming the mouth with food. Other sign configurations are gestural abstractions of some aspect of what the sign represents. The sign for "name," for example, is made by placing the index and middle fingers of one hand crosswise over the index and middle fingers of the other, thus forming an X configuration. Higgins traces the configuration back to the "mark X used by persons who cannot write their own names" (1942, p. 47). Other signs have been so changed in the course of time and use that it is difficult to trace their origins. There are also local signs, colloquial signs, slang signs, and "families" of signs. One such family involves the mind, and the family members all "have their locus on or about the forehead, i.e., think, forget, understand, remember, insane, wise, stupid, feebleminded, imagine, dream, idea" (Fusfeld, 1958b, p. 273).

Fant (1964) explains that these conventional configurations "express the noun, as it were, and the other parts of the body supply the modifiers" (pages unnumbered). Paramount among the modifiers is facial expression. "The face," says Fant, "functions for manual communication as the inflections of the voice for words" (pages unnumbered; see figure 4.3). Other important modifiers are shoulder movements, leg movements and positions, and even the "lowly feet" are sometimes involved. Added semantic distinctions and subtleties are conveyed by the vigor and speed with which a sign is made. It has been estimated that there are up to 2000 formal signs (Fant, 1964); but when joined with the various modifiers, each of the signs lends itself to a multiplicity of meanings that give surprising depth, dimension, and emotional tone to the communicative range of signed language, far more than for lipread language.

Bragg (1973) calls attention to the fact that Ameslan is seldom used in its purest form by the majority of deaf persons. "Our true vernacular is always made up of varying percentages of literal and nonliteral aspects of expression. . . . For some of us who are high verbal, it is always English that dominates over Ameslan, for others who are low verbal, it is the other way around" (p. 673). Bragg suggests that the term *Ameslish* (a combination of "Ameslan" and "English") presents a truer picture of communication by deaf people.

Figure 4.3.
Colloquialisms, demonstrated by Bernard Bragg, that give color and emphasis to Ameslish. Listed under each picture are possible verbal equivalents of the nuances captured by the accompanying facial expressions. The sign shown in the left group is derived from the basic sign for "finish," and the sign at right represents "what's up?" Although the intensities vary according to meaning, the signs remain broadly the same.
From Bragg (1973).

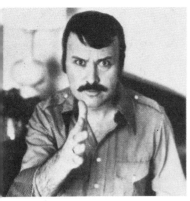

Cut it out, for once and all!
No monkey business, you dig?
I really mean it!

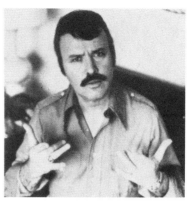

What's the big idea?
Why did it have to happen like that?
What the heck are you talking about?

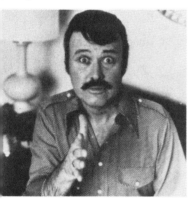

What shall I do, now that I know about it?
This is the end of the world, for sure!
Horror of Horrors!

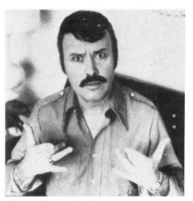

What's the matter?
Whatever has happened?
Why are you upset?

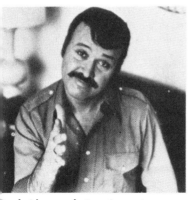

Look, I know what you're up to.
Oh, you'd not think me that naive.
Quit pulling my leg, will you?

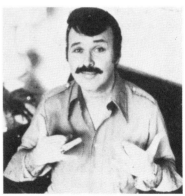

Just what did you do behind my back?
What are you up to?
What are you keeping from me?

Treasured though the language is by the deaf, various charges have been leveled against it. One is that it is a conspicuously unattractive form of communication. But as in spoken language, so in signed. There is elegant expression, as in deaf theater and on the lecture platform. There is informal everyday conversational expression that could be likened to the New Yorkese "Idowanna" meaning "I don't want to," and there is the sloppy casual exchange often used in the home, whose New Yorkese equivalents are exemplified by "Wa?" for "What do you want?" and "Jeet?" for "Did you eat?" Also, until recently, instruction in the sign language was banned in most schools for the deaf. As a result, signs were passed along from student to student, and in this "bootleg" process they suffered considerable deterioration. In consequence, signs are seldom seen in their pristine forms and beauty among the deaf at large.

A more serious charge made against the language is that it is simply an ungrammatical linkage of gestures whose effects on children, according to Van Uden, are that they are "educated directly for the deaf community, a ghetto apart from the dishumanizing influence of the signs themselves because a sign language is much too much a 'depicting language' keeping the thinking slow, much too concrete, and too broken in pieces" (1970, p. 103). Van Uden's abrasive comments express the feelings of most opponents of the use of Ameslan for instructional purposes.

These perennial debates over the instructional use of Ameslan have obscured an even larger linguistic issue: Is the American Sign Language a language at all? A chief argument against the "language" status is that Ameslan lacks the syntactic structure of English. This is, of course, an absurd criterion for establishing language status. The grammar of a language is derived not from the grammar of another language but from the way its building blocks have been put together in time and use by a particular language community. Every language has its own "personality" and its own rules of grammar. There is no universal syntax to which all must conform, least of all Ameslan, whose building blocks are concepts rather than words.

Ameslan has also been downgraded because of a number of linguistic lacks. Fant mentions a few: "There are no articles ('a,' 'an,' 'the') in Ameslan, . . . The verb "to be" does not exist in Ameslan. . . . There are no tenses in Ameslan" (1974–75, p. 2). There are undoubtedly other linguistic lacks as well, but not too dissimilar lacks are found in recognized languages.

Harold G. Henderson, an eminent translator of the Japanese form of poetry called *haiku,* writes, "First, there are no articles in the Japanese language, practically no pronouns, and in general no distinction between singular and plural. Japanese "prepositions" come after the word they modify and therefore are really "postpositions" (1959, p. vii). He continues, "the Japanese language is constructed differently from ours; there are, for example, no relative pronouns—any descriptive clause must precede its noun—and I was often confronted with the dilemma of whether to try to follow the strict grammatical form or whether to follow the order of thought, and to supply the comparatively unimportant intermediate words in accordance with English standards" (1959, p. viii). Yet none of these differences from English has been known to cause Japanese persons to lose face over their status as human beings or to suspect that their mother tongue did not qualify as a proper language.

An illustration of Henderson's dilemma is his word-for-word transcription from the Japanese, and his order-of-thought translation of a *haiku* (1959, p. 7):

Word-for-word transcription:	Tower / on / when-I-climb / cryptomeria's / top-twig / on / butterfly / one
Order-of-thought translation:	The tower high I climb, there, on that fir top sits a butterfly!

These are not too unlike Fant's transcription from Ameslan to English, which illustrates his theory that the order of signs follows the order of events and ideas as they occur in life (1974–1975, p. 2):

Sign-for-sign expression:	Now morning / sunrise / I-look-at / thrill
English equivalent:	It was a thrill to watch the sunrise this morning.

There is a striking similarity in feel and expression between Henderson's and Fant's examples, the one from a spoken language, the other from a signed language. It is not unlikely that similarities in word order will be found between the language of signs and other esoteric spoken languages in which expression, hence grammar, is governed by order of thought or events. We do not know. Studies of Ameslan are mainly involved with descriptive analyses and with comparisons of the syntax of Ameslan and spoken English (Bellugi, 1972; Schlesinger, 1971; Stokoe, 1974; Tervoort, 1961).

Regarding signs and syntax, I tend to view thinking in pure signs as resembling what Vygotsky calls "thinking in pure meanings" (1962, p. 149). The concept of "thinking" is itself beset by ambiguity (Thomson, 1959), but Lawrence Kubie's concept of what goes on in a person's mind at the initiation of creative thinking comes close to "thinking in pure meanings": "His brain is functioning as a communications machine, processing bits of information by scanning, ordering, selecting, etc. This is preconscious processing and it proceeds at extraordinary speed" (1965, p. 74). In Kubie's graphic illustration (figure 4.4), the "symbols shown on the screen represent a sampling of this preconscious activity. Here, our man is relating this sample to reality. His preconscious provides him with myriad bits; he samples these (a conscious activity), tests them, then back they go into the preconscious" (1965, p. 74).

The symbols, imagery, feelings, and other subliminal bits that bombard the mind during this preconscious phase of mental activity are not sequentially ordered. They come and go in flashes and bursts of "pure meaning" unhampered by strictures of language or rules of grammar. In fact, as Thomson observes, "We often have to struggle hard to find words to capture what our thinking has already grasped" (1959, p. 164).

Largely eliminated by Ameslan are the struggles to encage what goes on in the mind in rigid rules of English grammar. We may hypothesize that, with this obstacle eliminated, the "syntax" of unadulterated Ameslan is closer to the "syntax" of pure thought than is the syntax of verbal language. If so, there would be no need for articles, pronouns, tenses, or other linguistic clarifications of meaning. Meaning is directly imbedded in thought; and thought in turn is expressed as it flows through the mind. Over and above the influences of learned usage on Ameslan, the ordering of signs would thus be additionally influenced by (a) the signer's emotional investment in his message, and (b) the signer's perception of its impact on the receiver. In this hypothetical frame, investigations of the relationship between "thinking in pure meanings" and the expression of such thinking in signs, unhampered by linguistic restraints, offers a fertile area of research into the dynamics of thinking.

Obviously, Ameslan has provided scholars with highly complex problems, educators of the deaf with sharp differences of opinion, and numbers of literate deaf persons with the feeling that there is a need to "make it [Ameslan] and the deaf society it represents, more respectable" (Gustason, 1973, p. 89). But as Stokoe (1974, 1975) points out, in accordance with the principles of anthropological linguistics, Ameslan is already a "respectable" independent language with its own structure, vocabulary, and "personality" and, like all languages, is the possession and product of the people who fashioned it. The language does not denigrate its creators. Margaret Mead (1977), in fact, suggests that Ameslan could be developed into a worldwide common language. This is a major objective of the World Federation of the Deaf (Magarotto and Vukotic, 1959).

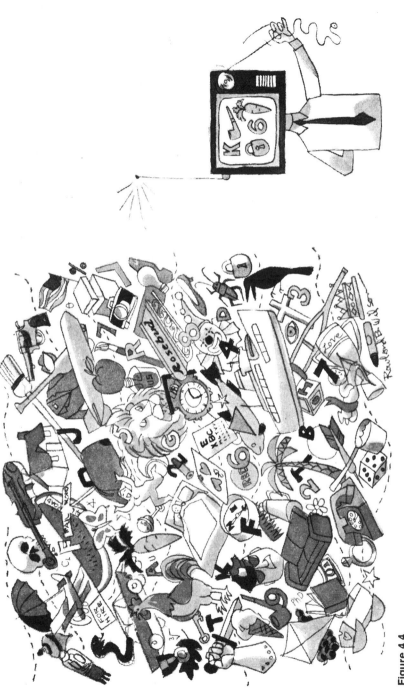

Figure 4.4.
The process of thought, as presented by L. S. Kubie (1956). Reprinted with permission of *Science and Technology.*

Methodical Signs

In recognition of the language-learning problems associated with the syntactic differences between signed language and the syntax of the verbal mother tongue, several systems have been devised in which manual symbols are used for expressing statements that are the syntactic parallels of their verbal counterparts (Bornstein, 1973; Cokely and Gawlik, 1973; Stack, 1972; Stokoe, 1974, 1975; Caccamise and Drury, 1976). The first approach to syntactically correct signing—a sign for every word of the mother tongue—was termed Methodical Signs. It had its beginnings in the heart and mind of one who referred to himself as "The Teacher of the Deaf and Dumb at Paris," Charles Michel, Abbé de L'Épée. In the early eighteenth century, moved by the plight of deaf twin sisters, the Abbé considered it "an indispensable obligation" (De l'Épée, 1860, p. 2) to bring all his exertions to their relief and to the relief of others like them. This he proposed to do by teaching the deaf "to think with order, and to combine their ideas" (1860, p. 2) as well as to "render them capable of perfecting their education themselves, by the perusal of good books" (1860, p. 5). This was a radical departure from the objectives of previous teachers of deaf pupils, such as Wallis of England and Bonet of Spain, as well as of de l'Épée's contemporaries such as Pereire in France and Heinicke in Germany. Their main objective was to teach the deaf to speak.

In preparation for his task, which was to become his life's work, the Abbé scrutinized all available literature on gestural language and on the methods used by other teachers. Of gestural language, especially as used by the uneducated deaf of the period, the Abbé concluded that while it was too meager in signs and substance to meet his objectives, it nevertheless had certain instructional possibilities for teaching concepts. Of speech objectives, the Abbé observed that

> it is not by the mere pronunciation of words, in any language, that we are taught their signification: The words *door, window*, etc., etc., in our own, might have been repeated to us hundreds of times, in vain; we should never have attached an idea to them, had not the object designated by these names been shown to us at the same time. (1860, p. 63)

His plan was to "show" meaning through methodical signs.

The plan grew out of the Abbé's belief that "to think with order" and "the perusal of good books" demanded expertise not only in the fluent use of verbal language but more particularly in understanding the *concepts* represented by the verbal forms; that without such understanding, language-learning was little more than a parrotlike exercise. The Abbé carried out his beliefs through the sequential use of fingerspelling and signs reinforced by writing. He used fingerspelling to teach the verbal components of language; but as each linguistic element was taught, its meaning was immediately demonstrated through methodical signs which the Abbé devised for the purpose. Reading and writing were taught at the same time.

A comprehensive description of de l'Épée's method is recorded in his book *The True Method of Educating the Deaf and Dumb; Confirmed by Long Experience,* published in French and Latin in 1784 and translated into English in 1860. Some of the section-headings are: "Of Articles, and the Signs corresponding to them," "Of Nouns Adjective in the Positive, Comparative, Superlative, and Excessive Degrees, and of the Signs corresponding to them," "Of Substantives formed from Adjectives termed Abstract Qualities, and of the signs agreeing to them," and so on through all the complexities and subtleties of syntax. On completing their instruction, the Abbé's pupils were able to read, write, and sign in well-ordered language with linguistic accuracy, and, more importantly, with conceptual understanding. The Abbé did teach some speech and lipreading, but for him these were minor considerations.

The furor generated by the Abbé's manual departure from the speech tradition has reverberated through the centuries as the "battle of methods." Nevertheless, the demonstrated success of his system was lauded by the French Academy, and the school he founded was eventually taken over by the state.

> The novelty of the undertaking exciting curiosity, and the public exercises of my pupils attracting notice . . . a continual confluence of persons of all conditions and of every country have been drawn to my lessons. I believe there is no part of Europe, with the exception of Turkey, whence strangers have not issued for the express purpose of ascertaining with their own eyes the reality of these matters. (De L'Épée, 1860, p. 84)

Among the visitors to de L'Épée's school was Thomas Hopkins Gallaudet, then a young theological student. In 1815 an association of Hartford residents who were concerned by the lack of educational facilities for deaf children in this country sent Gallaudet to Europe to learn about the methods used by foreign teachers, as preparation for founding a school for the deaf here. Strongly impressed with the "French" method, Gallaudet introduced it in the first school for the deaf in this country, the American School for the Deaf, founded in Hartford, Connecticut, in 1817.

The next 50 years witnessed a steady increase in the number of American schools for the deaf as well as the emergence of sharp differences of opinion among school heads concerning methods of instruction, with the teaching of speech and by speech gaining growing support (Schunhoff, 1957). As this happened, the sign language was gradually excluded from the instructional scene and forbidden in the classroom. It was kept alive through the love of the language by its deaf users, particularly those unable to profit from the speech approach. But without the necessary instruction in signs, departure from de l'Épée's high linguistic standards followed. There evolved an American Sign Language, fashioned by its users, with its "vocabulary" a possible mix and fusion of signs customarily used by the American deaf and of signs imported from France by Thomas Hopkins Gallaudet.

Manually Coded English

Despite the American rebuff to the language of signs, de l'Épée's vision of grammatical signing did not die. In the hope that the stubborn linguistic deficiencies of the deaf would yield to grammatical signing, it was revived in England by Paget (1954; Paget, Gorman, and Paget, 1969) in their Systematic Sign Language system; and in America by Stack (1972) and Bornstein (1973). Stack's Manual English system is "based primarily on the signed vocabulary of the American Sign Language used with fingerspelling in correct English syntactic and grammatical form, observant of verb tense, use of prepositions, and determiners, plurality and all word endings" (1972, p. iv). Bornstein's Signed English "is designed to cover the needs of the syntax and vocabulary used with the one to six year old child" and "substitutes American Sign Language words for English words without changing the form of the American Language to the form of the English word" (1973, p. 462).

In addition to these systems of grammatical signing, several other systems were devised, for which Brasel uses the umbrella term "Siglish" (Brasel, 1974; Caccamise and Drury, 1976). Their common goal was to develop "new sign languages," linguistically patterned on standard English. The best known were: Seeing Essential English or SEE 1 (Anthony, 1971, 1974–1975); Signing Exact English or SEE 2 (Gustason et al., 1975; Gustason, 1973, 1974–1975), and Linguistics of Visual English, LVE or LOVE (Wampler, 1971). Descriptions of the systems can be found in the cited references and current literature. Of SEE 1, Anthony explains, "SEE is an attempt to sign English, to *give* English, to make signs compatible with the English language as far as possible and as far as is practicable and practical" (1974–1975, p. 8). Gustason echos these sentiments for SEE 2: "English should be signed as it is spoken for the deaf child to have linguistic input that would result in his mastery of English" (1974–1975, p. 11).

The following excerpts from Bornstein's expert analyses briefly describe what is involved in operationalizing these systems. "SEE [1] signs actually stand for word forms or parts, i.e., word roots, prefixes, and suffixes. These are used in appropriate combinations to form any desired word" (1973, p.

454). He continues, "Because SEE treats word components, i.e., roots, prefixes, and suffixes, it uses a very large number of affixes. It has at least 22 adjective suffixes, 10 personal ending suffixes, 40 noun suffixes, and 11 verbal suffixes. . . . SEE 1 also has 35 general prefixes. . . . There are symbols for 43 handshapes, two hand positions, six directions for these hand positions, and a variety of placement explanations. The reader must learn the notations before he can understand how to form a SEE sign" (1973, p. 455). (One is reminded of the elaborate notation systems used by early educators for teaching sentence structure.) As a result of this process of sign transformation into English, SEE 1 signs bear little or no resemblance to the original source signs of the American Sign Language.

A chief difference between SEE 1 and SEE 2 is the much larger proportion of traditional signs in SEE 2.

The difference between the LVE and SEE systems is in the treatment of the word forms. Bornstein explains, "Rather than word root, prefixes, and suffixes, LVE signs are intended to represent morphemes . . . the smallest component of language sound which is meaningful" (1973, p. 460). Further, "LVE represents its sign word with a notation system which . . . consists of the manual alphabet and numbers one through eight, plus seven pages of symbols. The symbols represent 12 other handshapes, six palm directions, three hand directions, 12 positions, five position designations, 32 kinds of movements, and eight movement designations" (1973, pp. 460–61). Bornstein observes that LVE sign words bear less resemblance to signs of the American Sign Language than do SEE 1 or 2 sign words.

Lack of resemblance between "linguistic" signs and Ameslan signs is the difference between expressing a word and expressing a concept. For example, the "linguistic" sign for "butterfly" would be the traditional sign for the word "butter" plus the sign for the word "fly." Adding "fly" to "butter" to express "butterfly" strikes an Ameslan signer as hilarious. The Ameslan sign expresses the total concept "butterfly" and is made by crossing the hands at the wrists, palms facing the chest, thumbs interlocked, and fingers oscillating to convey the form and flutter of a butterfly's wings. Cokely and Gawlik (1973) give another example in the word "gravy." The linguistic sign in SEE 1 is the sign for "grave" plus the letter "y." To add "y" to "grave" and come up with "gravy" is also hilariously funny to the Ameslan signer. In Ameslan, gravy is signed as the concept "drippings-from-meat" and is made by grasping the lower edge of the left hand with the thumb and index finger of the right, and pulling down several times.

The language status of the new sign languages occupies an equivocal position in scholarly deliberations because of their composite manufacture out of already existing languages. "A real language," reflects George Steiner, "consists of far more than the sum of its words and grammatical rules. . . . No printout, no dictionary, no grammar, however exhaustive, are equivalent to a language as it is spoken, dreamt, thought, altered, lived by its native speaker'' (1977, p. 9). A language, in short, is fashioned by its users and their culture, not by linguists.

It is also questionable whether the bow to the American Sign Language will endear the new systems to the deaf at large. The late Frederick C. Schreiber, who was in the top ranks of distinguished deaf leaders, stated: ''While the new sign systems that developed are the products of deaf people, they were created by persons whose primary language was English. . . . But they were no linguists, and perhaps their very skills caused a complete disregard for rules upon which any system, be it language or auto mechanics, must be based'' (1974–1975, p. 5). Schreiber continues with the dismaying facts, ''Today in this country there are four major sign languages, and hundreds of people—both professional and nonprofessional—are busily adding to the confusion. . . . What matter that a teacher-training program needs to teach four different versions of sign language in order to be sure its graduates can be employed anywhere in the U.S., or that a family with a deaf child moving from one part of the country to another will have not only to learn a new system but also to unlearn the old? This is happening. To be precise, it has already happened'' (1974–1975, p. 6).

It seems that, another divisive battle of methods may be in the making, this time manual versus manual, sign versus sign. Anthony of SEE 1 finds great benefit in this, and offers the thought that this ''havering and palavering . . . is all to the good'' (1974–1975, p. 8). The reason? ''The more the public sees of signs, no matter the system, the less of a novelty will signs be'' (1974–1975, p. 8). Surely greater rewards than this are due deaf children who are experimental pawns in the new sign systems.

Interpreters and Interpreted Language

Bridging the linguistic gap between the deaf community and the hearing world is a unique group of communication mediators known as interpreters for the deaf. Until fairly recently, persons who interpreted for the deaf in most countries were generally volunteers who took the time to perform the service. They included children of deaf parents, religious workers, teachers of the deaf, and friends and relatives who were familiar with the language of signs. Rarely were they paid for their services. Steady jobs were unheard of. The only training available was offered by a handful of dedicated teachers of manual communication.

In this general no-status picture, an important breakthrough was made in Russia in the 1950s. Spearheaded by the All Russian Society of the Deaf, procedures were initiated to systematize and professionalize interpreting.

Standards of competence were established, training was instituted, and jobs were made available (Geylman, 1957).

In this country, the breakthrough occurred in 1964 at the Ball State Teachers College Workshop on Interpreting for the Deaf (J. M. Smith, 1964). The thrust came mainly from the unprecedented expansion of services for the deaf. In response to the related need for more interpreters, the Ball Workshop moved to establish a National Registry of Professional Interpreters and Translators for the Deaf. The purpose was "to promote the recruitment and training of an adequate supply of interpreters for the deaf, skilled in both manual and oral interpretation, and to maintain a list of qualified persons" (J. M. Smith, 1964, p. 3).

The registry's first task was to clarify the functions of "interpreters and translators" and to specify the qualifications of the "qualified persons" mentioned in the statement of purpose. A review of the literature on professional interpreting shows the following distinction between interpreters and translators. Interpreters deal mainly with oral verbatim reporting; they repeat in one language what a speaker is saying in another. They can do this in time with the speaker, as in simultaneous interpreting, or can wait until the speaker has completed a statement before proceeding, as in consecutive interpreting. Translators, on the other hand, are essentially writers whose main concern is with attaining meticulous equivalence in *meaning* between different languages. They are free to use whatever words they need and take all the time they require within reason, to attain this equivalence.

This distinction is not as finely drawn in interpreting for the deaf. As a rule, verbatim interpreting is used with the smallest segment of the deaf population—people with high linguistic attainments who do not want to miss a word of what the speaker says. But with most of the deaf, and particularly with those at low linguistic levels, interpreters function as translator and interpreter rolled into one. Their main concern is to convey *meanings*. To do this, they must make a rapid mental translation of a sender's statement into its basic meaning and then convey the meaning to the receiver in whatever communicative mode and concept level is best understood. A major skill of such interpreters is their ability, as Sussman would say, to "think deaf."

A common misconception is that anyone who knows the sign language can interpret for the deaf. This is not so. Interpreting, in any language, is one of the most demanding professions, as can be inferred from the following list of personal qualifications gleaned from Hendry (1969) and other sources in the profession:

1. *Stamina: independence of spirit.* A person who finds the way to link the people he is serving with a minimum of fuss and fluster; who is able to hold the reins no matter how rough the going becomes; who though caught

in a torrent of words, some of which seem to make no sense at all, refuses to panic.

2. *Empathy.* A person who possesses the art of "becoming" the personalities behind the statements he is interpreting and who is able to project their attitudes as well as their statements; who is able to quickly get the "feel" of speaker and receiver.

3. *Adaptability.* A person who is able to adjust to new and to unexpected situations, settings, ideas, and people with grace and flexibility while at the same time preserving his own identity and function.

4. *Broad interests.* A person who is interested in world events and people; who enjoys bringing people together in friendly relations; who derives satisfaction from serving as a link between different mentalities, cultures, and social systems.

5. *Outgoing personality.* A person who is more interested in others than in his own thoughts and feelings; a good listener as well as a good mixer; sensitive to his surroundings and to the feelings and attitudes of others; respected by others.

6. *Natural bent for languages and communication.* A person who enjoys communicating and does it well; who is language oriented to the point of continually seeking ways of perfecting himself in the languages of his expertise.

7. *Quickness of mind, retentive memory.* A person who is able to "think on his feet"; who does not get lost in the outpouring of words he is to interpret but is able to hold them in memory; who possesses the talent for immediate understanding.

Over and above these personal attributes are the technical competencies demanded of interpreters (see Appendix D). For those serving the manual-deaf, technical competencies include but are not limited to: (a) a high level of expertise in sending and receiving manually coded messages and in reverse interpretation; (b) an above-average level of linguistic expertise; (c) deep familiarity with the broad range and wide variety of life experiences and outcomes in the deaf population; and (d) a good educational background and scope of knowledge. Further, when interpreting takes place in special settings, such as legal, medical, psychiatric, or rehabilitation, the interpreter must be conversant with the technical language of the given setting. Finally, in certain situations, as in scholarly lectures and professional conferences, good hearing is important; in others, particularly in dealing with deaf individuals of low literacy, deaf persons can make superb interpreters when trained for the job, as can hearing persons who have been raised bilingually by deaf parents. Obviously, an interpreter for the deaf needs a great deal more than the ability to sign.

Interpreters are also available for the oral deaf who may be unfamiliar with signed language (Northcott, 1979). Oral interpreting is not "interpreting" in the customary sense, i.e., from one language or language form to another. The oral interpreter repeats a speaker's statement but in clear lip movements and without voice while standing about 4 to 6 feet from the receivers. This sounds like a simple enough procedure, but it is harder than it appears. The interpreter must keep pace with the speaker although, of necessity, "one word behind." My hard-of-hearing friends tell of oral interpreters who for one or another reason get far behind a speaker, and then try to make up for it in their own words while at the same time trying to catch up with the speaker's flow of discourse. The result can be a frustrating jumble for the receivers. As a rule, a special section of a lecture hall is reserved for persons requiring oral interpreters.

The deaf recipient of interpreted communication receives the messages second-hand, as it were; and their content is only as accurate as the interpreted language permits it to be. When the language is a "faithful echo" (Ekvall, 1960), then it has served its prime communicative function. But when interpreted language is ambiguous, distorted, or confusing, it simply adds to the communicative obstacles that bedevil the deaf. Unfortunately, not many receivers of interpreted messages are in a position to check for accuracy. They can only hope.

Compounding the problem of interpreting for the deaf is a critical shortage of expert interpreters, at a time when the demand for interpreters has increased markedly because of state mandates that deaf people must be provided with interpreters whenever their civil rights are involved (Dicker, 1976; Du Bow, 1979). In consequence, the need is filled by numbers of less than qualified interpreters, transmitting less than adequately interpreted messages.

Hope for improvement in the situation lies with the many interpreter training programs that are springing up throughout the country, and in the leadership of the Registry of Interpreters for the Deaf, which maintains a national office and provides information on request regarding interpreting services, training programs, and qualified interpreters (Caccamise, Stangarone, and Caccamise, 1978; Registry of Interpreters for the Deaf, 1978).

Summary

Perhaps a good way to bring home the message of this chapter is to count the ways born-deaf children would have to learn every word they know, in partial preparation for full and free communication with both deaf and hearing society. As an example we use the word "mother." The child must:

1. Learn the *concept* "mother."
2. Learn to *speak* the word "mother."
3. Learn to *lipread* "mother."
4. Learn the *sound* "mother" through the hearing aid.
5. Learn the *printed word* "mother."
6. Learn the *written word* "mother."
7. Learn to *spell* "mother."
8. Learn to *write* "mother."
9. Learn to *fingerspell* "mother."
10. Learn to *read-back* the *fingerspelled* word "mother."
11. Learn to *sign* "mother" in the *American Sign Language.*
12. Learn to *read-back* "mother" in the *American Sign Language.*
13. Learn to *sign* "mother" in the *Siglish* systems.
14. Learn to *read-back* "mother" as signed in the *Siglish* systems.

Accompanying this word-learning feat is the even more taxing one of learning the syntax of English as well as that of the American Sign Language. And this is not the end. Full communicative expertise also requires an understanding of the semantics of the nonverbal languages of social encounter—those characteristic of deaf society as well as those commonly used by the hearing; they are not always the same (Schiff and Thayer, 1974).

Congenitally and prelinguistically deaf persons who have mastered this tremendous communicative load, and there are those who have, are awesome human beings. Unfortunately, almost no research has been conducted to find out what combination of abilities, talents, and life circumstances has gone into their making. Many of them have weathered the same instructional experiences as their communicatively deficient peers. And yet they have come out whole. Why? There are opinions on the subject, but no definitive answers. All that is certain is that they are the "exceptional deaf" (Bowe and Sternberg, 1973; Crammatte, 1968). There is no doubt that they have something important to contribute to our understanding—if we would only ask.

For the "unexceptional" deaf, the deaf at large, another list could be compiled, a depressing list of deficits in all the verbally rooted links to the cultural milieu: deficiencies in vocabulary, syntax, reading, speech, lipreading, and fingerspelling. We do not yet know how the so-called Siglish systems will affect the picture, but Gustason's comment that "the variety of sign language modes being taught is wreaking havoc in sign language classes" (1973, p. 89) is not encouraging.

It is we the hearing who have created this language environment for the deaf; their linguistic deficits are largely the product of ineffective teaching and narrowed understanding. What we have created brings to mind the biblical Tower of Babel in which many languages were spoken but none were understood. The overworked accusing finger has been pointed in many directions. The heaviest blame has fallen on the practice of teaching *by* speech, and deservedly so. Generally under-recognized in this approach is the determining influence of *lipreading*. A deaf pupil is lost who lacks this gift but who nevertheless finds himself in a class in which instruction is conducted in speech. It is *lipreading* rather than speech-learning that is the fundamental problem of the pure-oral method.

But time brings hope; and hope now centers on two seemingly reasonable approaches to the teaching of language to deaf children: early auditory training and experiences on the one hand, and multimodal (total) communication on the other. It is likely that a well-conceived and expertly applied combination of the two holds the solution to the linguistic problems of the deaf.

References

Abernathy, E. R. 1959. An historical sketch of the manual alphabets. *American Annals of the Deaf,* 104: 232–40.

Anthony, D. 1971. *Seeing Essential English.* Anaheim, Calif.: Anaheim Union High School District.

Anthony, D. 1974–1975. Seeing essential English: SEE. *Gallaudet Today,* communication issue, 5(2): 6–10.

Bellugi, U. 1972. Studies in sign language. In T. J. O'Rourke, ed., *Psycholinguistics and Total Communication: The State of the Art.* Washington, D.C.: American Annals of the Deaf.

Bennett, C. 1974. Speech pathology and the hearing impaired child. *Volta Review,* 76: 550–58.

Berger, K., Garner, M., and Sudman, J. 1971. The effect of degree of facial exposure and the vertical angle of vision on speechreading performance. *Teacher of the Deaf,* 69: 222–326.

Berger, K. W., and Popelka, G. R. 1971. Extra-facial gestures in relation to speechreading. *Journal of Communication Disorders,* 3, 302–8.

Bernstein, B. B. 1971. Language and socialization. In N. Minnis, ed., *Linguistics at Large.* New York: Viking Press.

Bierwisch, M. 1969. Certain problems of semantic representations. *FL,* 5: 153–84.

Blair, F. 1957. A study of the visual memory of deaf and hearing children. *American Annals of the Deaf,* 102: 254–63.

Blanton, R. L. 1968. Language learning and performance in the deaf. In S. Rosenberg and J. H. Kaplan, eds., *Developments in Applied Linguistics.* New York: Macmillan Co. Pp. 121–76.

Bloomfield, L. 1933. *Language.* New York: Holt, Rinehart & Winston.

Boothroyd, A. 1975. Technology and deafness. *Volta Review,* 77: 27–34.

Boothroyd, A., Archambault, P., Adams, R. E., and Storm, R. D. 1975. Use of a computer-based system of speech training aids for deaf persons. *Volta Review*, 77: 178–93.

Bornstein, H. 1973. A description of some current sign systems designed to represent English. *American Annals of the Deaf*, 118: 454–63.

Bowe, F., and Sternberg, M. 1973. *I'm Deaf Too: 12 Deaf Americans*. Silver Spring, Md.: National Association of the Deaf.

Bowen, J. D. 1970. The Structure of language. In A. H. Markwardt and H. G. Rickey, eds., *Linguistics in School Programs*. Chicago: National Society for the Study of Education. Pp. 36–63.

Bragg, B. 1973. Ameslish: Our American heritage, a testimony. *American Annals of the Deaf*, 118: 672–74.

Braly, K. A. 1938. A study of defective vision among deaf children. *American Annals of the Deaf*, 83: 192–93.

Brannon, J. B., Jr. 1966. The speech production and spoken language of the deaf. *Language and Speech*, 9: 127–36.

Brasel, K. 1974. Total communication. *Deaf American*, 23: 36–37.

Bruhn, M. 1930. *Elementary Lessons in Lip Reading*. Lynn, Mass.: Michols Press.

Bunger, A. 1944. *Speech Reading Jena Method*. Illinois: Interstate.

Caccamise, F. C., and Drury, A. M. 1976. A review of current terminology in education of the deaf. *Deaf American*, 29: 7–10.

Caccamise, F., Stangarone, J., and Caccamise, M. 1978. *Interpreting Potpourri: Proceedings of the 1978 RID Convention*. Rochester, N.Y.: Registry of Interpreters for the Deaf.

Calvert, D. R. 1962. Deaf voice quality: A preliminary investigation. *Volta Review*, 64: 402–3.

Calvert, D. R., and Silverman, S. R. 1975a. Methods for developing speech (the auditory global method). *Volta Review*, 77: 501–11.

Calvert, D. R., and Silverman, S. R. 1975b. *Speech and Deafness*. Washington, D.C.: Alexander Graham Bell Association for the Deaf.

Campbell, R., and Wales, R. 1970. The study of language acquisition. In J. Lyons, ed., *New Horizons in Linguistics*. Baltimore: Penguin Books. Pp. 242–60.

Chomsky, N. 1957. *Syntactic Structures*. The Hague: Mouton & Co.

Chomsky, N. 1965. *Aspects of the Theory of Syntax*. Cambridge, Mass: M.I.T. Press.

Chomsky, N. 1968. *Language and the Mind*. New York: Harcourt, Brace & World.

Clarke, B. R., and Ling, D. 1976. The effects of using cued speech: A follow-up study. *Volta Review*, 78: 23–34.

Cokely, D. R. and Gawlik, R. 1973. A position paper on the relationship between manual English and sign. *Deaf American*, 25 (May): 7–11.

Connor, L. E. 1971. The president's opinion: Manpower shortages. *Volta Review*, 213–16.

Cooper, R. L., and Rosenstein, J. 1966. Language acquisition of deaf children. *Volta Review*, 68: 58–67.

Cornett, R. O. 1967. Cued speech. *American Annals of the Deaf*, 112: 3–13.

Cornett, R. O. 1975. Cued speech and oralism: An analysis. *Audiology and Hearing Education*, 1: 26–34.

Costello, M. R. 1958. Language development through speechreading. *Volta Review,* 60: 257–59, 272. Reprint no. 705, with unnumbered pages.

Council on Education of the Deaf. 1974. Standards for the certification of teachers of the hearing impaired. *Volta Review,* 76: 239–50.

Craig, W. N., Craig, H. B., and DiJohnson, A. 1972. Preschool verbotonal instruction for deaf children. *Volta Review,* 74: 236–46.

Crammatte, A. B. 1968. *Deaf Persons in Professional Employment.* Springfield, Ill.: Charles C. Thomas.

De l'Épée, Abbé Charles Michel. 1860. The true method of educating the deaf and dumb: Confirmed by long experience. Trans. from French and Latin. *American Annals of the Deaf and Dumb,* 12: 1–132. Originally published in Paris in 1784.

Delgado, G. L. 1973. A commentary on teacher preparation program review procedures: Council on Education of the Deaf. *American Annals of the Deaf,* 118: 667–69.

Dettering, R. W. 1970. Language and thinking. In A. H. Marckwardt and H. G. Richey, eds. *Linguistics in School Programs.* Chicago: National Society for the Study of Education. Pp. 275–301.

Dicker, L. 1976. Intensive interpreter training. *American Annals of the Deaf,* 121: 312–19.

Downs, M. P. 1968. Identification and training of the deaf child: Birth to one year. *Volta Review,* 70: 154–58.

Du Bow, S. 1979. Federal actions on interpreters and telecommunications, *American Annals of the Deaf,* 124: 93–96.

Eisenberg, D., and Santore, F. 1976. The verbotonal method of aural rehabilitation: A case study. *Volta Review,* 78: 16–22.

Eisenberg, R. B. 1976. *Auditory Competence in Early Life: The Roots of Communicative Behavior.* Baltimore: University Park Press.

Ekvall, R. N. 1960. *Faithful Echo.* New York: Twayne Publishers.

Erber, N. P. 1971. Effects of distance on the visual reception of speech. *Journal of Speech and Hearing Research,* 14: 848–59.

Erber, N. P. 1977. Developing materials for lipreading evaluation and instruction. *Volta Review,* 79: 35–42.

Espeseth, V. K. 1969. An investigation of visual sequential memory in deaf children. *American Annals of the Deaf,* 114: 786–89.

Ewertsen, H. W, Nielsen, H. B., and Nielsen, S. S. 1970. Audio-visual speech perception. *Acta Oto-Laryngologica,* Suppl. no. 263: 229–30.

Fant, L. J. 1964. *Say It with Hands.* Washington, D.C.: Gallaudet College.

Fant, L. J. 1974–1975. Ameslan. *Gallaudet Today,* communication issue, 5(2): 1–3.

Farwell, R. M. 1976. Speech reading: A research review. *American Annals of the Deaf,* 121: 19–30.

Fay, E. A., ed. 1889. Miscellaneous. "Speech-Reading." *American Annals of the Deaf,* 34: 81–82.

Fay, E. A., ed. 1896. Methods of instruction and industries taught in American schools. *American Annals of the Deaf,* 41: 36–48.

Fay, G. O. 1889. A week at Rochester. *American Annals of the Deaf,* 34: 241–62.

Fellendorf, G. W., ed. 1977. *Bibliography on Deafness: 1847–1976.* Washington, D.C.: Alexander Graham Bell Association for the Deaf.

Fellendorf, G. W., ed. 1980. *Supplement to Bibliography on Deafness: 1977–1979.* Washington, D.C.: Alexander Graham Bell Association for the Deaf.

Fillenbaum, S. 1971. Psycholinguistics. In P. H. Mussen and N. R. Rosenzweig, eds., *Annual Review of Psychology.* Palo Alto, Calif.: Annual Reviews. Pp. 251–80.

Fitzgerald, E. 1926. *Straight Language for the Deaf.* Staunton, Va.: McClure Co.

Furth, H. G. 1961. The influence of language on the development of concept formation in deaf children. *Journal of Abnormal and Social Psychology,* 63: 386–89.

Furth, H. G. 1964. Research with the deaf: Implications for language and cognition. *Psychological Bulletin,* 62: 145–64.

Fusfeld, I. S. 1955. Suggestions on causes and cures for failure in written language. Paper presented at the 37th Regular Meeting of the Convention of American Instructors of the Deaf, West Hartford, Connecticut, June 1955. Mimeographed.

Fusfeld, I. S. 1958a. Factors in lipreading as determined by the lipreader. *American Annals of the Deaf,* 103: 229–42.

Fusfeld, I. S. 1958b. How the deaf communicate: Manual language. *American Annals of the Deaf,* 103: 264–82.

Fusfeld, I. S. 1958c. How the deaf communicate: Written language. *American Annals of the Deaf,* 103: 255–63.

Galloway, J. H. 1964. The Rochester method. In *Proceedings of the International Congress on Education of the Deaf and of the Forty-First Meeting of the Convention of American Instructors of the Deaf.* Washington, D.C.: United States Government Printing Office.

Geylman, I. 1957. *The Hand Alphabet and Speech Gestures of Deaf Mutes.* Transl. by Joseph and Tunya Ziv. Moscow: Soviet Cooperative Publishing Co.

Griffiths, C. 1975. The auditory approach: Rationale, techniques, and results. *Audiology and Hearing Education,* 1: 35–39.

Groht, M. A. 1958. *Natural Language for Deaf Children.* Washington, D.C.: Alexander Graham Bell Association for the Deaf.

Gruver, H. H. 1955. The Tadoma method. *Volta Review,* 57: 17–20.

Guberina, P. 1964. Verbotonal method and its applications to the rehabilitation of the deaf. In *Report of the Proceedings of the International Congress on Education of the Deaf.* Washington, D.C.: Government Printing Office. Pp. 279–99.

Gustason, G. 1973. The languages of communication. *Deafness Annual,* 3: 83–93.

Gustason, G. 1974–1975. Signing exact English. *Gallaudet Today,* communication issue, 5(2): 11–12.

Gustason, G., Pfetzing, D., Zewalkow, E., and Norris, C. (illustrator). 1975. *Signing Exact English.* Rev. and enlarged ed. Modern Signs Press. (1st ed., Silver Spring, Md.: National Association of the Deaf, 1972.)

Hardick, E. J., Oyer, H. J., and Irion, P. E. 1970. Lipreading performance as related to measurements of vision. *Journal of Speech and Hearing Research,* 13: 92–100.

Heider, F. 1943. Acoustic training helps lip reading. *Volta Review,* 45: 135, 180.

Heider, F. K., and Heider, G. M. 1940a. A comparison of sentence structure of deaf and hearing children. *Psychological Monographs,* 52(1): 42–103.

Heider, F. K. and Heider, G. M. 1940b. An experimental investigation of lipreading. *Psychological Monographs,* 52(1): 124–53.

Heidinger, V. 1972. An exploratory study of procedures for improving temporal features in the speech of deaf children. Ed.D. diss., Columbia University.

Henderson, H. G. 1959. *An Introduction to Haiku.* Garden City, N.Y.: Doubleday Anchor Books.

Hendry, J. F. 1969. *Your Future in Translating and Interpreting.* New York: Richards Rosen Press.

Hester, M. S. 1964. Manual communication. In *Proceedings of the International Congress on Education of the Deaf and the Forty-first Meeting of the Convention of American Instructors of the Deaf.* Washington, D.C.: United States Government Printing Office. Pp. 211–21.

Higgins, D. D. 1942. *How to Talk to the Deaf.* Chicago: J. S. Paluch Co.

Hiskey, M. S. 1950. Determining mental competence levels of children with impaired hearing. *Volta Review,* 52: 430–32.

Holm, A. 1972. The Danish mouth-hand system. *Teacher of the Deaf,* 70: 486–90.

Hudgins, C. V. 1936. A study of respiration and speech. *Volta Review,* 38: 341–43, 373.

Hudgins, C. V. 1937. Voice production and breath control in the speech of the deaf. *American Annals of the Deaf,* 82: 338–63.

Hudgins, C. V. 1946. Speech breathing and speech intelligibility. *Volta Review,* 48: 642–44.

Hudson, P. L. 1979. Recommitment to the Fitzgerald Key. *American Annals of the Deaf,* 124: 397–99.

Israel, R. H. 1975. The hearing aid. *Volta Review,* 77: 21–26.

Johnson, E. H. 1948. The ability of pupils in a school for the deaf to understand various methods of communication. *American Annals of the Deaf,* 93: 194–213, 258–314.

Johnson-Laird, P. N. 1974. Experimental psycholinguistics. In M. R. Rosenzweig and L. W. Porter, eds., *Annual Review of Psychology.* Palo Alto, Calif.: Annual Reviews. Pp. 135–60.

Jordan, I. K., Gustason, G., and Rosen, R. 1979. An update on communication trends at programs for the deaf. *American Annals of the Deaf,* 124: 350–57.

Kates, S. L. 1972. *Language Development in Deaf and Hearing Adolescents.* Northampton, Mass.: Clarke School for the Deaf.

Kubie, L. S. 1965. Blocks to creativity. *International Science and Technology,* June 1965 (No. 42): 69–78.

Laird, C. 1953. *The Miracle of Language.* New York: World Publishing Co.

Larkin, W. D. 1976. The CCR program in speech training: An analysis and approach. In *Proceedings of the Forty-eighth Meeting of the Conference of Executives of American Schools for the Deaf, Inc.* Rochester School for the Deaf, National Technical Institute for the Deaf. Rochester, N.Y. Pp. 32–47.

Lenneberg, E. H. 1964. A biological perspective of language. In E. H. Lenneberg, ed., *New Directions in the Study of Language.* Cambridge, Mass: M.I.T. Press. Pp. 65–88.

Lenneberg, E. H. 1967. *Biological Foundations of Language.* New York: John Wiley and Sons.

Lewis, D. N. 1972. Lipreading skills of hearing impaired children in regular schools. *Volta Review,* 74: 303–11.

Lilly, J. C. 1967. *The Mind of the Dolphin: A Nonhuman Intelligence.* New York: Doubleday & Co.

Ling, D. 1976. *Speech and the Hearing Impaired Child: Theory and Practice.* Washington, D.C.: Alexander Graham Bell Association for the Deaf.

Lloyd, L. L, and Dahle, A. J. 1976. Detection and diagnosis of hearing impairment in the child. In R. Prisina, ed., *A Bicentennial Monograph on Hearing Impairments: Trends in the U.S.A.* Washington, D.C.: Alexander Graham Bell Association for the Deaf. Pp. 12–23.

Lowell, E. L. 1959. Research on speechreading: Some relationships to language development and implications for the classroom teacher. In *Report of the Proceedings of the Thirty-ninth Annual Meeting of the Convention of American Instructors of the Deaf.* Pp. 68–73.

Lyons, J., ed. 1970. *New Horizons in Linguistics.* Baltimore: Penguin Books.

McNeill, D. 1966. The capacity for language acquisition. *Volta Review,* 68: 17–33.

Magarotto, C. and Vukotic, D. 1959. *First Contribution to the International Dictionary of Sign Language, Conference Terminology.* Rome: World Federation of the Deaf.

Mandelbaum, D. G., ed. 1956. *Edward Sapir: Culture, Language and Personality.* Berkeley, Calif.: University of California Press.

Markides, A. 1970. The speech of deaf and partially-hearing children with special reference to factors affecting intelligibility. *British Journal of Disorders of Communication,* 5: 126–40.

Markwardt, A. H., and Richey, H. G., eds. 1970. *Linguistics in School Programs.* Chicago: National Society for the Study of Education. Distributed by University of Chicago Press.

Marshall, J. C. 1970. The biology of communication in man and animals. In J. Lyons, ed., *New Horizons in Linguistics.* Baltimore: Penguin Books. Pp. 229–41.

Mason, M. K. 1943. A cinematographic technique for testing visual speech comprehension. *Journal of Speech Disorders,* 8: 271–78.

Mead, M. 1977. Unispeak: The need for a universal second language. *Deaf Spectrum,* 1977 issue: 8–9. (5070 SW Menlo Drive, Beaverton, Oregon 97005.)

Miller, G. 1951. *Language and Communication.* New York: McGraw-Hill Book Co.

Moores, D. F. 1969. Cued speech: Some practical and theoretical considerations. *American Annals of the Deaf,* 114: 23–33.

Morkovin, B. V. 1960. Experiment in teaching deaf preschool children in the Soviet Union. *Volta Review,* 62: 260–68.

Morkovin, B. V., and Moore, L. M. 1948–1949. *A Contextual Systematic Approach for Speech Reading.* Los Angeles: University of Southern California. (Manual accompanying a training film.)

Myklebust, H. R. 1960. *The Psychology of Deafness.* New York: Grune & Stratton.

National Joint Committee on Infant Hearing Screening. 1971. Policy statement issued jointly by the American Speech and Hearing Association, American Academy of Ophthalmology and Otorhinolaryngology, and the American Academy of Pediatrics.

National Joint Committee on Infant Hearing Screening. 1973. Supplementary statement re: Infant hearing screening, issued jointly by the American Speech and Hearing Association, American Academy of Ophthalmology and Otorhinolaryngology, and the American Academy of Pediatrics.

Nelson, M.S. 1949. The evolutionary process of methods of teaching language to the deaf with a survey of methods. *American Annals of the Deaf*, 94: Pt. I, 230–86; Pt. II, 354–96; Pt. III. 491–511.

New, M. C. 1940. Speech for the young deaf child. *Volta Review*, 42: 592–99.

New, M. C. 1949. Speech in our schools for the deaf. *Volta Review*, 51: 61–64.

New, M. C. 1954. The deaf child's speech vocabulary. *Volta Review*, 56: 105–8.

Newsounds. 1977. 1977–78 conferences throughout the nation aim for improved teaching methods. Vol. 2, No. 10. (Newsletter, Alexander Graham Bell Association for the Deaf.)

Neyhus, A. I. 1969. *Speechreading Failure in Deaf Children*, Washington, D.C.: Office of Education, Department of Health, Education, and Welfare. P. 169.

Nickerson, R. S. 1975. Characteristics of the speech of deaf persons. *Volta Review*, 77: 342–62.

Niemann, S. L. 1972. Listen! An acoupedic program. *Volta Review*, 74: 85–90.

Nitchie, E. B. 1930. *Lip-reading Principles and Practice*. New York: Frederick A. Stokes Co.

Northcott, W. 1979. Guidelines for the preparation of oral interpreters: Support specialists for hearing-impaired individuals. *Volta Review*, 81: 135–45.

O'Neill, J. J., and Davidson, J. L. 1956. Relationship between lipreading and five psychological factors. *Journal of Speech and Hearing Disorders*, 21: 478–81.

O'Neill, J. J., and Oyer, H. J. 1961. *Visual Communication for the Hard of Hearing*. Englewood Cliffs, N.J.: Prentice-Hall.

Paget, R. n.d. *The New Sign Language: Notes for Teachers*. London: Phonetics Department, University College.

Paget, R. 1954. Preface to K. W. Hodgson, *The Deaf and Their Problems*. New York: Philosophical Library. Pp. ix-xvii.

Paget, R., Gorman, P., and Paget, C. 1969. *A Systematic Sign Language*. London.

Peck, A. W., Samuelson, E. E., and Lehman, A. 1926. *Ears and the Man: Studies in Social Work for the Deafened*. Philadelphia: F. A. Davis Co.

Pei, M. *The Story of Language*. 1949. Philadelphia: J. B. Lippincott Co.

Peterson, G. E. 1962. Technological frontiers in communication. *Volta Review*, 64: 369–74.

Pickett, J. M. 1976. Speech-processing aids: Some research problems. In R. Frisina, ed., *A Bicentennial Monograph on Hearing Impairments: Trends in the U.S.A.* Washington, D.C.: Alexander Graham Bell Association for the Deaf. Pp. 82–87.

Pintner, R. 1929. Speechreading and speechreading tests for the deaf. *Journal of Applied Psychology*, 13: 220–25.

Pollack, D. 1964. Acoupedics: A uni-sensory approach. *Volta Review*, 66: 400–409.

Pollack, D. 1970. *Educational Audiology for the Limited Hearing Infant*. Springfield, Ill.: Charles C. Thomas.

Popelka, G. R., and Erber, N. P. 1971. Gestures and visual speech reception. *American Annals of the Deaf*, 116: 434–36.

Prall, J. 1957. Lipreading and hearing aids combine for better comprehension. *Volta Review,* 59: 64–65.

Pronovost, W. L. 1978. Programs in action: Speech-processing aids for the deaf: International research. *Volta Review,* 80: 41–45.

Quigley, S. P. 1969. *The Influence of Fingerspelling on the Development of Language, Communication, and Educational Achievement in Deaf Children.* Urbana, Ill.: Institute for Research on Exceptional Children.

Quigley, S. P., Power, D. J., and Steinkamp, M. W. 1977. The language structure of deaf children. *Volta Review,* 79: 73–84.

Registry of Interpreters for the Deaf. 1978. *American Annals of the Deaf,* 123: 284–86.

Reid, G. W. 1947. A preliminary investigation of the testing of lipreading achievement. *Journal of Speech and Hearing Disorders,* 12: 77–82.

Risberg, A. 1971. A critical review of work on speech analyzing hearing aids. *Volta Review,* 73: 23–32, 33–35.

Robson, E. M. 1959. *The Orchestra of the Language.* New York: Thomas Yoseloff.

Roche, T. F., Sheehan, P., Lydia, M., Walsh, J., and Macairt, J. 1971. A study of handicaps and their effect on lipreading among rubella-deaf girls. *Developmental Medicine and Child Neurology,* 13: 497–507.

Rosenthal, R. 1975. *The Hearing Loss Handbook.* New York: St. Martin's Press.

Ross, M. 1976. Verbal communication: The state of the art. *Volta Review,* 78: 324–28.

Ross, M., and Calvert, D. R. 1977. Guidelines for audiology programs in educational settings for hearing-impaired children. *Volta Review,* 79: 153–61.

Russell, W. K., Quigley, S. P., and Power, D. J. 1976. *Linguistics and Deaf Children.* Washington, D.C.: Alexander Graham Bell Association for the Deaf.

Sanders, J. W., and Coscarelli, J. E. 1970. The relationship of visual synthesis skill to lipreading. *American Annals of the Deaf,* 115: 23–26.

Sapir, E. 1921. *Language: An Introduction to the Study of Speech.* New York: Harcourt, Brace & World.

Schiff, W., and Thayer, S. 1974. An eye for an ear? Social perception, nonverbal communication, and deafness. *Rehabilitation Psychology,* 21: 50–70.

Schlesinger, I. M. 1971. The grammar of sign language and the problem of language universals. In J. Morris, ed., *Biological and Social Factors in Psycholinguistics.* London: Logos Press. Pp. 98–121.

Schmitt, P. J. 1966. Language instruction for the deaf. *Volta Review,* 68: 85–105.

Schreiber, F. C. 1974–1975. New signs . . . and the cons. *Gallaudet Today,* communication issue, 5 (Winter): 5–6.

Schunhoff, H. F. 1957. *The Teaching of Speech and by Speech in Public Residential Schools for the Deaf in the United States, 1815–1955.* Romney, W.V.: West Virginia School for the Deaf and the Blind.

Scouten, E. L. 1964. The place of the Rochester Method in American education of the deaf. In *Proceedings of the International Congress on Education of the Deaf and of the Forty-first Meeting of the Convention of American Instructors of the Deaf.* Washington, D.C.: U.S. Government Printing Office. Pp. 429–32.

Scouten, E. L. 1967. The Rochester Method, an oral multi-sensory approach for instructing prelingually deaf children. *American Annals of the Deaf,* 112: 50–55.

Scouten, E. L. 1969. The influence of fingerspelling in early language training of the deaf. Erwin Kugel Lecture, New York Society for the Deaf, New York City, November 1969.

Sharp, E. Y. 1972. Relationship of visual closure to speechreading. *Exceptional Children*, 38: 729–34.

Siegenthaler, B. M., and Gruber, V. 1969. Combining vision and audition for speech reception. *Journal of Speech and Hearing Disorders*, 34: 58–60.

Simmons, A. A. 1959. Factors related to lipreading. *Journal of Speech and Hearing Research*, 2: 340–52.

Simmons, A. A. 1962. A comparison of the type–token ratio of spoken and written language of deaf children. *Volta Review*, 64: 417–21.

Simmons, A. A. 1968. Content subjects through language. *Volta Review*, 70: 481–86.

Simmons-Martin, A. 1972. The oral/aural procedure: Theoretical basis and rationale. *Volta Review*, 74: 541–52.

Smith, C. R. 1972. Residual hearing and speech production in deaf children. Ph.D. diss., City University of New York.

Smith, J. L. 1897. Characteristic errors of pupils. *American Annals of the Deaf*, 42: 201–10.

Smith, J. M., ed. 1964. *Workshop on Interpreting for the Deaf*. Muncie, Ind.: Ball State Teachers College.

Stack, A., ed. 1972. *An Introduction to Manual English*. Vancouver, Wash.: Washington State School for the Deaf.

Steiner, G. 1977. The Tongues of Men: Part II: A World Language? BBC and WGBH, Boston: WGBH Educational Foundation. NOVA transcript No. 415.

Sternberg, M. L. 1981. *American Sign Language: A Comprehensive Dictionary*. New York: Harper & Row.

Stockwell, E. 1952. Visual defects in the deaf child. *AMA Archives of Ophthalmology*, 48: 428–32.

Stokoe, W. C. 1974. *Sign Language Studies*. The Hague: Mouton.

Stokoe, W. C. 1974–1975. The view from the lab: Two ways to English competence for the deaf. *Gallaudet Today*, communication issue, 5(2): 31–32.

Stokoe, W. C. 1978. *Sign Language Structures*. Rev. ed. Silver Spring, Md.: Linstock Press.

Strong, W. J. 1975. Speech aids for the profoundly/severely hearing impaired: Requirements, overview, and projections. *Volta Review*, 77: 536–56.

Stuckless, E. R., and Pollard, G. 1977. Processing of fingerspelling and print by deaf students. *American Annals of the Deaf*, 122: 475–79.

Tato, J. M., and Arcella, A. I. 1955. The percentage of intelligibility of speech in deaf-mutes. In *Proceedings of the Second World Congress of the Deaf*. Belgrade: Central Committee of the Yugoslav Federation of the Deaf. Pp. 157–65.

Tervoort, B. T. M. 1961: Esoteric symbolism in the communication behavior of young deaf children. *American Annals of the Deaf*, 106: 436–80.

Thomson, R. 1959. *The Psychology of Thinking*. Baltimore: Penguin Books.

Tiffany, R., and Kates, S. 1972. Concept attainment and lipreading ability among deaf adolescents. *Journal of Speech and Hearing Disorders*, 27: 265–74.

Trybus, R. J., and Karchmer, M. A. 1977. School achievement scores of hearing impaired children: National data on achievement status and growth patterns. *American Annals of the Deaf,* 122: 62–69.

Upton, H. W. 1968. Wearable eyeglass speechreading aid. *American Annals of the Deaf,* 113: 222–29.

Utley, J. A. 1946. A test of lipreading ability. *Journal of Speech and Hearing Disorders,* 2: 109–16.

Van Uden, A. 1970. *A World of Language for Deaf Children.* Rotterdam: Rotterdam University Press.

Vernon, M. 1972. Mind over mouth: A rationale for "total communication," *Volta Review,* 74: 529–40.

Von Frisch, K., and Lindauer, M. 1965. The "language" and orientation of the honeybee. In T. E. McGill, ed., *Animal Behavior.* New York: Holt, Rinehart, & Winston.

Vorce, E. R. 1974. *Teaching Speech to Deaf Children.* Washington, D.C.: Alexander Graham Bell Association for the Deaf.

Vygotsky, L. S. 1962. *Thought and Language.* Ed. and trans. by E. Hanfmann and G. Vakar. Cambridge, Mass.: M.I.T. Press.

Wampler, D. 1971. *Linguistics of Visual English.* Santa Rosa, Calif.: (2322 Maher Drive #35, Santa Rosa, California 95405).

Whatmough, J. 1956. *Language: A Modern Synthesis.* New York: St. Martin's Press.

Wilbur, R. B. 1977. An explanation of deaf children's difficulty with certain syntactic structures of English. *Volta Review,* 79: 85–92.

5 Educational Environments: Options and Issues

The way a person responds to a situation is often a better clue to what his teaching has been than to what his personality is.
Linton, *The Cultural Background of Personality*

FOR A small deaf child, a first look at the school environment has little meaning. To be sure, the ultimate goals of education are firmly fixed in the hopes of teacher and parent. But the child has no such image in his mind's eye. All he knows is what he sees, that this is a different place, another unknown. He fears he may be banished to this place away from home and family. Again, he knows not why. For some children it takes months before the accustomed routines, activities, and companions of school overcome initial anxieties and the child is ready to accept instruction. Others never fully overcome resentment.

In view of the incredibly difficult learnings that lie ahead for a deaf child, the key imperative, particularly at the beginning level, is to make the child *want* to learn. Latent mental hungers must be rekindled; the push to environmental exploration revived; the longing to communicate, satisfied. One of the great talents of master teachers is their ability to make learning an exciting experience at all age levels, but especially at the youngest level where the foundations are laid. As expressed by Hart and Cory, "we want [our pupils] to be curious and ingenious explorers, eagerly pursuing interests and knowledges, uncovering facts, evaluating them and using them, and even sometimes deliberately discarding them in favor of fantasy and creativity" (1968, p. 462).

The question is how to achieve this goal in the education of deaf children.

Unresolved Determinants

As matters stand the answer to the question involves other questions, beginning with

1. *Where* to teach: is it or is it not to a deaf child's advantage to be educated along with other deaf children in a school or class specifically designed and staffed for the purpose, and, if not, what is the best possible alternative?

2. *When* to begin: what is the optimum age at which auditory amplification and instructional practices should commence?

3. *How* to teach: through what system of instruction is communication, hence education, best effected?

4. *What* to teach: what curricular content and programming are best suited to the needs of deaf children for personal development and for adaptation to the networks of society?

And underlying these is the all-embracing and perhaps most important question:

5. *Who* is to teach: what combination of personal traits, special abilities and experiences, and level of training qualify a person to teach deaf children?

The issue that has generated the hottest and longest debate is how to teach. Better known as the "methods controversy," the differing viewpoints and biases concerning the methods of communication to be used in instruction have commanded the major portion of field interest and energies for centuries. Other issues have been left more or less on the sidelines, except when scattered voices call attention to one or another from time to time or when a debatable innovation makes its appearance. However, the accountability mandated in 1975 by the Education of All Handicapped Children Act, PL 94-142 (U.S., Congress, 1975) and particularly its Individualized Education Program section implies extensive changes from this traditional pattern.

Mandated Planning and Accountability

The Education of All Handicapped Children Act was conceived to protect the rights of these children to (1) an education; (2) a free education; (3) an appropriate education; (4) an education conducted in the least restrictive environment; (5) parental challenge through due process; (6) confidentiality; and (7) nondiscriminatory testing. To guard these rights, each state is required to set up procedures whereby handicapped children are, to the maximum appropriate extent, educated with the nonhandicapped except when the handicapping condition is such that education in the regular classes cannot be satisfactorily achieved even with the use of supplementary aids and devices. The act became fully operative for handicapped children of ages 3 to 18 years in October 1977 (Buscaglia and Williams, 1979; Martin, 1979).

The Individualized Education section of the law requires that education programs be specifically designed for each handicapped child by a team consisting of a representative of the local school agency, the child's teachers, the child's parents or parent surrogates, the child when appropriate, and such other individuals as may be deemed necessary by parents or agency. Also required is a written document of agreement among all team members. The document must include: (1) a statement of the child's present educational level; (2) annual as well as short-term instructional goals; and (3) a statement of the specific educational services to be provided and the extent to which the child will be able to participate in regular educational programs. The broad aim of these mandates is to assure placement for handicapped children in a setting that is least restrictive to educational progress. For further assurance, accountability and due-process procedures are built into the law, whereby parents may challenge placement, evaluation, and instruction through special grievance procedures.

The mandate to fit the needs of deaf children into the framework of PL 94-142 has raised vexatious problems for educators. Particularly sensitive issues are the conceptualization of "least restrictive" environment and the associated issue of mainstreaming, which is discussed later (Conference of Executives of American Schools for the Deaf, 1977; Council on Education of the Deaf, 1976; Nix, 1977a,b; *PL 94-142 and Deaf Children,* 1977). Through what procedures are "restrictive" evaluations to be made? At what point does a "least restrictive environment" for a deaf child of one age level become "restrictive" for the same child when it is older? What are the adjustment hazards for such a child when a midstream change must be made from one type of educational setting to another?

A particularly provoking issue is that of psychological assessment, and allied to it is the problem of prediction. Assessment and prediction are the two main pillars on which decision-making rests in fashioning individualized programs and in determining school/class placement. However, the shortage of psychologists who are trained, qualified, or otherwise prepared to evaluate deaf children is a matter of dismal record, as is the lack of tests and other instrumentation on which to base predictive judgments (Levine, 1971, 1974, 1977). As Bruce sums up the situation, "by our own admission, we have far to go in perfecting our ability to predict and prescribe the auditory, educational, and communicative futures of our young charges" (1976, p. 322).

For parents, PL 94-142 offers an unprecedented opportunity to participate in educational decision-making and to demand accountability (Kidd, 1977).

This is a giant step forward from the traditional role of parents, which, as Danahy observes, "has been confined to a peculiar form of participation which has allowed a degree of identification, but hardly the degree of involvement necessary in the education of the handicapped child" (1970, p. 154).

However, this new role places a heavy responsibility on parents, the responsibility for recognizing which is the "least restrictive" educational environment for their child among the mass of options, issues, unresolved questions, and technical problems that bedevil the field. As described by Denton (1971), these "educational crises" include: (1) the communication crisis; (2) crisis in family involvement; (3) crisis in morality, in sensitivity to spiritual needs and values; (4) crisis in teacher education; (5) crisis in curriculum; and (6) crisis in educational programs.

Parent leaders are keenly aware that, in order to carry out these new responsibilities, parents must function as *informed* participants in the decision-making process (Allen, 1977; Champ-Wilson, 1977; Moses, 1977); and that to do so requires a clear understanding of what is involved in the various options and crises, and of what coping abilities are required of the child. Toward this end, new impetus has been given to parent education programs and parent organizations (Grisham, 1974). But even so, these measures cannot erase the traditional fear of parents of deaf children—the fear of making a wrong decision. If anything, the weight of the new responsibilities may heighten anxiety as parents become more knowledgeable about the variety of education options available, the pros and cons of each, and the divisive issues that plague the field.

Educational Settings

The historical background of educational settings for deaf children has been comprehensively reviewed in the literature (Bender, 1960; Di Carlo, 1964; Hodgson, 1953), and details concerning current special-education settings and programs in the United States are summarized in the annual Directory Issue of the *American Annals of the Deaf*. Here we shall briefly scan the options facing parents in deciding which is the best educational setting for their children. The following are among the options open to them.

1. *Correspondence courses.* The most famous of these, the John Tracy Correspondence Course (Tracy, 1968), is designed to help parents home-teach deaf children in the age range of 2–5 years. The course consists of 12 lessons and includes first lessons in sense training, lipreading, language, auditory training, and speech preparation. There is also a pre-correspondence course called "Letters to the Parents of Deaf Babies."

2. *Classes for parents.* In line with the thought that education of a deaf child begins with the education of the child's parents, numerous facilities and parent associations offer both formal and informal opportunities for parents to become more knowledgeably involved in the education of their deaf children.

3. *Parent–infant programs.* As described by Connor (1976), such programs are designed for deaf infants (from birth to 3 years) and involve parent–teacher collaboration in speech, listening, and language activities. "Parent–teacher interactions are classroom-oriented, with the teacher of the deaf intent on having the parent understand and apply the 'lessons' to be practiced with the child at home (see Tracy Clinic curriculum)" (Connor, 1976, p. 9). Parent–infant programs are conducted at various schools for the deaf and at certain speech and hearing centers. Their major emphasis is on the use of residual hearing, language development, and communication, with numerous programs also stressing the socializing aspects of child–family relations (Northcott, 1972), and increasing numbers focusing on total communication.

4. *Demonstration-home programs.* Demonstration homes are actual residences set up by a host facility and furnished as ordinary living quarters in which a mother and her deaf child live for specified periods, with the mother carrying out her usual, home-making activities. While the mother is so engaged, a teacher of the deaf is at hand to show her how she can use these activities to develop the child's language and lipreading skills. The best-known demonstration homes are those conducted by the John Tracy Clinic (Tracy, 1968) and the Bill Wilkerson Hearing and Speech Center (McConnell, 1968).

5. *Speech and hearing centers.* There are hundreds of speech and hearing (or hearing and speech) centers, throughout the country, that provide diagnostic, clinical, and/or habilitative and rehabilitative services in the area of impaired hearing. (See the *Guide to Clinical Services in Speech Pathology and Audiology,* published by the American Speech and Hearing Association.) Many of these centers have tutoring and class-instruction programs for hearing-impaired children, and/or conduct parent education and parent–infant programs.

6. *Residential schools.* Publicly and privately funded residential (boarding) schools grew mainly out of the need to provide special-education services for the comparatively small and geographically scattered population of deaf children who live too far away to use services in metropolitan areas. The advantage claimed by residential schools is that having been founded, designed, and staffed for the exclusive benefit of a deaf pupil population, they are in an exceptional position to serve the children by way of teachers and staff trained for work with the deaf, through familiarity with the special-

ized instructional techniques and technologies required, and by providing a broad range of special programs, such as career development (Twyman and Ouellette, 1978), and planned extracurricular activities.

7. *Day schools.* Day schools are public schools established to serve a pupil population of deaf children who live at home. The advantages claimed are that such schools avoid the separation of child from family that occurs with residential placement, support family living, and promote the child's integration with the everyday hearing community while at the same time providing for the special-education needs.

8. *Day classes.* Day classes are special-education classes for deaf children in regular "hearing" schools. Parents select such placement for various reasons: they oppose child–family separation and special school segregation; they live too far away from a day school; they feel that a day-class setting will eventually enable the child to enter and succeed in a regular class as an integrated pupil. The quality of day-class education varies widely and depends in large measure on teacher qualifications, support services afforded teacher and child, the number and homogeneity of deaf pupils in the class, and the receptiveness of the school and its population to deaf pupils.

9. *Integrated programs.* The move to identify the "least restrictive" learning environment for deaf pupils has resulted in a number of programs in which deaf pupils are partially integrated into regular school programs. They spend part of the school day in specified classes and/or activities with hearing pupils, and part of the school day, as needs require, in a special-education class for the deaf.

10. *Mainstream programs.* A complete mainstream program is one in which a deaf pupil "pursues all or a majority of his education within a regular school program with non-handicapped students" (Clark, 1975, p. 2), with some support services to teacher and pupils. Some deaf children begin their education as mainstreamed pupils; others are mainstreamed after special-education foundations are laid. In the writer's experience, mainstreamed deaf children, particularly in the pre- and elementary-school range, rely more or less heavily on outside tutorial assistance.

For an uninitiated parent of a first deaf child to make a choice among these 10 options is taxing enough; but the difficulties do not end here. Imbedded in the options are still other options that demand appraisal. Possibly the most sensitive involves the communication philosophy of a given setting. For example, some parent and parent–infant programs espouse the unisensory auditory approach, others the global-auditory, and still others the use of one or another variety of the language of signs. Which is the "right" choice? At the school level, some schools and classes for deaf pupils are committed to the oral/aural system of instruction, others to a combined system or to total communication, and a few to the Rochester method or a modification thereof. Again, which is the "right" choice? And beyond variations in philosophy of education and systems of instruction there are variations in the caliber of a setting. Some function at a superior level, others are mediocre, and still others are downright poor. How is an uninitiated parent to know? Added to the decision-making burden are field issues such as mainstreaming, total communication, the "Siglish" explosion, to be discussed in the next section, that tend to focus the attention of many parents on the issue rather than the child.

The anguish of decision-making is described as follows by one concerned parent of a deaf child:

> Each family . . . had a different decision to make when it came time to do something about the child's education. For some there were schools or facilities close enough to use without a major disruption of the family. But even then there was the question of whether those facilities were right for you and your child. Some families decided on the oral method of learning, while others chose the manual. For some the answer was the residential schools and some preferred day programs. This decision, of course, did not involve only what was best for the child with the hearing impairment, but what was best for the whole family. In some cases the decision involved a move to a different place, and this added more problems to an already major decision. In choosing between oral and manual communication, residential and day classes, whether to move to enroll in classes or stay home and work through correspondence, the various professional people can point out the advantages and disadvantages, but they cannot tell the parents exactly what to do. At this point, the whole decision that will control someone else's life for years to come is difficult, especially when there are so many choices and each so far reaching and different. Around you go, pro and con until finally you make the decision, but occasionally the nagging question returns—are we doing the right thing? (Williams, 1970, p. 305)

Like parents, many conscientious professional persons frequently wonder, Are we doing the right thing?

Educational Issues

Educational issues are no novelty in the field of the deaf. Some are ingrained in tradition; others thrive on change and innovation. Occasionally an issue instigates volcanic debates that rock the field. Two such are reviewed here—mainstreaming and total communication—along with the less spectacular but possibly more important issue of curriculum.

Mainstreaming

Although the term "mainstream" is a recent addition to the glossary of "deaf education," the idea of educating deaf children in the regular schools is far from new. It was given an intensive trial over a century ago, and we are told that "Graser and Stephani in Bavaria, Daniel in Wurtemberg, Arrowsmith in England, Blanchet in France, and others, have advocated it warmly, and in some cases so effectively as to make converts of men in authority, and cause the experiment to be fully and fairly tried" (Fay, 1875, p. 116). So enthusiastic, in fact, were the French "converts" and advocates of the period that they formed a sponsoring organization to promote the practice of mainstreaming—the Société pour l'enseignement simultané des sourds-muets et des entendants-parlants.

To facilitate the instruction of deaf pupils in regular classes, an ingenious system was devised by M. Augustin Grosselin in the mid-nineteenth century—the phonomimic method (Bourguin, 1871). It was based on a "phonomimic" alphabet of 32 gestures, each representing one of the 32 sounds of the French language. These phonetic gesture symbols accompanied spoken language in much the same way that phonetic hand-position symbols accompany speech in the mouth–hand and cued speech systems of more recent vintage.

The "full and fair" trials given to these mid-nineteenth-century educational innovations yielded disappointing results. Of mainstreaming, we are told that

> even under the most favorable circumstances, the experiment has never proved a success.
>
> Teachers could not give the few deaf-mute children placed under their charge the time and attention necessary for imparting even the rudiments of an education without doing injustice to the hearing children who formed the great majority of their pupils, and the result has been that the deaf-mute sat in school neglected and alone, acquiring, doubtless, some useful habits of order, learning the alphabet and perhaps a few words, but gaining nothing that could really be called an education or form a preparation for the duties of life. In most of the countries of Europe the experiment was long ago abandoned; in France, while some deaf-mute children are still taught in the public schools, they are grouped in classes by themselves, under special teachers, so that there also the experiment is virtually abandoned. (Fay, 1875, pp. 116, 117)

Regarding the phonomimic method which had been tested under the auspices of the French Ministry of Public Instruction, we are told:

> Of the result of these two experiments on a larger scale than had been attempted before, we are not informed; but from the somewhat guarded manner in which the conductors of the *Bulletin* speak of the method we infer that they do not esteem it very highly, and that it is not now practised in the National Institution. (Fay, 1875, p. 119)

The unsuccessful outcomes of European experiments in mainstreaming discouraged organized moves toward the practice in this country until the

latter half of the twentieth century. Of course, there were various instances
in which mainstreaming was carried out with deaf children before this time,
and presumably they included successes as well as failures. But these cases
were largely undocumented. One such effort was conducted in the early
1950s with several elementary-level pupils of the Lexington School for the
Deaf who were congenitally hearing-impaired as a result of maternal rubella
(Levine, 1951). All had substantial amounts of residual hearing, superior
mental and scholastic abilities, and exceptional oral communicative skills. In
addition to these advantages, the criteria for mainstreaming included: the
children's emotional stability and stamina, social patterns and adaptability,
and their wishes in the matter of being mainstreamed; the nature of the
transfer hearing school; and the parents' views on the proposed transfer. The
transfer schools were carefully selected; they included several innovatively
inclined private schools interested in trying out the mainstream experiment
and one similarly inclined public school, all with small classes. Orientative
conferences were held with the school personnel to explain the special needs
of hearing-impaired pupils, and with the parents to ascertain their wishes in
the matter and their ability to provide emotional and tutorial support. Where
all circumstances appeared favorable, mainstreaming was carried out and
proved successful in every case, as indicated by follow-up.

I have also encountered numerous mainstream failures over the years
who, while just as capable as this success group scholastically, were unable
to cope with the tensions and burden of work involved in toeing the ''hearing'' mark, particularly in an indifferent school and with over-anxious, driving parents. Most if not all such cases have also gone undocumented.

By contrast, the mainstream injunction inherent in PL 94-142 produced an
avalanche of documented reaction. While no quarrel is reported among educators with the concept of placing a deaf child in an educational environment
that offers the least restrictions to progress and enrichment, opinions differ
concerning the *type* of setting that is ''least restrictive,'' particularly during
the formative years of a deaf child's life.

Speaking in behalf of the mainstream trend in education is Ewald B.
Nyquist, Commissioner of Education of the State of New York:

> educators are showing an increased interest in programs that encourage the edu-
> cation of handicapped and nonhandicapped children together. There are a
> number of reasons for this preference. First, studies done of the effectiveness of
> special class vs. regular class placement have failed to reveal any conclusive
> results. Secondly, many educators are concerned about civil rights issues in
> school districts with high enrollments of handicapped children in separate facili-
> ties. Also, the benefits to the handicapped children of contact with nonhan-
> dicapped children are increasingly evident. Studies show dramatic improve-
> ments in coping and in interpersonal relationships for children in mainstreamed
> settings. Finally, many educators are convinced that the nonhandicapped child

makes important gains in understanding and values by having the opportunity to grow up with handicapped children. Each of these reasons for mainstreaming underlines the values and importance of this trend in education. (Nyquist, n.d., p. 4)

Much of the evidence noted by Nyquist in support of mainstreaming comes from the field of mental retardation.

The wisdom of mainstreaming a deaf child is, however, open to challenge. A prominent educator of the deaf, a deaf leader, and the parents of a deaf child speak their doubts on the subject. The educator maintains that

> the typical deaf child with a tremendous communication handicap is not best placed in a regular classroom. The teacher in the regular classroom does not have the competencies to meet this child's needs. Placement of one deaf child in a class of hearing children precludes his receiving the proportionate amount of time he needs even from the best intentioned teacher. (Brill, 1975, p. 180)

The deaf leader warns

> The deaf (and their friends) should be aware of this threat to quality and meaningful education of the hearing impaired through the "back door" approach of mainstreaming. If this "pie in the sky" philosophy becomes widespread, billions of dollars will need to be appropriated for rehabilitation a few years hence. (Smith, 1974, p. 2)

The parents of a deaf child sum up their experiences with mainstreaming:

> In the situation of "mainstreaming," we as parents feel the hearing world is not being realistic with the deaf. We are expecting too much of them, when placing them in the same educational situation with a hearing handicap. There are many times the deaf need extra or special attention in their school work and social life. This the regular school doesn't have time for. The competition is very great when a deaf person is placed in a large school for hearing children. . . . "Mainstreaming" doesn't give the deaf the feeling of "being in" like hearing people (who are for mainstreaming) think it does. (Van Engen, 1977, p. 3)

The problem facing educators of the deaf is how to meet the special needs and unique problems of deaf children while at the same time bowing to mainstream philosophy. Some see partial integration as the way. In certain programs, deaf children occupy a home- or resource-room and are mainstreamed only for special subjects or activities; in others, team teaching is the practice, or special tutoring and support services are provided as required. McGee (1976) describes eight different kinds of integration strategies used with hearing-impaired children. In addition, there is a growing trend to integrate deaf pupils by teaching the sign language to their hearing classmates and/or by providing interpreters for class activities (Cooney, 1977). Eloise

Leitzow, director of deaf services for the Iowa State Department of Health is quoted as saying that "the idea of mainstreaming with an interpreter at younger levels really is exciting and a growing trend" (Cooney, 1977, p. 1). One might look upon this as a kind of reverse integration.

But here too there is no agreement among educators of the deaf about the benefits of partial integration. Brill voices an opposing view:

> Special supportive services in an integrated program generally mean some individualized tutoring. This is not sufficient for the typical prelingual deaf child. He needs a constant total program and he needs to associate with other children in the class who are truly his peers if he is going to learn to get along in society. (1975, p. 381)

Opinions and program-experiments could be more soundly assessed if based on firm research evidence. But as yet there is no such body of data. Most of the literature consists of articles on programs in action, various mainstream techniques, individualized education programming (e.g., Ling, Ling, and Pflaster, 1977), survey data (e.g., Craig and Salem, 1975; Craig, Salem, and Craig, 1976), plus a wide assortment of views, opinions, and proposals. Noteworthy are several publications covering significant aspects of mainstreaming (Nix, 1976, 1977a; Northcott, 1973; Paul, Turnbull, and Cruikshank, 1979).

The few reported studies are what Reich, Hambleton, and Houldin (1977) would probably call the "snapshot" variety as opposed to the badly needed longitudinal studies. Some of the "snapshots" show deaf mainstreamed children able to keep up scholastically with their hearing classmates (Kennedy et al., 1976; Reich, Hambleton, and Houldin, 1977; Rister, 1975; van den Horst, 1971); others show a failure to keep pace (Fisher, 1971; Peckham, Sheridan, and Butler, 1972). A number of studies suggest that the pressures of mainstreaming adversely affect emotional adjustment (Craig, 1965; Reich, Hambleton, and Houldin, 1977; Shears and Jensema, 1969; van den Horst, 1971). Ross (1978) in particular deplores the lack of attention paid to the personal/social implications of mainstreaming.

In short, the philosophy of mainstreaming deaf children is going through another experimental trial more than a century after its initial test. As yet, the practice is still at the "unresolved issue" stage. But even so, certain understandings and clarifications are gradually emerging. A parent who has coped with the mainstream problem tells about some of the determinants he has observed:

> we have learned that success is dependent upon receptive and supportive professionals, committed and involved parents, and, above all, fully prepared children.

We learned the necessity of constant monitoring of our children's placement.

We learned the need for proper preparation of both the teacher and the other students when a deaf child is to be part of a class.

And most important of all, we learned that the child—not the professional or the parents—is probably the best judge of whether an educational situation is providing successful social living. *Thus, we learned to rely on the children's signals.* There is no doubt that a child must be emotionally ready for mainstreaming. (Meltzer, 1978, pp. 110–11)

The problem is how to prepare a child emotionally for such personal and social problems of mainstreaming as those reported by parents to Greenberg and Doolittle (1977):

No matter which kind of integration was mentioned, both deaf children and their parents contradicted the glowing hope of theoreticians and the picture presented so compellingly on the recent public-television special "Including Me." . . . The picture we got from parents was one of consistent loneliness, isolation and social loss:

"If they can, they find other deaf kids and stay with them."

"The others don't tease them [the deaf students], they just ignore them." . . .

After school, the loneliness of the day only deepens:

"Oh, yes, on the surface there is communication, a greeting when he comes in—a sign or two that the kids learned or picked up from him. It isn't enough for real social contact; it's strictly a token thing. He's a curiosity."

"No one understands her speech. She is continually frustrated."

"The kids have 'friends' from 8 to 4," a teacher says. "After that they sit at home alone." (Greenberg and Doolittle, 1977, pp. 80, 82)

These statements recall the failure of the nineteenth-century experiment in mainstreaming. Yet there are some remarkable successes too. With compelling arguments on both sides of the issue, again parents ask: What is the right choice for my child?

Total Communication

In Total Communication as in mainstreaming, the roots extend well back into the previous century. At that time, total communication was not the seething issue it later became. Nor was it called "total communication." In fact, it had no special name but was classified as one of the many variations of the Combined System, the one in which "The sign language, the manual alphabet, writing, articulation, and speech reading are all used as means of instruction by the same teachers with the same pupils" (Fay, 1889, p. 68). The rationale for using the "total" approach therefore followed that of the combined system, namely:

Articulation and speech-reading are regarded as very important, but mental development and the acquisition of language are regarded as still more important. It is believed that in many cases mental development and the acquisition of language can be better attained by some other method than the Oral, and, so far as circumstances permit, such method is chosen for each pupil as seems best adapted to his individual case. (Fay, 1889, pp. 65–66)

However, side by side with this statement was a growing conviction among educators of the period that strong efforts should be made to teach every deaf schoolchild how to speak and read the lips (Schunhoff, 1957, p. 28). So strong was the belief that an advocacy organization, The American Association to Promote the Teaching of Speech to the Deaf, was founded in 1890. Largely through its efforts, the percentage of pupils being taught speech in schools for the deaf jumped from 27.2 in 1884 to 63 in 1900. Eventually instruction included not only the teaching *of* speech but teaching *through* speech; a 1954–1955 survey of the 72 public residential schools for the deaf in the country showed that 55.9 percent of the 62 responding schools were conducting all instruction through speech, 38.6 percent used speech all or part of the time, plus some fingerspelling and signs, and only 5.5 percent conducted programs of "no speech" (Schunhoff, 1957, p. 79).

In the course of time, it became increasingly evident that the growth in speech statistics was not matched by growth in speech intelligibility. Nor was it matched by growth in language acquisition or in level of scholastic achievement. The deaf pupil population proved deficient in all these areas. Speech proponents now shifted the emphasis from "more" speech to "better" speech, while those concerned less with speech than with scholastic attainment and social development voiced increasingly outspoken denunciations of the time consumed through instruction by speech at the expense of "mental development and the acquisition of language."

Matters reached a climax with the Babbidge indictment of the education of the deaf (*Education of the Deaf,* 1965). More and more concerned professionals held that education's failures were due to the strictures of teaching *by* speech (Vernon, 1968). They demanded that manual methods, in particular the outlawed language of signs, be included in the instruction of deaf pupils. Their stand was supported by the results of a number of studies comparing deaf children reared in the sign language through having deaf parents, with deaf children of hearing parents. The studies included: comparison of the educational achievement of deaf children of deaf parents with that of deaf children of hearing parents (Stevenson, 1965); the influence of early manual communication on linguistic development (Stuckless and Birch, 1966); comparison of deaf children of deaf parents with deaf children of hearing parents in intellectual, social, and communicative functioning (Meadow, 1968);

comparison of intelligence quotients of deaf children of deaf parents with those of deaf children of hearing parents (Brill, 1969); the influence of fingerspelling on language, communication, and educational achievements (Quigley, 1969); comparison of the educational achievements of deaf children of deaf parents with those of deaf children of hearing parents (Vernon and Koh, 1970); the effects on educational achievement of oral preschool education, early manual communication, and no preschool education but hearing parents (Vernon and Koh, 1971); and a series investigating the influence of early manual communication on achievement, communication, and adjustment (Schlesinger and Meadow, 1972). The overall finding of these studies indicated the general superiority of deaf children who had been exposed to early manual communication.

The studies did not go unchallenged. Conscientious reviews by Owrid (1971) and by Nix (1975) disclosed various procedural weaknesses. Quigley (1969) pointed out that in several studies (Meadow, 1968; Quigley, 1969; Stuckless and Birch, 1966) the differences obtained between the groups "were not large even when statistically significant," while Levine (1976) made a similar observation in regard to the Brill (1969) study. Finally, Messerly and Aram report the results of their investigation of hearing-impaired (HI) students, "in which HI students of hearing parents were superior to a group of HI students of HI parents" (1980, p. 26).

There is, however, a noticeable scarcity of research in support of oral education. Its success is documented in studies by Lane and Baker (1974) and Lane (1976), and Jensema (1975) provides some support in a review of the exceptional achievements of members of the Oral Deaf Adults Section (ODAS) of the Alexander Graham Bell Association for the Deaf, nearly half of whom received their education in oral schools for the deaf. Much of the justification for oralism takes the form of position papers rather than research; and in view of education's failures with the deaf under the oral system, these do not offer convincing rebuttal to the sign language studies, certainly not enough to slacken the sign language momentum.

As the "manual" momentum increased, the need for a more systematized thrust soon became evident. The syntactic deficiencies of the deaf had to be tackled, and the benefits of other communicative modes had to be woven into the evolving pattern of manual instruction. In answer to the syntactic problem, sign-coded straight language systems were devised, as discussed in chapter 4; and in answer to the instructional challenge, there developed the philosophy of total communication (Garretson, 1976).

The terms "total communication" and "total approach" are credited to Roy K. Holcomb, himself a deaf person and supervisor of programs for the hearing impaired. Holcomb describes the terms as indicating a philosophy, not a method:

The Total Approach is using everything and anything that will help the children here and now. Among the many factors which make up the Total Approach are the parents, the hearing children, the community, extra-curricular activities, the curriculum, the teacher and Total Communication. . . . While all things in the Total Approach are vital, Total Communication is basic. (1972, pp. 523–24)

In keeping with this belief, Holcomb describes total communication as "using all means of communication with the children, especially at the earliest possible age" (1972, p. 524). These would include speech, lipreading, cued speech, amplified audition, fingerspelling, the various sign language systems, writing, printing, appropriate gestures, and possibly more. When operationalized, total communication has been said to bear a striking resemblance to the Simultaneous Communication method (Caccamise, 1978; Dale, 1974; Lloyd, 1975). However, since *all* means of communication obviously cannot be rendered "simultaneously," total communication can be conceptualized as calling for an orchestrated rather than a simultaneous input of the various communication modes, such that each contributes to mutual reinforcement and total understanding. I term the system "Multimodal Communication."

The concept of total communication was introduced into the educational scene in the late 1960s and quickly captured the interest of educators of the deaf. The spread was rapid. A national survey of schools and classes for the hearing impaired that was conducted less than a decade later, during the 1975–1976 school year, showed that 64% of the 796 responding programs (which represented 82% of the total surveyed) were using some form of total communication (Jordan, Gustason, and Rosen, 1976). A breakdown of the number of classes for each method disclosed: cued speech, 37; oral/aural, 2,370; Rochester method, 155; total communication, 4,619. Accompanying these remarkable statistics was an equally revolutionary shift from previous educational policy—the burgeoning of formal classes in fingerspelling and signs for parents as well as hearing-impaired pupils. The favored signs taught at preschool and elementary levels were reported to be the newer systems of manual English. A 1978 update of communication trends in the schools showed a continuing shift to total communication and manual English sign systems, in particular Signing Exact English (Jordan, Gustason, and Rosen, 1979).

This shift in instructional communication was accompanied by one in the focus of research. Whereas the focus had been on comparisons of deaf pupil-groups (those with deaf parents versus those with hearing parents), research attention was now directed to comparisons of the various communication modes. A number of early studies of the "total communication" era are cited in table 5.1. Because they deal with experimental subjects of different ages, instructional backgrounds, and communicative experiences,

Table 5.1. Efficiency-Comparisons of Communication Modes

Investigator	Modes Compared	Most Efficient
Klopping (1972)	speechreading with voice, Rochester method, total communication	total communication
Higgins (1973)	Rochester method, Ameslan, "Siglish"	"Siglish"
White and Stevenson (1975)	total communication, manual communication, oral communication, reading	reading, manual communication
Luterman (1976)	visual/oral method, auditory/oral method	auditory/oral method
Beckmeyer (1976)	oral, signs, fingerspelling, oral + sign language, oral + fingerspelling (with oral- and manual-preference subjects)	oral (for oral preference) manual (for oral and manual preference) manual (for manual preference)
Moores, Weiss, Goodwin (1974)	sound alone, sound + speechreading, sound + speechreading + fingerspelling, sound + fingerspelling + signs, the printed word	simultaneous use of residual hearing + speechreading + fingerspelling + signs
Reich and Bick (1976)	investigation of claims in support of fingerspelled English superiority	no superiority of fingerspelling noted
Caccamise, Blasdell, Heath-Lang (1977)	live, televised, and rear-screen projection conditions	live presentation
Caccamise and Blasdell (1977)	oral-manual direct simultaneous communication and oral-manual interpreted communication	oral-manual direct communication
Murphy and Fleischer (1977)	Ameslan versus Siglish	No difference

and with comparisons of different communication modes, they cannot be expected to point to any definitive disclosure of a "best method"; but there seems to be an undercurrent in favor of manual methods.

Alerts were also sounded about various questionable aspects of multimodal communication. For example, Lloyd wants to know "just how one goes about combining the various modes for communication"; this, he remarks, is "not specified" (1975, p. 13). In the same connection, Reich and Bick (1976) report the problem of "mismatch" between fingerspelled items and the corresponding spoken items. A likely explanation for the mismatch is that "many teachers who are starting to use Total Communication . . .

are woefully inept'' (Moores, 1972, p. 8). So too, it may be assumed, are most hearing parents of deaf children, as well as dormitory counselors. It can be further assumed therefore that mismatch is not an uncommon occurrence in multimodal communications. The question arises: How does a deaf receiver of mismatched communication cope with the problem?

In addition, Beckmeyer cautions that although total communication serves the needs of some hearing-impaired persons, ''It would be well to consider the possibility that it may actually be reducing communication efficiency for others'' (1976, p. 572). As Drumm explains, ''People not fluent in the silent deaf language are distracted by gestures interfering with perception of speech, and speech efforts distract deaf signers'' (1972, p. 565). Individual differences must be taken into account. Alexander reviews other cautions that should be exercised and notes particularly that ''when some of these [total communication] programs are laid bare, and the 'label' is not there, it is certain one would be hard pressed to 'label' the program 'total communication' '' (1978, p. 21). Alexander stresses that such mislabeling not only defeats the purpose of total communication but also threatens the validity of research.

Ling points to the dangers of sensory overload through total communication:

> ''total communication'' has still never been defined as a simultaneous or successive thing or both; I've been told what is used, but I've not been told or shown adequately how it's used. It appears though that it's a simultaneous sort of thing where information in numerous modalities is thrown at a child all at the same time. We have to figure that a whole lot of children are not going to be able to process such information because of sensory overload. I myself have done an experiment using fingerspelling, lipreading, and the two combined; and the scores for the two combined are not superior to the scores for straight fingerspelling alone. (1972, p. 560)

Could it be that despite multimodal input, the deaf receiver gains information mainly from one preferred mode while more or less blocking out the others?

A member of the Oral Deaf Adults Section of the Alexander Graham Bell Association for the Deaf calls attention to the different brain paths taken by seen and heard communication:

> The spoken language is normally perceived by ear and the silent deaf language by eye. They are also quite different in their values of sound and sight and their sum-total pattern-of-thought. Plus, we have the third language in there, lipreading (speechreading), a sight language which parallels spoken language, with constant translation to and from auditory and visual values and terms. . . .
> Language learning by eye utilizes different areas of the brain from those used

when an individual learns through auditory means and we are just beginning to explore the resulting differences in language-thought processes. (Drumm, 1972, pp. 565, 568)

Drumm also urges that research be conducted with orally successful deaf adults to find out how they managed to make the "hearing" grade:

> I say we've looked at this problem from the wrong end of the telescope—from the point of view of school children—not regarding the contributions adult deaf persons can make if located and called upon. I suspect that there are many more proficient speakers as deaf as I am, who've long ago slid into the hearing/speaking majority. I challenge you to find these deaf adults, who probably don't consider themselves deaf but "hard of hearing," and who would certainly resist being labeled "deaf," with its present connotation of incapability, by their peers and employers. (1972, p. 567)

Other problems stemming from the rapid and unsystematized spread of total communication, combined with the new sign systems, are noted in the following resolution submitted by the Resolutions Committee to the Conference of Executives of American Schools for the Deaf at its forty-eighth meeting:

> *RESOLUTION NO. 8*   (not approved)
> WHEREAS each program for the deaf utilizing manual communication as an instructional media appears to be developing within its sphere of influence the new manual signs to meet instructional needs; and
> WHEREAS, there appears to be little or no common ground for the development or creation of new manual signs to deal with the various linguistic features of communication; and
> WHEREAS, deaf students of a given geographic area may find it difficult to communicate accurately and decisively with those of another geographic area if the divergent trends of sign development continue; and
> WHEREAS those programs for the deaf utilizing total or manual communication find themselves actually teaching manual communications for the first time; and
> WHEREAS it would appear appropriate and beneficial to maintain an up-to-date inventory of new signs to be disseminated to all programs utilizing them; therefore
> BE IT THEREFORE RESOLVED that the Conference of Executives of American Schools for the Deaf go on record as supporting the interest of the Colorado School for the Deaf and Blind and the University of Colorado in their intent to submit a request to the U.S. Office of Education to call for a meeting of those individuals presently engaged in the development of systems and approaches to new manual signs, to the end that some common approach and methodology be utilized by all to the advantage of those individuals who rely totally or partially upon manual communication. (Peck, 1976, p. 278)

An important, albeit seemingly ignored, point of inquiry in multimodal communication is the question of the equivalence in meaning among statements with similar intent but expressed in different communicative modes. A very interesting series of studies on the subject was conducted by Anderson (1966, 1968) with nondeaf persons, using experimentally equated messages presented through pictorial, aural, and print media. Anderson found that "the results presented demonstrate that statements equated in content and complexity but presented in different media evoke *different* connotative meanings" (1966, p. 503; italics added). To my knowledge, this question of meaning-equivalence among different communicative modes has not yet been raised in connection with total communication. It should be.

A final point is Newman's (1973) observation of the resemblance between failures in the education of the deaf and failures in current bilingual education for non-English-speaking hearing children, which, as Herbert (1977) remarks, seems to be "missing the mark" (p. 8). Newman quotes the administrator of one bilingual program as attributing much of its failure to the simultaneous input of the children's first language, second language, and academic concepts. The result is a child "who ends up barely functioning in either language" (Newman, 1973, p. 12). This outcome is in line with Ruesch's psychiatric dictum, "One thing at a time," for children in the formative years. Applying this to language learning, Ruesch states: "when at the time of his mastery of the basic vocabulary a child is exposed to two languages . . . the impact may be serious enough to retard his language development" (1957, p. 64). Whether this observation has relevance to total communication's multimodal form of instruction remains to be explored. In regard to "first language," Newman expresses the conviction of "many" deaf people that "the failure in the education of the deaf can be traced to the failure to accept manual communication as the deaf people's first language and, on this basis, to designate educational programs for them" (1973, p. 12).

In the midst of all the inquiry and debate sparked by total communication is the unspoken plea of the deaf child. The late Frederick C. Schreiber, himself a deaf person, interprets the child's plea as follows:

I need more than anything to be able to understand you and to make you understand me. I need to be able to sit with you and ask you why? To ask you to help me explore the universe around me. To understand the do's and don'ts of everyday living. These are hard things to learn—don't make them any harder for me than they already are. Give me the freedom to ask and understand in the easiest way possible—if there is an easy way.

Talk to me, yes, but give me the help that I get from signs and finger spelling. Remember, I don't speak or lip read well. . . . Communication is my greatest need. Given adequate means of free and easy communication I can acquire language and possible speech as well. I will also acquire the things I need to know that are not formally taught in school and that will help me to grow up to be a well adjusted citizen, able to handle the demands of the world around me. (1969, p. 6).

Drumm, also a deaf person, places his emphasis differently:

most deaf persons, myself, your deaf child, who don't hear some supposedly essential speech sounds, can learn to *feel,* visualize, and project spoken language quite effectively as adults. This is especially true now that early training with hearing aids can stimulate auditory perception even with 100 db. deafness. . . . So what is it that we want? We want *more* of our deaf children to achieve success as adults in a predominantly hearing/speaking world. . . . This we can do for our children NOW, to prepare them for the reality of a long adulthood. Whether they later live in a minority world, or in the world of the majority, or both, is up to them—but let us at least give deaf children thorough training in the basic terms and nuances of the spoken language of the majority, so they will have a wider choice as adults. (1972, pp. 568–69)

Schreiber's child stresses the urgency of the need of all children, whether deaf or hearing, to know "here and now" in order to understand and assimilate the realities of the world in pace with maturational imperatives; Drumm's child, the need for training in the "basic terms and nuances of the spoken language" in preparation for a long period of adulthood in a hearing-speaking world, training that thus far has proved unsuccessful for the large majority of deaf adults.

Again, the question facing uninitiated parents charged with decision-making responsibilities is: Which is the right choice?

Curriculum: State of the Art

Although discussed here under Educational Issues, the status of the curriculum in the education of deaf children has actually aroused little active concern. To call it a "side-issue" would probably be nearer the mark. The reason lies not in the lesser importance of the curriculum, but rather in its overwhelming complexity. The task of designing a flow of studies that will build psychologically viable and culturally compatible human beings out of communicatively isolated small deaf children is herculean enough to intimidate the stoutest heart.

In the early days of deaf education, it seemed feasible to model curricula for deaf children along the 3-R lines then used with hearing children. The pioneers had to begin somewhere, and this seemed as good a place as any. However, in the course of time and social change, it became increasingly evident to the regular "hearing" schools that pupils raised on a 3-R diet were ill-prepared to cope with the wider alphabet of societal demands.

School administrators began to press for curricular reform. As Dyer (1966) relates, eventually the regular schools were swamped with more devices, strategies, and curricular materials than educational systems were prepared to absorb or evaluate. The reform watchword was for innovation and experimentation, learning through discovery, and a realistic emphasis on what a pupil needs to know, namely, "what kind of world he is living in, how his future in this world may be shaped, and how he can help shape it" (Panel on Educational Research and Development, 1964, p. 33).

Together with these reform moves, there appeared a growing awareness of the need for what Ellis (1972) calls "emotional education in the classroom," with a strong focus on the feelings that underlie interpersonal relations, on their meanings, their effects on the self and on others, and on their healthy management.

A common belief is that emotion is a kind of "natural" phenomenon, an entity apart from learning. But Hallowell, quoting Landis (Goodman, 1967), rejects this notion: "Emotional life is modified more rigorously in the growth and education of an individual than perhaps any other variety of human experience" (p. 178); this statement is supported by abundant psychological, psychiatric, and cross-cultural evidence. Thus, argue the reform educators, if emotional patterns are learned, then emotional insights can be taught; and a number of demonstration programs in affective education are now showing the way in regular school settings, beginning as early as the preschool years (Bessell, 1968; Ellis, 1972; Timmerman, 1970). A major purpose of such programs is to free cognitive functioning, as far as possible, from disruptions caused by adverse emotional interference.

At about the time that reform recommendations were sweeping through "hearing" education circles, there appeared the Babbidge Report on the education of deaf children (Education of the Deaf, 1965). Its first sentence read: "The American people have no reason to be satisfied with their limited success in educating deaf children and preparing them for full participation in our society" (p. xv). The statement came as no shock to educators of the deaf. They had long been dissatisfied with the state of their art and of the outcomes. In the discussion of responsible factors, the surprising omission in the Report was any mention of the outmoded design, inadequate content, and unsystematized application of curricula in most schools and classes for the deaf. Nor was any recommendation made for a panel of experts in curriculum design to study the problem, to deliberate on what must be imparted to deaf children both cognitively and affectively to bring them closer to the multiple realities of life.

However, curricular inadequacies in the education of deaf children had not gone unnoticed. As early as 1957, Streng sought to raise the level of field awareness concerning these inadequacies with a survey of 75 public and private residential schools; she found that in most schools the curriculum was just as subject-centered as it had been 100 years before, *"with the emotional and social aspects of the learner's development . . . minimized or neglected"* (1957, p. 294; italics added). A decade later, Behrens and Meidegeier noted the same pattern: "A realistic content curriculum is in itself a rare item in most schools for hearing-impaired children" (1968, p. 412); and Gough exhorted "the various groups that aspire to a better education for the deaf [that] the time was never more propitious for joining forces to forge new curricula, breaking the chains that have fettered the deaf too long" (1968, p. 459). Still more recently, Bowe reminded educators that "work on the question of what to teach, in curriculum and content, appears to be lagging behind that in communication methodologies" (1974, p. 11).

This lag has always hampered curricular reform in schools for the deaf. As Leitman (1968) remarks, forces are at work in the schools that "unintentionally limit the scope of educational experience of the deaf child." He explains: "The countless hours spent by the deaf child sitting in groups and drilling on language and speech skills tend to foster a kind of passivity in the child. The passivity runs counter to the need of a child to explore the world."

From the deaf pupil's point of view, however, there is little incentive to explore a world that is hemmed in by fixed routines, compartmentalized subjects, predigested information, unexpressed feelings, and incessant correction—the need to explore indeed exists, but not the appropriate environment. As Rosenstein states, "For curriculum, the design of environment becomes one of the most pressing tasks of the present. Here the design activity must focus on the creation of a personal space where an individual can seek the new ways of behaving that are necessary to his experience and thus find his relationship with the various aspects of the curriculum a meaningful one" (1971, p. 494). In the context of educational reform philosophy, a school's learning environment should represent a microcosm of societal reality; the curriculum should provide the ways and means for acquiring and assimilating the multiple aspects of that reality in order to fit comfortably and knowledgeably within its sociocultural frame.

The traditional criterion of a small deaf child's progress—the number of words he knows as compared with his hearing peer—has no place in current special-education thinking. The real test matches experience to experience, not word to word. How many of the *experiences* necessary for healthy development are provided a deaf child in pace with need, and how do these compare in range and variety with the cognitive and affective experiences that supply the developmental and maturational needs of hearing children? A deaf child's lack of words does not hamper learning through experience. Experiences have their own semantics; and, in fact, the concepts thus acquired are a deaf child's strongest motivation for learning the matching words and language. For deaf children, a curriculum based on experiential requirements is "better than any other, because it holds the greatest promise for providing the kinds of experiences consistent with what is known about learning and growth needs of children" (Streng, 1957, p. 295).

This criticism of the curricula to which deaf children are exposed does not mean that educators have been entirely passive about seeking educational reform. To counteract the ingrained priority of method over content, Simmons urges that "teachers first know *what* they want to teach, then *why* they want to teach it, before they begin to think of *how*" (1968, p. 463). One basic problem is a lack of consistency: the "what" to teach varies from school to school and from teacher to teacher, as do both the "why" and the "how." Reeves questions "whether any method can flourish in an adverse climate" (1977, p. 54); while Streng sums up in the statement, "The big issue is not really that of oralism versus manualism, but what is best for what child" (1967, p. 100).

Within their own classrooms, many creative teachers have successfully experimented with experiential learning and discovery techniques (Kopp, 1968). But again, there are wide gaps from school to school and even, as Rosenstein comments, a "wide gap between teachers in the same school" (1971, p. 495). Some teachers have ventured into the curricular area (Grammatico and Miller, 1974; Maxwell, 1979), but their efforts have not inspired a systematized total school approach.

By and large, innovation in schools for the deaf is represented mainly by educational technology (Symposium on Research and Utilization of Educational Media, 1969, 1974, 1978). The emphasis is still on the "how." Calvert amusingly predicts, "We will see increasing 'media complexity' with the teacher facing myriad of switches, dials, meters, knobs, and buttons as she operates overhead, opaque, movie, filmstrip, and slide projectors, and plays magnetic tape, records, and videotape" (1970, pp. 17–18). If the focus of all this hard- and soft-ware remains fixed on the "how" of teaching, the deaf child will not be much farther along the road to the experiential "what" and "why" of curricular enrichment.

In all fairness, curricular reform of the extensive type deemed necessary in the education of deaf children is a tremendous undertaking. It cannot be done in isolated bits and pieces: one class here, one group there; a new idea or fad foisted upon a reluctant teacher; a doctoral dissertation; a short-term grant project. Clues may indeed emerge from such approaches, but extensive change demands total immersion, total reorientation, and total involvement. And what school is in a position to lend itself to total reformation even if there were a promising curricular guide to follow, which there is not.

Furthermore, where will the funds come from to devise such radically different curricula and support the lengthy research needed for evaluation? Granted an expert panel of specialists, the minimum time required would be at least 10 years. But the usual funding patterns do not allow for anywhere near such lengthy time schedules. A possible solution comes from D. Allen's proposal (1971) for legislation to authorize individual schools to set aside a certain portion of their budgets for the support of experimental schools. As yet, the suggestion is in the dream stage.

In the meanwhile, most deaf children remain trapped in obsolete curricular philosophy, outmoded practices, or the curricular patchworks common to many integrated programs. A hearing child in the same position has the advantage of much informal, out-of-school input. But the deaf child is heavily dependent on school. Whereas a hearing child acquires considerable flexibility in thinking, feeling, and doing from the many challenges and confrontations of everyday encounters, the deaf child's "informal" learning is sharply limited. A paramount limitation is in opportunities for independent thinking and for developing mental initiatives and controls.

This thinking-limitation was noted and deplored as long ago as 1896 by Putnam in his complaint that deaf children are not trained to think. "The child's brain is treated as a receptacle of facts, rules, etc. The pupil religiously fills it daily, and almost as rapidly unloads it" (1896, p. 268). Putnam's thoughts are echoed in the present by Kopp: "No student should be permitted to operate only as a follower of directions or as a passive recipient of facts. . . . To be skilled at inducing the learner to think is the fundamental goal of the teacher" (1972, pp. 270, 272). One of the most passionate advocates of teaching deaf children to think is Hans Furth (1966), who brought thinking directly into the classroom by way of a workbook of Piagetian thinking games, in collaboration with Wachs (Furth and Wachs, 1974).

Possibly the least-recognized omission in curricula for deaf children is emotional education. As noted, Streng long ago pointed out that the emotional aspects of a deaf pupil's development were neglected, and Blanton remarked on the singular deficiency of affective vocabulary in "deaf language" (Streng, 1957; Blanton, 1968). The seriousness of the implication seems to have escaped general field notice, with the outstanding exception of Joanne G. Schwartzberg, a physician and mother of a deaf child. Schwartzberg (1976) says:

> we want for our deaf children the same things that we want for our hearing children: to be able to understand, express and control their own feelings, to be able to understand the feelings and expressions of others, not only to tolerate but to be able to reach out and help others in need. We teach these things to our hearing children very casually through daily living experiences. As parents we are sometimes unaware that we *are* teaching. Our deaf children can share the same daily living experiences, but we, parents and teachers alike, must become

more conscious of how and what we teach so that our deaf children will be able to develop normally. . . . With pictures and pantomime and patience we can bridge the communication gap with the preverbal very young deaf child and make sure that he perceives and learns the patterns and values of human emotions as well as any hearing child his age. (p. 17)

That these recommendations can be successfully carried out through teaching procedures is demonstrated by Schwartzberg herself, combining the use of stick figures and faces with her own sensitive perceptions (1969).

The importance of emotional enculturation for deaf children cannot be overstressed. Emotions, as we are told by Freud and other eminent psychiatrists, are rooted in hearing. We do not expect deaf children to fend for themselves in the cognitive area; we dare not in the affective area. To do so would be to endanger healthy psychological development, unhampered cognitive functioning, and healthy adaptations to the feelings and values of the human community. As Schwartzberg points out, "Decreased understanding of an emotional stimulus may lead to both (a) decreased reactions and (b) inappropriate behavior" (1976, p. 15). It is more than likely to lead to emotional immaturity and to the excessive prevalence of emotional disturbance among deaf pupils as reported by Schlesinger and Meadow (1972).

In my opinion, a sound curriculum in tune with reality is the best mental health safeguard that can be offered deaf children by the schools, and would in all probability lead to a perceptible decrease in the later need for psychiatric services and mental health clinics.

Summary

Children are sent to school to acquire the knowledge, insights, and what Whitehead (1953) calls "the art of utilization of knowledge" for healthy participation in the networks of society. For a school to discharge this responsibility is no simple matter even under the best conditions. To carry it out with children who cannot hear is a highly complex task that has not yet been mastered. As summarized by Denton (1971), there are "crises" in methods of communication, in family involvement, teacher education, in curriculum, and in educational programs. The options and issues spawned by these crises have produced an educational environment for deaf children that is rent by sharp dissension, untested advocacies, and clashing practices. In the Babbidge committee's judgment, "the American people have no reason to be satisfied with their limited success in educating deaf children" (Education of the Deaf, 1965, p. xv).

Failure in educating the deaf is a composite of many failures. Not the least is the failure to relate the content of education to the bio-psychological "hungers" and needs that underlie normal development, to extrapolate the

kinds of cognitive and affective experiences that satisfy maturational imperatives, and to use them as framework for a consistent flow of curricular input
through all age levels.

Instead, the deaf child's developmental needs are parceled into methods
and subjects. The child cannot hear; he is supplied with hearing aids and auditory training. He cannot speak; the method is speech therapy. Speech is
too slow to meet communicative need; manual methods come to the rescue.
Scholastic competencies must be provided; the 3 Rs are called into service.
And so on through the school years. When the time comes for pupils to
leave school and "go out into the world," the method for many is represented by the well-trodden path to the rehabilitation counselor's office. It is
an unhappy commentary on the education of the deaf when habilitation must
be followed by rehabilitation.

The greatest methods fixation by far is on methods of communication. In
the flurry of debate, it has escaped the notice of advocates of all communicative persuasions that the term "method," no matter in what connection it is used, simply indicates a means to an end. It is not an end in itself.
In the habilitation of deaf children, methods of communication can be conceived as the utensils—the knife and fork—which the children are taught to
use as the *means* for getting at the substance of education. But given the
means, the children must also be provided with educational food, and this is
represented by the psycho-educational sustenance and sociocultural experiences of which they are deprived by reason of deafness. No matter how ef-
ficiently the knife and fork are used, if there is not enough of this food on
the plate, the result is psycho-educational malnutrition. If in addition to lack
of sufficient food, the utensils themselves are ineffective, the result is starva-
tion. And this tells much of the story underlying the poor showing of the
deaf pupil population. A scan of the state of the educational art indicates that
the utensils have generally proved less than adequate; the diets, monotonous;
the food sparse, limited in variety, poorly prepared, and even more poorly
served.

In protest against this methods fixation, J. K. Reeves, editor of the British
publication *The Teacher of the Deaf,* expresses his opinion that "the method
of communication to be used in the classroom is not a broad educational
matter but rather a peripheral affair which is of secondary or even tertiary
importance to major issues" (1977, p. 43). Among the "far more fundamental issues" mentioned by Reeves are: the provision of good teaching,
an adequate supply of good teachers, and improved training for teachers. To
these admittedly critical essentials, I would add a sound experientially based
curriculum and knowledgeable parent participation in the education process.

References

Alexander, K. R. 1978. Forgotten aspects of total communication. *American Annals of the Deaf*, 123: 18–30.

Allen, D. 1971. The seven deadly myths of education and how they mangle the young. *Psychology Today*, 4: 70–72.

Allen, J. C. 1977. A challenge to parents. *Volta Review*, 79: 297–302.

Anderson, J. A. 1966. Equivalence of meaning among statements presented through various media. *Communication Review*, 14: 499–505.

Anderson, J. A. 1968. More on the equivalence of statements presented in various media. *Communication Review*, 16: 25–32.

Babbidge Report, see *Education of the Deaf*, 1965.

Beckmeyer, T. 1976. Receptive abilities of hearing impaired students in a total communication setting. *American Annals of the Deaf*, 121: 569–72.

Behrens, T. R., and Meidegeier, R. W. 1968. Social studies in the education of deaf children. *Volta Review*, 70: 410–14.

Bender, R. E. 1960. *The Conquest of Deafness*. Cleveland: Press of Western Reserve University.

Bessell, H. 1968. The content is the medium: The confidence is the message. *Psychology Today*, January 1968 (reprint).

Blanton, R. I. 1968. Language learning and performance in the deaf. In S. Rosenberg and J. H. Kaplan, Eds., *Developments in Applied Linguistics*, pp. 121–76. New York: Macmillan.

Bourguin, L. A. 1871. *Manuel complet de la phonomimie*. Paris: Alphonse Picard.

Bowe, F. 1974. National trends in the education of deaf children. *Deaf American*, 26: 11–12.

Brill, R. G. 1969. The superior I.Q.'s of deaf children of deaf parents. *California Palms* (reprint).

Brill, R. G. 1975. Mainstreaming: Format or quality? *American Annals of the Deaf*, 120: 377–81.

Bruce, W. T. 1976. Trends in education. *Volta Review*, 78: 318–23.

Buscaglia, L. F., and Williams, E. H., Eds. 1979. *Human Advocacy and PL 94-142: The Educator's Roles*. Thorofare, N.J.: Charles B. Slack.

Caccamise, F., Ed. 1978. Sign language and simultaneous communication: Linguistic, psychological, and instructional ramifications. *American Annals of the Deaf*, 123: 798–877.

Caccamise, F., and Blasdell, R. 1977. Reception of sentences under oral-manual interpreted and simultaneous test conditions. *American Annals of the Deaf*, 122: 414–21.

Caccamise, F., and Blasdell, R., and Heath-Lang, B. 1977. Hearing-impaired persons' simultaneous reception of information under live and two visual motion media conditions. *American Annals of the Deaf*, 122: 339–43.

Calvert, D. R. 1970. The deaf child in the seventies. *Volta Review*, 72: 14–20.

Champ-Wilson, A. 1977. Parent advocacy: Being a part of the team. *PL 94-142 and Deaf Children*, Special Issue, *Gallaudet Alumni Newsletter*, p. 16.

Clark, G. M. 1975. Mainstreaming for the secondary educable mentally retarded: Is it defensible? *Focus on Exceptional Children*, 7: 2.

Conference of executives of American Schools for the Deaf. 1977. Statement on "least restrictive" placements for deaf students. *American Annals of the Deaf,* 122: 70–71.

Connor, L. 1976. New directions in infant programs for the deaf. *Volta Review,* 78: 8–15.

Cooney, P. 1977. A new deal for deaf children. *Iowans at Home,* Nov. 13, p. 1.

Council on Education of the Deaf. 1976. Resolution on individualized educational programming for the hearing impaired (deaf and hard-of-hearing). *Volta Review,* 78: 302 (news note).

Craig, H. B. 1965. A sociometric investigation of the self-concept of the deaf child. *American Annals of the Deaf,* 110: 456–74.

Craig, W. N., and Salem, J. M. 1975. Partial integration of deaf with hearing students: Residential school perspective. *American Annals of the Deaf,* 120: 28–36.

Craig, W. N., Salem, J. M., and Craig, H. B. 1976. Mainstreaming and partial integration of deaf with hearing students. *American Annals of the Deaf,* 121: 63–68.

Dale, D. 1974. *Language Development in Deaf and Partially Hearing Children.* Springfield, Ill.: Charles C. Thomas.

Danahy, R. 1970. A parent's challenge to educators and parents. *Volta Review,* 72: 153–55.

Denton, D. M. 1971. Educational crises. *Operation Tripod.* Northridge, Calif.: Department of Special and Rehabilitative Education, San Fernando Valley State College. Pp. 32–37.

Di Carlo, L. M. 1964. *The Deaf.* Englewood Cliffs, N.J.: Prentice-Hall.

Drumm, P. R. 1972. "Total Communication" *Volta Review,* 74: 564–69.

Dyer, H. S. 1966. The discovery and development of educational goals. Paper presented at the Educational Testing Service Invitational Conference on Testing Problems, New York City, October 29, 1966.

Education of the Deaf: A Report to the Secretary of Health, Education, and Welfare by His Advisory Committee on the Education of the Deaf. 1965. Washington, D.C.: U.S. Government Printing Office.

Ellis, A. 1972. Emotional education in the classroom: The living school. *Journal of Clinical Child Psychology,* 1 (Fall): 19–22.

Fay, E. A., Ed. 1875. Notice of publications. *American Annals of the Deaf,* 20: 116–20.

Fay, E. A., Ed. 1889. Methods of instruction in American schools. *American Annals of the Deaf,* 34: 64–69.

Fisher, B. 1971. Hearing impaired children in ordinary schools. *Teacher of the Deaf,* 69: 161–74.

Furth, H. G. 1966. *Thinking without Language.* New York: Free Press.

Furth, H. G., and Wachs, H. 1974. *Thinking Goes to School: Piaget's Theory in Practice.* New York: Oxford University Press.

Garretson, M. D. 1976. Total communication. In R. Frisina, Ed., *A Bicentennial Monograph on Hearing Impairment: Trends in the U.S.A.* Washington, D.C.: Alexander Graham Bell Association for the Deaf. Pp. 88–95.

Goodman, M. E. 1967. *The Individual and Culture.* Homewood, Ill.: Dorsey Press.

Gough, J. A. 1968. View from the foot of the hill. *Volta Review,* 70: 458–59.

Grammatico, L. F., and Miller, S. D. 1974. Curriculum for the preschool deaf child. *Volta Review,* 76: 280–89.

Greenberg, J., and Doolittle, G. 1977. Can schools speak the language of the deaf? *New York Times Magazine,* December 11, 1977, pp. 50ff.

Grisham, J. 1974. Parent organizations: Six important questions. In P. M. Culton, Ed., *Operation Tripod: Toward Rehabilitation Involvement by Parents of the Deaf.* Washington, D.C.: U.S. Government Printing Office. Pp. 54–58.

Hart, B. O., and Cory, P. B. 1968. The contribution of library resources to academic curriculum. *Volta Review,* 70: 460–64.

Herbert, W. 1977. Bilingual education missing the mark? *APA Monitor,* 8 (Sept./Oct.): 8.

Higgins, E. 1973. An analysis of the comprehensibility of three communication methods used with hearing impaired students. *American Annals of the Deaf,* 118: 46–49.

Hodgson, K. W. 1953. *The Deaf and Their Problems.* New York: Philosophical Library.

Holcomb, R. K. 1972. Three years of the total approach: 1968–1971. *Proceedings of the Forty-fifth Meeting of the Convention of American Instructors of the Deaf.* Washington, D.C.: U.S. Government Printing Office. Pp. 522–30.

Jensema, C. 1975. A deaf adult speaks out: A note on the educational achievement of ODAS members. *Volta Review,* 77: 135–37.

Jordan, I. K., Gustason, G., and Rosen, R. 1976. Current communication trends at programs for the deaf. *American Annals of the Deaf,* 121: 527–32.

Jordan, I. K., Gustason, G., and Rosen, R. 1979. An update on communication trends at programs for the deaf. *American Annals of the Deaf,* 124: 350–57.

Kennedy, P., Northcott, W., McGauley, R., and Williams, S. M. 1976. Longitudinal sociometric and cross-sectional data on mainstreaming hearing impaired children: implications for preschool programming. *Volta Review,* 78: 71–81.

Kidd, J. 1977. Parents and Public Law 94-142. *Volta Review,* 79: 275–80.

Klopping, H. W. E. 1972. Language understanding of deaf students under three auditory-visual stimulus conditions. *American Annals of the Deaf,* 117: 389–96.

Kopp, H. G., Ed. 1968. Curriculum: Cognition and content. *Volta Review,* 70: 372–516.

Kopp, H. G. 1972. Cognition and curriculum. In *Report of the Proceedings of the Forty-fifth Meeting of the Convention of American Instructors of the Deaf.* (1971 proceedings.) Washington, D.C.: U.S. Government Printing Office. Pp. 268–72.

Lane, H. S. 1976. The profoundly deaf: Has oral education succeeded? *Volta Review,* 78: 329–40.

Lane, H. S., and Baker, D. 1974. Reading achievement of the deaf: Another look. *Volta Review,* 76: 489–99.

Leitman, A. 1968. The workshop classroom. Paper presented at the Symposium on Research and Utilization of Educational Media in Teaching the Deaf, Lincoln, Nebraska, February 1968.

Levine, E. S. 1951. Psychoeducational study of children born deaf following maternal rubella in pregnancy. *A.M.A. American Journal of Diseases of Children*, 81: 1–9.

Levine, E. S. 1971. Mental assessment of the deaf child. *Volta Review*, 73: 80–96, 97–105.

Levine, E. S. 1974. Psychological tests and practices with the deaf: A survey of the state of the art. *Volta Review*, 76: 289–319.

Levine, E. S. 1976. Psychological contributions. In R. Frisina, Ed., *A Bicentennial Monograph on Hearing Impairment: Trends in the USA*. Washington, D.C.: Alexander Graham Bell Association for the Deaf. Pp. 23–33.

Levine, E. S. 1977. *The Preparation of Psychological Service Providers to the Deaf*. PRWAD Monograph No. 4. *Journal of Rehabilitation of the Deaf*.

Ling, D. 1972. Statements of panel of reactors on oralism/auralism and "total communication." *Volta Review*, 74: 552–63.

Ling, D., Ling, A. H., and Pflaster, G. 1977. Individualized educational programming for hearing-impaired children. *Volta Review*, 79: 204–30.

Linton, R. 1945. *The Cultural Background of Personality*. New York: Appleton-Century-Crofts.

Lloyd, G. T. 1975. Total communication: Some perspectives and potential problems. *Deaf American*, 27: 13–15.

Luterman, D. M. 1976. A comparison of language skills of hearing impaired children trained in a visual/oral method and an auditory/oral method. *American Annals of the Deaf*, 121: 388–93.

McConnell, F. E. 1968. The Bill Wilkerson hearing and speech center. In M. V. Jones, Ed., *Special Education Programs within the United States*. Springfield, Ill.: Charles C. Thomas. Pp. 224–37.

McGee, D. I. 1976. Mainstreaming problems and procedures: Ages 6–12. In G. Nix, Ed., *Mainstream Education for Hearing Impaired Children and Youth*. New York: Grune & Stratton.

Martin, R. 1979. *Educating Handicapped Children: The Legal Mandate*. Champaign, Ill.: Research Press Company.

Maxwell, M. M. 1979. A model for curriculum development at the middle and upper school levels in programs for the deaf. *American Annals of the Deaf*, 124: 425–32.

Meadow, K. P. 1968. Early manual communication in relation to the deaf child's intellectual, social, and communicative functioning. *American Annals of the Deaf*, 113: 29–41.

Meltzer, D. R. 1978. Mainstreaming: As the parent sees it. *Volta Review*, 80: 109–11.

Messerly, C. L., and Aram, D. M. 1980. Academic achievement of hearing-impaired students of hearing parents and of hearing-impaired parents: Another look. *Volta Review*, 82: 25–32.

Moores, D. F. 1972. Communication: Some unanswered questions and some unquestioned answers. In T. J. O'Rourke, Ed., *Psycholinguistics and Total Communication: The State of the Art*. Washington, D.C.: *American Annals of the Deaf*. Pp. 1–10.

Moores, D. F., Weiss, K. I., and Goodwin, M. W. 1973. Receptive abilities of deaf children across five modes of communication. *Journal of Exceptional Children, 1973,* 22–28.

Moses, C. 1977. Parent advocacy subcommittee. *PL 94-142 and Deaf Children,* Special Issue, Gallaudet Alumni Newsletter, p. 16.

Murphy, H. J., and Fleischer, L. R. 1977. The effects of ameslan versus siglish upon test scores. *Journal of Rehabilitation of the Deaf,* 11: 15–18.

Newman, L. 1973. Bilingual education. *Deaf American,* 25: 12–13.

Nix, G. 1975. Total communication: A review of the studies offered in its support. *Volta Review,* 77: 470–94.

Nix, G. W. 1976. *Mainstream Education for Hearing Impaired Children and Youth.* New York: Grune & Stratton.

Nix, G. W. 1977a. The least restrictive environment. *Volta Review,* 79: 287–96.

Nix, G., Ed. 1977b. The rights of hearing-impaired children. *Volta Review,* 79, Monograph 349.

Northcott, W., Ed. 1972. *Curriculum Guide: Hearing Impaired Children—Birth to Three Years and Their Parents.* Washington, D.C.: Alexander Graham Bell Association for the Deaf.

Northcott, W., Ed. 1973. *The Hearing Impaired Child in a Regular Classroom: Preschool, Elementary and Secondary Years.* Washington, D.C.: Alexander Graham Bell Association for the Deaf.

Nyquist, E. B. n.d. *Mainstreaming: Idea & actuality.* An Occasional Paper. Albany, N.Y.: University of the State of New York, The State Education Department.

Owrid, H. L. 1971. Studies in manual communication with hearing impaired children. *Volta Review,* 73: 428–38.

Panel on Educational Research and Development: A Progress Report. 1924. Washington, D.C.: U.S. Government Printing Office.

Paul, J. L., Turnbull, A. P., Cruickshank, W. M. 1979. *Mainstreaming: A Practical Guide.* New York: Schocken Books.

Peck, B. J., Chairman. 1976. Report of the Resolutions Committee. *Proceedings of the Forty-eighth Meeting of the Conference of Executives of American Schools for the Deaf.* Rochester, N.Y.

Peckham, C. S., Sheridan, M., and Butler, N.Y. 1972. School attainment of seven-year-old children with hearing difficulties. *Developmental Medicine and Child Neurology,* 14: 592–602.

PL 94-142 and Deaf Children. 1977. Special Issue, Gallaudet Alumni Newsletter.

Putnam, G. H. 1896. How to study. *American Annals of the Deaf,* 41: 265–74.

Quigley, S. P. 1969. *The Influence of Fingerspelling on the Development of Language, Communication, and Educational Achievement in Deaf Children.* University of Illinois, Institute for Research on Exceptional Children.

Reeves, J. K. 1977. Scope for oralism. *Volta Review,* 79: 43–54.

Reich, C., Hambleton, D., and Houldin, B. K. 1977. The integration of hearing impaired children in regular classrooms. *American Annals of the Deaf,* 122: 534–43.

Reich, P. A., and Bick, M. 1976. An empirical investigation of some claims made in support of visible English. *American Annals of the Deaf,* 121: 573–77.

Rister, A. 1975. Deaf children in mainstream education. *Volta Review*, 77: 279–290.

Rosenstein, J. 1971. Curriculum and cognition. *Volta Review*, 73: 481–96.

Ross, M. 1978. Mainstreaming: Some social considerations. *Volta Review*, 80: 21–30.

Ruesch, J. 1957. *Disturbed Communication*. New York: W. W. Norton & Company.

Schlesinger, H. S., and Meadow, K. P. 1972. *Sound and Sign*. Berkeley, Calif.: University of California Press.

Schreiber, F. 1969. Feature of the Month: The deaf adult's point of view. Paper presented at the Teacher Institute, Maryland School for the Deaf, Frederick, Maryland. Pp. 5–8.

Schunhoff, H. F. 1957. *The Teaching of Speech and by Speech in Public Residential Schools for the Deaf in the United States, 1815–1955*. Romney, W.V.: West Virginia Schools for the Deaf.

Schwartzberg, J. 1969. A young deaf child learns emotional concepts from stick figures and faces. *Volta Review*, 71: 228–32.

Schwartzberg, J. 1976. Affective education: Ways to help a deaf child learn about his own emotions. *Hearing Rehabilitation Quarterly*, 2(Fall): 15–17.

Shears, L. N., and Jensema, C. J. 1969. Social acceptability of anomalous persons. *Exceptional Children*, 36: 91–96.

Simmons, A. A. 1968. Content subjects through language. *Volta Review*, 70: 481–86.

Smith, J. M. 1974. The Editor's Page. Mainstreaming. *Deaf American*, October, p. 2.

Stevenson, E. A. 1965. A study of the educational achievement of deaf children of deaf parents, Berkeley: California School for the Deaf, 1964. *Maryland Bulletin*, February.

Streng, A. 1957. Curriculum in schools for the deaf. *Volta Review*, 59: 291–96.

Streng, A. 1967. The swing of the pendulum: A critique of the education of the deaf. *Volta Review*, 69: 94–101.

Stuckless, E. R., and Birch, J. W. 1966. The influence of early manual communication on the linguistic development of deaf children. *American Annals of the Deaf*, 111: 452–460, 499–504.

Symposium on Research and Utilization of Educational Media for Teaching the Deaf. 1969, 1974, 1978. *American Annals of the Deaf*, 114: 814–937; 119: 452–656; 123: 624–774.

Timmermann, W. 1970. Communicating feeling: A how-to-do-it program for teachers. *UCLA Educator*, 12: 12–13.

Tracy, Mrs. Spencer. 1968. John Tracy Clinic. In M. V. Jones, Ed., *Special Education Programs within the United States*. Springfield, Ill.: Charles C. Thomas. Pp. 155–78.

Twyman, L. H., and Ouellette, S. E. 1978. Career development programs in residential schools for the deaf: A survey. *American Annals of the Deaf*, 123: 10–17.

U.S., Congress. 1975. Education of All Handicapped Children Act of 1975. Public Law 94-142. November 27, 1975.

Van den Horst, A. P. J. M. 1971. Defective hearing, school achievements, and school choice. *Teacher of the Deaf,* 69 (Nov.): 398–414.

Van Engen, J. 1977. In the real meaning of "least restrictive environment" (Melda E. Alber). *Rushmore Beacon,* October, p. 3.

Vernon, M. 1968. The failure of the education of the deaf. *Illinois Advance,* 101: 1–4.

Vernon, M., and Koh, S. D. 1970. Early manual communication and deaf children's achievement. *American Annals of the Deaf,* 115: 527–36.

Vernon, M., and Koh, S. D. 1971. Effects of oral preschool compared to early manual communication on education and communication in deaf children. *American Annals of the Deaf,* 116: 569–74.

White, A. H., Jr., and Stevenson, V. M. 1975. The effects of total communication, manual communication, oral communication and reading on the learning of factual information in residential deaf children. *American Annals of the Deaf,* 120: 48–57.

Whitehead, A. N. 1953. *The Aims of Education and Other Essays.* New York: New American Library, Mentor Book.

Williams, P. 1970. The fears we face. *Volta Review,* 72: 303–9.

Part Three
PRODUCTS OF THE "SOUNDLESS WORLD"

6 Sketches from Life

WE TURN now from the fashioning environments of deaf persons to the "products of environment," from influences to outcomes. We recall that environmental psychologists and culture-pattern theorists tend to view the human "products" as genetically conditioned microcosms of the influencing environment, whose behavior is programmed in accordance with the overall design of culture-input. Chapters 6 and 7 examine the postulate from two perspectives. In this chapter, the behavior of deaf persons is scanned from real life samplings. The focus is on the population at large and its exceptional heterogeneity as illustrated by selected rehabilitation clients; on aspects of community living and life-styles; and on deaf leadership. Chapter 7 focuses on the "products" as seen from the perspectives of personality research and theory.

Population Heterogeneity

We begin with an overview of the deaf population. A common misconception about prelinguistic deafness is that it reduces all its victims to one common personality denominator. This is not the case; far from it. Apart from innate variables, the range of differences in educational experiences and communicative exposures could alone be expected to produce exceptional variations among the deaf. The expectation is borne out in life.

For example: there are deaf persons who can speak and read the lips with exceptional proficiency; others who can speak but are only indifferent lip-readers; still others who can read the lips fairly well but whose speech is barely comprehensible; and some deaf persons can do neither. There are deaf individuals who are masters of all forms of communication and can move as easily in deaf as in hearing society; and at the other extreme, there are some who have never acquired any conventional mode of communication and must convey messages through pantomime and home-made signs and gestures. Then, there are deaf persons whose education has been more or less appropriate to their needs and others whom education has badly failed. There are those whose oral skills are inferior but whose language abilities are exceptional, and conversely there are others with excellent oral expression but with limited language resources.

To continue: there are deaf persons whose school-life contacts with their families have been restricted to weekend and holiday visits, and others who have lived with their families throughout their school years, sometimes for better and sometimes for worse. Some deaf persons have no contact whatsoever with other deaf individuals because of family prohibition, lack of opportunity, or personal preference; and others live a full rich life with both deaf and hearing friends. There are deaf persons who cannot communicate freely with members of their hearing families for lack of a mutually understood method, and others who cannot communicate with certain of their own deaf peers for the same reason. Finally there are the emotionally adjusted and the emotionally disturbed; the mature and the incredibly immature; those of high mental endowment and those with limited capacity. There are the sick and the well. There are the multihandicapped. And between the extremes are countless variations and combinations of ability, achievement, and adjustment.

It is truly said the deaf population makes up in heterogeneity what it lacks in size.

Principal Groupings

To reduce this complex heterogeneity to manageable proportions is a practical necessity in many phases of work with the deaf. The sketches that follow provide a rough classification of the principal groups that make up the deaf population.

Exceptional. The exceptional group includes deaf persons of high mental capacity, superior functioning intelligence, exceptional achievement, and superior linguistic abilities. Their speech may or may not be intelligible, but the best oral communication is to be found in this group. So too is the finest manual communication. Members of the group are not necessarily good lipreaders. Those who are not manage through excellent written communication as required. Many are graduates of colleges for the deaf or of regular colleges and universities, and form the backbone of the deaf professional community (Crammatte, 1968). A goodly number owe their educational foundations to special schools for the deaf; others have succeeded in regular schools. Among the members of the group are deaf persons who can move as easily in hearing as in deaf society. The group also includes unknown numbers of deaf persons who live entirely in the hearing world and do not associate with any deaf groups or persons.

Above Average. Above average deaf persons have good and sometimes superior functioning and innate intelligence but less than matching linguistic and scholastic achievements. Verbal language level as measured by reading achievement is generally at about 6th to 9th grade, and written language reflects these grades. There are some in the group with college ambitions, but they are unable to meet college admissions standards. Nevertheless, many deaf leaders come from the group, and many group members own their own homes and businesses or hold responsible positions. They may or may not have intelligible speech or good lipreading ability, but they manage through good written communication when need dictates. Ameslish is the favored method for intragroup communication.

Average. The average group encompasses the deaf-at-large. The chief handicaps are scholastic retardations, linguistic deficiencies, and related conceptual gaps and limitations. Nevertheless, innate mental endowment is average and not infrequently better than average. The bulk of the group represents education's failures. There are deficits in all forms of verbal expression and reception, with reading levels at about 4th grade and sometimes less. Ameslan is the favored communicative mode. Communication with hearing society is severely handicapped. Yet despite the handicaps, most of these persons acquire a variety of vocational skills in which they equal or surpass their hearing peers. They live a good life, raise fine families, and form the backbone of the deaf community at large.

Below Average. Persons in this category function at drastically retarded levels scholastically, conceptually, and in social knowledge and awareness. The causes vary. Some are education's most extreme failures. In others, retardation may be due to innate mental limitation, an exceptionally late school start or no schooling at all, brain damage, or serious chronic psychopathology. Whatever the cause, they cannot catch up. Reading level is generally at 2nd grade or even less, sometimes despite years of schooling. They are also deficient signers. Those who make good vocational adjustments are found in the unskilled occupational category.

Marginal. The marginal deaf have not been able to reach the communicative and adjustment levels of even the below-average group. Most are completely illiterate even though they may have attended school for a time. Many are unschooled or practically so and have no ability to read, write, sign, or communicate in other than pantomime, self-devised gestures, or debased signs. Some are multihandicapped. Yet interestingly enough, numbers of these impoverished beings are animated persons with strong communicative drives and a lively interest in the passing scene. But they cannot break through. Some respond well to rehabilitative efforts.

It is important to bear in mind that the preceding groupings are not based on innate mental potential, but rather on *functioning* intelligence—the intelligence that ''shows'' in life performance and achievements. This is not always consonant with innate endowment. For example, a number of persons in the below-average and even in the marginal categories are of average innate endowment and sometimes even better, and there are persons in the average categories who are of superior mental potential. But the weight of adverse life and educational circumstances depresses the development and expression of original potential. Hence the lowered intellectual functioning. Environmental psychology would point to these persons as evidence that the individual is more a product of environmental influences than of innate endowment, and so it appears to be.

Deaf Clients: The Counselor's Dilemma

For closer acquaintance with some of the people who compose the preceding groupings, let us pay a visit to the office of a vocational rehabilitation counselor. Here we see not only representative deaf persons coming for assistance of one kind or another, but also the dilemmas of a counselor serving his first deaf clients. The following sketches are drawn from life.

John

John S. arrives at the counselor's office for help. He is a nice-looking, congenitally deaf young man of 24, neatly dressed, with a pleasant, alert air about him. The records show that he graduated from a school for the deaf a few years ago, and that he decided to continue his education at Gallaudet College for the deaf. Actually, his decision reflected more the wishes of his hearing family, in which he was the only child, than any burning ambition of his own. He was never an outstanding student, and just managed to get by. Nevertheless, he insisted on taking the college entrance examinations. He failed. Now he wants a job.

John has already had some work experience, thanks to concerned relatives who "took him into the business." But even with their indulgence, he couldn't make the grade. He has had no job training or occupational orientation, and the records hint that he did not get along well with his hearing co-workers.

The counselor to whom John turns for help has had only hearsay knowledge of deaf clients. John, in fact, is his first one. The counselor has heard from his colleagues something of their difficulties with the deaf; but he has also read that the general principles of job placement for the disabled are similar to the placement principles for the nondisabled. He is therefore not overly concerned about his ability to handle the case.

The counselor proceeds according to accepted practice. In order to find the right job for John, he must know (a) the job applicant, namely John; (b) the job requirements; and (c) how well the one will fit the other. To know John involves knowing his mental ability, personality, scholastic attainments, emotional stability, vocational training and job experiences, special skills and aptitudes, and the selective factors that severe deafness may introduce into the picture. To know the job involves knowing the skills and abilities the work requires, the attributes needed by the worker, the physical requirements necessary for job performance, and the special environmental factors associated with the job that may have an adverse effect on a deaf worker. When all this information is eventually assembled, the counselor will be prepared to match job to client.

John's counselor begins the task of getting to know John. The first step is the interview; the first goal, winning the client's trust and confidence. Toward this end, the counselor tries to create a relaxed interview situation in which he will listen to what the client has to say in a calm, composed way and in a completely nonpunitive frame in which the client feels safe to explore plans and problems. He encourages John to tell his own story in his own words as if to a friend.

John proceeds to do so. But as he talks, the counselor finds to his great embarrassment that he understands very little of what his client is saying. John's speech happens to be mediocre deaf speech, and the counselor's ear is not attuned to any deaf speech, even good speech. To ease the situation, the counselor nods and smiles as John talks pretending to understand. He even throws in a question now and again. Embarrassment approaches consternation when he realizes that not only does he not understand John, but obviously neither does John understand him. It so happens that John is an indifferent lipreader, over and above which the counselor's language is beyond him.

To overcome this inauspicious beginning, the counselor turns from oral to written communication. He remembers having heard other counselors say that this was how they handled similar situations. And sure enough, things seem to improve. Short written communications that involve brief answers present no great difficulty. Then, hoping to use this communicative approach to learn more about the client, the counselor asks John to write about himself. This is what he receives in answer:

> Their mother and father wanted their deaf children to go to school. Because they get more education when they finish their school. Some of them can find a job for their life. Some of them can go to Galluet College. If they can passed, then they can go there. They wanted get more education. They get their lesson and study every night. When they finish their College. Their mother and father were proud of their children.
> Many people in different states and countries choose them to go to their job. They were happy that they can find job. (Excerpted from Fusfeld, 1955, p. 71.)

The counselor's bewilderment on reading this communication is entirely understandable. One counselor has said of his first experience with a deaf client:

> I am sure on my first encounter with a deaf person, I was cured of ever using the term "deaf and dumb," so great was *my* sense of inadequacy. I remember resorting to the use of paper and pencil when I discovered my client did not read the lips. Somehow I started the interview. My client, however, wrote without logical sequence and with a shorthand type of communication. Fortunately, I remembered reading of such cases, and began to compare the sentences, ultimately making some sense of the "hodge-podge." We communicated, but the eliciting of information, evaluation of the client, assessing his abilities, capacities, training and general alertness became prolonged and difficult. (Personal communication)

To return to John's counselor: After bypassing the oral barrier by substituting written for oral communication, the counselor now finds himself facing this new barrier of "hodge-podge" language. What does this kind of language betoken? Is this an outcome of deafness or could there be other responsible factors present? If so, what could they be? Brain damage? Mental retardation? Aphasia?

To add to the counselor's dilemma, he notices that John has responded to various noises during the course of the interview. This seems a surprising phenomenon. Evidently John can hear even though he wears no hearing aid. What does this mean? Could it be that John is not as deaf as has been supposed? Or that his hearing has improved since the last hearing test, or that he is psychogenically deaf? And if John can hear, why can't he understand what is said to him?

As the questions crowd in on the counselor's thoughts, so does the unusual challenge of the mystery that John presents. But there is work to be done, a job of counseling to carry out. John is referred for psychological evaluation in the hope of clearing up some of the questions. At the same time, the counselor takes steps to prepare himself for the next deaf client. He starts reading the literature concerning deaf persons, and arranges to be tutored in manual communication.

Norma

A few months later, another deaf client arrives at the counselor's office. The counselor feels himself better prepared for this one. He is now able to use some manual communication and looks forward to the interview with anticipation, albeit mixed with some anxiety.

Norma B. now enters the office. She is a lovely young woman of 20. Like

John, she wants to continue her education at Gallaudet College, having recently graduated with honors from a school for the deaf. And, like John, she is congenitally deaf with no deaf relatives and no siblings.

The counselor proceeds to break the ice by meticulously signing, "Hello. I am happy to meet you. My name is Mr. X. What is your name?" He is proud of himself for having signed so well. He smiles. Norma returns his warm greeting with a cold stare. She speaks, informing him, "I do not understand signs and I do not use signs. I am an oralist. I use only speech." Counselor X is dismayed. He feels he has committed a faux pas and, judging by Norma's expression, a serious one. Despite his earnest preparation for a deaf client, he was not prepared for this. The interview takes an oral turn.

Fortunately, the interview goes well. Norma soon gets over her initial annoyance and "converses as if with a friend." Her speech is easier to understand than John's, and her language is impeccable. Her needs are for some financial assistance to see her through college and for educational advice. In the course of the interview, Norma's special interests and hobbies come into the frame of inquiry. She confides that her chief "hobby" is writing poetry. She is persuaded to give a sample. She writes:

I am deaf
  That is true,
And yet I can hear.

I can hear with my eyes
  And with my eyes I can hear
Music, Sound, Harmony.

See that yonder robin soaring
  It is music in motion.
Look over there, children playing at tag,
  That is sound at play
Read this poem by Shelley,
  That is harmony to my eyes.

With all the sounds I can hear
  With my eyes
How can I be deaf?

The beauty of the lines and the poignancy of the theme are a moving experience for the counselor. He is deeply touched. He is also deeply bewildered. Comparing the beauty of these lines with the "hodge-podge" writing of his previous deaf client multiplies the questions and increases his dilemma. What now, he wonders, and what next?

Roberto

Next comes Roberto B. Also congenitally deaf and, like John and Norma, the only deaf member of his family, Roberto comes from a foreign-language home. However, he was born in this country and attended school for the deaf since early childhood. He is now seventeen and has completed "schooling." He comes to the counselor for vocational guidance. He needs to be prepared for the world of work.

The counselor has carefully reviewed the background summary which, fortunately, arrived before Roberto did, and from the highly unsatisfactory nature of the report he assumes that it is safe to use signs for this interview. As Roberto enters the office, the counselor again breaks the ice with his careful little sign-introduction: "Hello. I am happy to meet you. My name is Mr. X. What is your name?" Roberto's response is a pleasant smile. The counselor repeats his speech. Roberto continues to smile, adding a nod or two. He obviously does not understand the counselor's signs.

Remembering Norma, the counselor tries the oral approach, both in English and in Roberto's home language. Roberto looks distressed, pantomiming that he can neither hear nor read the lips. The counselor resorts to writing. Roberto's distress increases. At this point, the counselor resorts to intuition and reduces his introduction to two signs: "Name, you." Roberto's face lights up. He utters something imcomprehensible. He is provided with a pencil and paper and told in panto-signs, "Write name." In large childish script and with much pleasure, Roberto complies.

Having finally gotten this far in the interview, the counselor now has to figure out how to proceed. At his wit's end, he pantomimes to Roberto to write more. Roberto happily does so, and painstakingly produces the following:

Dear:
I am sorry "you "wrong" "why!.
the to Read learned before long.
"please", ask I sings conversation
two with that office for.
He is writing on paper   A B C D
A, B, C, D alphabet worng good   ′ ′ ′ ′
or Bad Both Low.   ′ ′ ′ ′
I patient Learn can't me think.   ′ ′ ′ ′
it is a paper alphabet A. B, C, D,   ′ ′ ′ ′
gone *pictures* Book not think. I
meeting you conversation as "o.k."
                    Thank
                    Roberto

Roberto looks up from his writing with pleading eyes. Buried somewhere in the linguistic jumble is a wish that he prays will be granted. He pins his hopes on the counselor. The counselor, reading the message, now realizes that John's language was not nearly the hodge-podge he first thought. Roberto's language is the real thing. At this point, the counselor feels that he needs help as desperately as does his client.

Eventually, the skills of an interpreter are brought to bear on the problem. Communication is carried out in a mixture of pantomime and debased, colloquial signs, which are the only ones Roberto knows. It turns out that Roberto's perceptions of his needs are considerably sharper than his communicative skills would lead one to believe. Roberto wants interpersonal relations, and for this he needs to know "conversation," specifically conversation in the sign language ("sings"). Books are not useful for the purpose. They are only "paper alphabet." He learned this alphabet long ago, and still does not know conversation or how to think. He begs to be taught to sign.

What Roberto's future holds when he does learn to sign is an open question for the counselor. But tutoring in manual communication is at least a good starting point. So Roberto's wish is granted.

Susan

Susan R. is our counselor's next client. She comes to his office with a diploma from a vocational high school and a psychiatrist's diagnosis of "unresponsive, semiliterate, mentally retarded." This paradoxical combination is not uncommon for young deaf people exposed to specialists unfamiliar with deafness and its implications. Here, for example, is Susan. Even though she accomplished the feat of graduating from a regular high school, she is pronounced "mentally retarded" by a specialist who neither had the wit nor would take the time to see beyond the confines of his professional rut.

Like our counselor's previous clients, Susan is also congenitally deaf, the only deaf member of a family that includes two hearing siblings. A graduate of a school for the deaf as well as of a "hearing" vocational high school, Susan, aged 23, was employed as a garment machine operator, and later as an office worker. After the loss of her last job through no fault of her own, she became moody and irritable. Psychiatric help was sought; the diagnosis of mental retardation was the outcome. The indignant family decided to send Susan to the local Office of Vocational Rehabilitation for help. She agreed to go, but this time prepared herself for the interview with a written account of her experiences. She submitted the following:

MY LIFE

I was a really deaf in all my life and how came from birth. When I was six years old, my mother did not know where school for the deaf is. Then she saw a deaf woman, our former neighbor, who lived in next apartment. She came to meet her and asked her where deaf school is. She taught her, but she did not understand what she say when she spoke her. She did not know how to use the deaf people. They were both writing notes to tell her everything about deaf schools. There are many deaf schools in New York City. My mother would not want me to attend X school. She wanted me to come home from school every days. I attend Y school. I stayed school for 12 years until graduation. At three years later when I was in 2nd grade I read the blackboard by my eyes were tears and burn that I cannot see, when I read it. My mother came to school for parent's meeting. A teacher told her all about my eyes. She bought me a new glasses. I wored it and it felt much better to see, no hurt my eyes. It had many kinds of academic subject, that I studied was a good in report card. Then grew up, when I was in 7th grade, my class and I went to vocational dept for one and helf hour at sewing room. We had to learn how to sewing. I liked sewing very much. It was interesting to me. I planned to go to high school for needle trade after graduated. I learned more and more sew and sewing machine in three times in 7th and 9th grades. Then I graduated. I received a diploma of studies courses and won a prize of General Improvement.

I came to Vocational High School to learn trade for jobs as soon as I graduated. I was in third term, I understood the working, but I watched a teacher's lips that I did not understand and misunderstood. Every morning I went to trade room to sewing and sewing. When my mother came to school for meeting and she met the teachers. I was good reports in 3rd, 4th, and 5th terms, but I was in 6th term, it was too hard for me to study chemistry. It was failing in first and mid-term report and in final report was pass. A teacher from Y school came to Z school to help deaf girls. If the girls were in trouble with working, she helped us. I went to operating room to learn how to work operating. A operating teacher was a nice, but she was least not much to help and show me the working. She talked and talked too much to hearing girls about operating machines. I made three smocks for third termers girls. When I finished the working I called the girl to show me working on the machine. At final time before promoting to next term, I did not finish another smock. After promoting to 7th term in another trade of dressmaking, I left back to 6th term trade in the morning. I was really in 7th term in the afternoon. I dropped from academic subjects to trade for all day, because it was too hard for me to understand what the teachers say and teach in the working. At 8th term, I worked a trade of dressmaking all day and then I graduated.

I had a job with operating of skirts, and helped me by school guidence. I worked there for four weeks and later I was layed off and left it. I had much trouble with operating. The thread was broken all the time. Some of the dark color threads that I cannot see it. I had another job of operating. I was in trouble again and the same liked the last time. I left. It was too hard for me. My mother and I went to have an interview about my jobs, and they helped me to find a nice job in an office. I liked it very much. I liked the people, good friendly, to me. I was filing clerk. I undrstood the working well and good skillful mind. I was happy. Then the place where I worker was moving away. They said no more working anymore. I lost it. I rather decided to work on operating machine again.

My home life is good and my parents are both kind to me.

Such is the story of Susan's "MY LIFE." Its course of events is not uncommon among deaf youth. The struggle to get into the mainstream of living and the frustrations encountered along the way are hard to take. Susan retreated for a while to give her bruised ego a chance to recover. Her counselor's wise understanding and gentle help bring her to life again to continue the struggles; but this time she has "guidence" on her side, and this means half the battle won.

To sum up: the few clients sketched here show something of the extraordinary range of extremes in the deaf population, with Norma at the upper end, Roberto at the lower end, and John and Susan representing the average–above-average in between. Despite the sharp differences among these persons, all are united by an underlying tie—the fortitude it takes to be deaf and yet survive. A deafened member of the American Professional Society of the Deaf expresses it this way:

> The self-discipline—patience to recover, patience to learn sign language, patience to lipread, courage to overcome self-doubt, courage to overcome put-down after put-down, courage to continue despite prediction of failure, courage to attempt the unknown—together with the incentive required to compete with the physically-able peers are all exploitable characteristics which should be looked upon favorably by anyone seeking high quality performance. The handicapped minority is the quiet minority; perhaps what it needs is a very loud spokesman to change the attitude of "normal" society. (Keller, 1978, p. 4)

Robert G. Sanderson, a distinguished deaf leader, calls deaf adults who have successfully survived their confrontations with the world "the Gallants." He says:

> To me it is something of a miracle that a few have survived this constant assault on their self-images for so long, and have risen above the rank and file. They are the Gallants in the finest sense of the word. Yet it is also true that far too many deserving and talented young deaf people have not developed self-images strong enough to withstand the test of competition, of adversity and defeat, and I am led to wonder whether our school administrators are conscious of the vital need of young students for ego support. It would seem that in some cases the self-image is being unwittingly *destroyed* rather than built up. (Sanderson, 1969, p. 13)

Sanderson's observations can be construed as a reflection of the splintered-education theme previously reviewed, in particular the lack of sensitivity to

the critical need of deaf pupils for what has been called "emotional education in the classroom," including what Sanderson terms "ego support."

Community Living

A question of compelling interest concerns the nature of the communities
that are formed from such diverse members as characterize the deaf population. Numbers of studies and workshops have been conducted to get a closer
look at such communities (Community Organization with the Deaf, 1967;
Community Responsibilities, 1964; Crammate and Schreiber, 1961; Furfey
and Harte, 1968; Lloyd, 1972; Schein, 1964; Schein and Delk, 1974). The
findings supply interesting data, discussion and valuable demographic details. What seldom emerge are pictures of the actual life-styles of deaf population clusters, or of the cohesive forces that fuse the clusters into communities. The discussion that follows is an attempt to impart some "real life" to
the demographic statistics.

Community Communication-Links

The ability to hear the acoustic signals that regulate the routines of everyday living is a major link in maintaining normal community cohesion. If the
signals were suddenly to go dead, the result in hearing communities could
be bedlam. A homely example: there would be no alarm-clock assault to
rouse the sleeping wage-earner; there would be no telephone ring from an
irate boss demanding to know where he is; no doorbell ring from a concerned co-worker; and no telephone ring back to the irate boss to let him
know the sleeper is finally on the way. The result of such mutings on a
grand scale would be pandemonium. Yet the hearing simply take such signals for granted.

Deaf persons have managed to survive the absence of everyday acoustic
signals in a variety of ingenious ways. One of the earliest and still most
common is to substitute light signals for acoustic ones. More recently, varieties of sophisticated systems and devices have been pressed into service to
enrich community living and enable deaf persons to maintain closer community ties (Gendel, 1974).

Household Devices. Numerous relatively simple devices are used by deaf
persons to help carry out the routines of everyday living and safeguard the
household. These include wake-up signals that serve alarm-clock functions
and signaling devices for such sounds as baby cries, doorbell, and telephone; there are also prowler alerts. Visual and/or vibratory signals are used
in these devices as substitutes for acoustic signals. In the alarm-clock, for
example, a time-activated flasher device switches a bedside lamp on and off
about 80 times a minute. This works well for light-sensitive sleepers. For

those who are not, there are time-activated vibrating mechanisms that can be placed under a pillow or mattress, or mounted on the head- or base-board of a bed, to vibrate a sleeper awake. For very heavy sleepers whom the gentle vibrations would simply lull into a deeper sleep, there is a device that gives the bed a vigorous shaking that would be difficult for any sleeper to ignore.

A close friend and colleague, Max Friedman, tells of his early experiences with household devices:

> The telephone and doorbell lights we had put up about 28 years ago are a tangle of wires and fixed lamps attached to our walls. Between the two we have 10 bulbs. I have my system and know which is which, but my wife, Fran, is sometimes confused. Our new home will be without all these wires. We will go wireless. No knocking holes in our walls. Just a transmitter and three or four portable receivers, and Fran won't be confused. We had one of the first baby-cry signals when Michele was a baby. It was so sensitive that it went off every time a bus or truck passed on the street. We had to get rid of it. (Personal communication)

Household devices are much improved now, with one particular "device" long used by many deaf people now gaining increased recognition as a communication alert. This is man's best friend, the dog. Hearing Ear dogs are being trained to serve deaf persons, as Seeing Eye dogs serve the blind (Lawrence, 1979).

Telephone Communication Devices. Rapid distance-communication is another of the major links that hold community members together. The prime medium is the telephone. Although it was undreamed in the past that deaf persons would actually communicate by telephone, this too has come to pass (Castle, 1977; Jamison and Crandall, 1974). The first major breakthroughs were Visible Speech, developed by the Bell Telephone Laboratories in the early 1940s; and the tactile receiver for coded signals, designed by Bell Laboratories for the deaf-blind.

Visible Speech is produced by an intricate piece of machinery that transforms the flow of speech uttered by the message-sender into moving sound-wave patterns which the person on the receiving end sees on a small screen attached to the telephone, and which he must be able to translate back into their verbal equivalents. Obviously this is an extremely difficult operation for most persons, whether deaf or hearing.

In the coded signal method, the message sent can be tapped out on the mouthpiece of a telephone in an agreed upon code (such as the Morse code). The recipient gets the message by placing a finger on a vibrating button on the telephone's dial-face. Again, a difficult method for persons unfamiliar with the Morse or any other tappable code. This I found out for myself when trying it out with a deaf friend and colleague, Martin Sternberg, after a deaf-blind friend, Robert Smithdas, brought it to our attention. When Levine telephoned to Sternberg, or Sternberg to Levine, there was a mad scramble for the Morse code cards, an ensuing confusion and errors in message exchange, and great joy when even the tiniest message finally came through; the memory still brings on bursts of hilarity.

Although neither Visible Speech nor the tapped code seemed to have any practical value for deaf persons, the idea of telephonic communication for the deaf was not abandoned. Joining me in the search for a feasible alternative was the late Jean Leigh, mother of a deaf son, wise and knowledgeable in matters relating to the deaf, and a gracious, warm-hearted philanthropist. Realizing the need for an organizational base for further exploration, Jean established and funded Telephonic Communication for the Auditorially Disabled, Inc., in the early 1960s. The ensuing search led to the Electrowriter, the teletypewriter, and was climaxed by the Picturephone.

The Electrowriter and the teletypewriter are systems based on Data-Phone service, developed by the Bell System, in which messages written (Electrowriter) or typed (teletypewriter) on one of these units are automatically transmitted to the receiving mate by the data facilities over the regular telephone network exactly as written or typed. As described by the Bell System, the procedure for use is as follows: First, a regular telephone call is made. Then, the person at the receiving location manually activates the equipment by pushing a button. The person at the sending location then writes a message on a roll of paper in the device. The information automatically passes to the data set, which converts it to tones suitable for transmission over telephone lines. At the receiving end an identical data set converts the incoming tones to a form that can be fed to the connecting writing machine. This unit then duplicates the message sent, completing transmission within seconds after the message has been written or typed.

Thanks to the organization founded by Jean Leigh and the cooperation of the manufacturing concerns, it was possible to test the machines by placing them in the homes of selected deaf persons (Friedman, 1964a). Of the two, the Electrowriter was preferred since it simply required writing and did not tax the typewriting skills of sender or receiver. However, the costs proved prohibitive for general use.

Even more exciting to deaf persons than the Electrowriter was the Picturephone. Simply stated, the Picturephone is a telephone instrument that transmits visual images of sender and receiver over great distances, rather like a television picture. Through the generosity of the American Telephone and Telegraph Company, in 1964 I was able to arrange a demonstration for Picturephone communication between one group of deaf persons located at the National Geographic Building in Washington, D.C., and another group at Grand Central Station in New York City (Friedman, 1964b). A deaf participant in the momentous occasion expressed his reaction as follows:

The Picturephone demonstration was the high point of the 1964 convention of the National Association of the Deaf. It evoked the most profound reaction of pleasure I have ever observed in a group of deaf people. Even the most sophisticated were open-mouthed. You yourself saw the wide eyes, you heard the squeals of happiness, you observed the boundless surprise when two friends, both without hearing, communicated across the miles. . . . For the deaf it was as new an experience as landing on the moon—and as exciting! (Personal communication)

The television-like pictures transmitted by the Picturephone presented no difficulties in either reading signs or reading the lips, and this fact inspired my later efforts in television for the deaf. Unfortunately, telephonic communication via Picturephone was prohibitively expensive.

However, once having tasted the joys of telephonic communication, the deaf did not give up. The teletypewriter was the instrument of choice. Beginning with the least costly reconditioned models, this instrument (popularly known as TTY), has become standard equipment in professional offices of deaf persons, in organizations of and for the deaf, and in many homes. Some deaf people hesitate to use the instrument because of poor typing ability and/or poor language which they do not wish to expose. But for growing numbers, the TTY acts as a valued means of distance communication.

Notable confirmation of its practical communicative value was the installation of TTY equipment in the New York City office of the Social Security Administration in June 1978 to facilitate providing deaf persons with answers to inquiries and other needed information. Similar moves are spreading through other government agencies as well as banks, business concerns, and various professional organizations such as the American Psychological Association.

Another contribution of telephonic communication for deaf persons is the Code-Com attachment, made available through the New York Telephone Company, by which hearing-impaired persons can alert the telephone operator in an emergency. Information on further advances and current devices can be found in articles and the advertising sections of The Deaf American, the journal of the National Association of the Deaf.

Captioned Films and Telecommunications. A major expansion of community ties and resources for the deaf came with the passage in 1958 of Public Law 85-905, "to provide in the Department of Health, Education, and Welfare for a loan service of captioned films for the deaf" (Carpenter, 1967, p. 1). Heretofore, deaf movie-goers had customarily attended foreign film showings because of the English captions. To follow the story line of domestic films through lipreading was a hopeless task, even for experts. With the passage of PL 85-905, the film medium took on exceptional value in the service of deaf children and adults. As set forth by this Law, the purposes of the Captioned Film program are:

> (1) to bring to deaf persons understanding and appreciation of those films which play an important part in the general and cultural advancement of hearing persons;
> (2) to provide, through these films, enriched educational and cultural experiences through which deaf persons can be brought into better touch with the realities of their environment; and
> (3) to provide a wholesome and rewarding experience which deaf persons may share together.

The functions authorized by the law are to:

> (1) Acquire films (or rights thereto) by purchase, lease, or gift.
> (2) Provide for the captioning of films.
> (3) Provide for distribution of captioned films through State schools for the deaf and such other agencies as the Secretary may deem appropriate to serve as local or regional centers for such distribution.
> (4) Make use, consistent with the purposes of this Act, of films made available to the Library of Congress under the copyright laws.
> (5) Utilize the facilities and services of other governmental agencies.
> (6) Accept gifts, contributions, and voluntary and uncompensated services of individuals and organizations. (Carpenter, 1967, p. 1)

These basic purposes and functions were gradually enlarged by successive amendments to the law. Provisions were made for: (1) research in the use of educational and training films for the deaf: (2) the production and distribution of educational media for the deaf, for parents of deaf children, and for other persons who are involved in service to the deaf or who are actual or potential employers of deaf persons; and (3) training persons in the use of educational media for the instruction of the deaf.

With these expansions, the original Captioned Film project, begun in 1950 as a private, nonprofit venture at the American School for the Deaf, has taken prodigious strides in both organizational stature and funding. From a beginning allocation of $78,000 in 1958, it grew to a projected allocation for 1975 of $13.5 million. From its original status as the Captioned Films for the Deaf project of the Division of Educational Services of the U.S. Office of Education, it became the Captioned Films and Telecommunications Branch of the Division of Media Services of the Bureau of Education for the Handicapped in the U.S. Office of Education, with a nationwide regional network (Du Bow, 1979; Craig and Craig, 1978; Hairston, 1974).

A sampling of some of the early projects in deafness of the Division of Media Services includes: a project (LIFE) to develop better methods and facilities for teaching language to deaf children; a project to produce a series of films in total communication to facilitate language growth, communication, and child–parent interaction in young deaf children; the development of computerized speech-training aids for the deaf; a number of projects involving the use of media in the training of teachers of the deaf; an educational theater project to promote drama as an educational and creative force in schools and in other programs for the deaf; and ongoing projects to evaluate, acquire, and caption general interest and feature films for use by deaf audiences (Hairston, 1974).

One of the most exciting outcomes of the original captioning idea was the inroad made into television for deaf viewers. Shortly after the Picturephone demonstration cited above, I called together a group of some 20 prominent deaf figures in New York City for an informal conference on their television viewing habits and experiences and those of their deaf friends. The general response was that television designed for the hearing was a lost cause for the deaf, except for sports programs, captioned silent films and captioned foreign films, and the few religious programs that had simultaneous-interpretation (Ameslan) insets on the viewing screen. An appeal was made to several major television companies for similar insets in news programming, but it met polite but firm refusals. Evidently a great deal more than the small voice of this group was needed to make an impression.

Thanks to more powerful voices, television finally found its way into the silent world (Television and Deaf Persons, 1973, 1978; Workshop II, 1969). Three of the early projects of the Division of Media Services in the mid-1970s were studies concerned with captioned network newscasts and captioning techniques for hearing-impaired television viewers, conducted respectively by the WGBH Educational Foundation of Boston and the Public Broadcasting Service in Washington, D.C. A major project of the Public Broadcasting Service was the testing of a "decoder" to enable hearing-impaired viewers to elicit captions for their own viewing that are not visible to hearing viewers. Information on other and current projects for deaf viewers can be obtained on request from the Captioned Films and Telecommunications Branch of the Bureau of Education for the Handicapped, U.S. Office of Education, Washington, D.C.

Concurrently with these developments, studies were begun of the viewing habits and preferences of deaf television viewers (Freebairn, 1974; Jackson and Perkins, 1974; Sendelbaugh, 1978). An interesting finding is that captioned broadcasts are preferred over interpreted ones. This is perhaps surprising in view of the poor reading abilities of the deaf. However, in interviews with a number of subjects, Sendelbaugh found three major objections to interpreted broadcasts: "(1) the interpreter was comparatively small in relation to the size of the screen; (2) the vocabulary of signs used by interpreters was different from what was used in some classrooms; and (3) the speed of sign communications was too fast" (1978, p. 529). Sendelbaugh adds, "it was indicated by those interviewed that, although the vocabulary used [in captioning] was often difficult, the picture offered along with the written message allowed subjects to 'figure out' unknown terms" (1978, pp. 539, 540). It may be that captioning will stimulate interest among the deaf in improved reading. As to program preferences, action-type programs were the favorites for the obvious reason that the action is the message.

Among the foremost leaders in television for the deaf is the Office of Educational Technology of Gallaudet College and its gifted staff of deaf and hearing television experts (Leon, 1978). One of them, Earl Higgins, remarks:

> The growing indication of deaf people's interest in their own culture, as evidenced by thoughts of deaf pride, or awareness, or even deaf power, should also be an indication that deaf persons care about communication in the form of television. . . . Deaf people, like television, should be visible. (1973, p. 7)

Possibly the most impressive and beautiful forms of visibility thus far televised are the talents of deaf theatrical performers. They more than justify deaf pride, and serve an unforgettable advocacy function among nondeaf viewers. On the more practical side was the ruling of the Federal Communications Commission in 1977 that all television emergency messages be transmitted visually as well as aurally for the protection of persons with impaired hearing.

Community Life-Styles

The many problems encountered by deaf persons might be expected to cast a depressing pall over their lives and communities. Such, however, is not the case. In his classic *Deafness and the Deaf in the United States,* Best sees deaf persons from the following perspective:

> While their inability to hear (and to an extent to speak) must always be a serious and distressing affliction, and even handicap and burden as well, and while they must often bemoan their fate, it yet seems to be true that the deaf as a lot are not unhappy. They are not morose, sullen, discontented. They remain undismayed. They are good-natured, see the world from an odd angle sometimes, yet are as much philosophers as the average man. . . . All things considered, cheerfulness may be said to be an attribute of the larger number of the deaf. (1943, p. 336)

The same cheerful animation generally characterizes groups and clubs of deaf persons, together with high enthusiasms and occasional displays of temper and temperament. It is when faced with persistent downgrading by hearing society that this animation is stilled, and deaf groups become a bitter "silent minority" (Stewart, 1972).

In the following personal communication, Max Friedman, distinguished "elder statesman" in deaf affairs, and his equally gifted wife Frances, supply a glimpse of the actual happenings in deaf circles when the deaf are in the company of their own deaf peers:

Before one can know what the deaf community cultural and social life is, one must know what it is not. It is not opera and the ballet. It is not concerts, radio, and recorded music. It is not the live theater as the general public know it, and, as to television and the usual run of motion pictures, deaf people can enjoy these only within rather restricted limitations. One unfamiliar with the resourcefulness of the deaf would think that, fenced in as they are, they would lead a rather bleak social and cultural life.

But that is not the case. Their ability to adjust and to cope is rather remarkable. It is true they miss out on things musical, on those avenues of information, pleasure and culture that depend solely upon hearing. But they make up for it, at least in their own estimation (and what else counts), by their increased enjoyment of those activities in which hearing is not a factor or a very limited one.

Take the ordinary community of hearing folk. Affinity groups are formed by bonds of family relationship, neighborliness, employment, or the sharing of common interests. Deaf people, on the other hand, may be scattered over tens or scores of miles. But for the most part they have been classmates or attended the same schools, sharing similar experiences. Because they are so few and so scattered, their need for companionship is intensified, and there is scarcely a town of any size in the country that does not have its clubs, churches, or tightly knit social groups that cater to their common interests with regular programs and activities. In some of our larger cities deaf people even own their own clubhouses. And they enjoy a wide variety of activities.

For example: the National Fraternal Society of the Deaf, which offers its members of both sexes insurance and health and accident benefits, has more than 150 divisions throughout the country. These local lodges meet ten times a year and hold national conventions every three years. Further, in many states, school alumni associations are very active and periodically run affairs and functions to supply gifts and other contributions to their alma maters. Deaf people also form clubs which concern themselves with civic matters, consumerism and protection of their civil rights. These local clubs in turn band together into state associations, affiliated with the National Association of the Deaf which counts 47 state associations in its membership. The National Association of the Deaf also sponsors a Junior Association with a very popular summer camp in Minnesota. These Junior Associations have been formed in most of the residential schools in the country and provide their members with a center of activities while training them for future citizenship and leadership. For the more athletically inclined young adults there is the American Athletic Association of the Deaf with about 120 member clubs which hold state and regional tournaments climaxing in annual national tournaments in basketball, softball, and volleyball. The American Athletic Association of the Deaf is a member of the World Games for the Deaf, which holds winter contests and Olympic-type competition every four years.

Since the use of teletypewriters has become increasingly widespread, the deaf have found another excuse for forming local clubs as well as a national organization of TTY owners. Those engaged in servicing TTYs have also formed local groups which in turn has become the nationwide Teletypewriters for the Deaf, Inc. This group holds biennial national gatherings attended largely by persons engaged in servicing and selling these machines and other household communication devices.

Besides the national organizations which also include the religious denominations, the deaf manage to find every imaginable excuse for holding large gatherings. In addition to the tournaments sponsored by the American Athletic Association of the Deaf, there are state and regional contests in golf and bowling for both men and women. There are regional and even a national gathering of ski enthusiasts which meet to hold contests lasting several days. And deaf owners of campers from over a wide area will assemble at a public campground at a pre-arranged time to enjoy vacations in common with friends and families. Deaf people also gather regularly during appropriate seasons at beaches, lakes, and picnic areas.

In the more densely populated areas it is usually the clubs which assume the lead in providing for the social lives of their members. They hold frequent affairs at which captioned films and games, such as cards and bingo, are offered. Occasionally, there are what are called literary nights at which speakers tell stories and present song and poetry recitals in signs. Some clubs have drama groups which offer presentations of varying degrees of competence. More and more, local community colleges are offering special programs for the deaf. The subjects may include consumerism, hobbies, and basic education courses. These programs are becoming increasingly popular as deaf adults discover that they are profitable and enjoyable ways to spend idle evenings. And more and more Golden Age clubs are springing up everywhere, usually sponsored by the churches.

In the rural areas where the deaf population is more thinly spread, it is generally the church which is the center of deaf community life. Like the circuit riders of old, clergymen, both hearing and deaf, travel on fixed schedules over wide areas, appearing at each town once or twice a month. But that does not necessarily mean that the parishioners gather only when their clergymen appear. In between are meetings of men's and women's clubs with their specific interests, church suppers, socials, and showings of captioned films. Deaf people travel 30 and 40 miles each way even in inclement weather to hear their clergymen and to socialize. Truth to tell, though, deaf people living in isolation from other deaf people or in semi-isolation will often pull up stakes and move to localities where they can enjoy a more active community life.

Perhaps the most popular recreation, avenue of relaxation, and excuse for getting together are the captioned films. Besides showings at clubs and churches, deaf people form groups which meet in turn at members' homes. The only costs to viewers are for the projectors, screens, and return postage. These private ''movie clubs'' often form card clubs as well. Sometimes a club fee is charged, and when enough money is raised in the treasury, the members go off on a trip, an excursion, or on a binge in a fancy restaurant.

The Friedman account gives a vivid picture of the bustle and activities that animate the silent minority. The nature of activity in a particular group reflects the interests and levels of group membership; and here, too, a picture of considerable heterogeneity prevails. Jacobs provides another perspective:

In nearly every large city there is at least one club for the deaf. Although some of these clubs own their premises, most of them rent halls. Some pay monthly rent for the full use of their quarters, but the others meet only once or twice a month. These [latter] organizations usually have a difficult time meeting their expenses, for their deaf members on the average cannot afford to pay dues large enough to take care of all the desired expenditures. In addition, the "gimme" attitude of many of them has not accustomed them to taking up their fair share of the burden if it means making some personal sacrifices. Therefore except for a few which are endowed, these clubs usually have to be content with inadequate facilities in undesirable neighborhoods. Since the only qualification for membership in these clubs is deafness, all kinds of people congregate there. This tends to discourage some types of deaf people from patronizing the clubs, for they know that they are sure to find some undesirable characters in attendance. (1974, p. 42)

But by and large, at whatever the level of club organization, deaf persons are ardently club-oriented, are great travelers, enjoy a good gossip or a good card game, and are always ready for new and exciting experiences. If, as Best remarks, they see the world from an odd angle sometimes, they generally enjoy the view and "move in and out of the larger culture according to their needs of the moment but always have available a complex of their own resources that enables them to live happy, reasonably balanced and profitable lives" (Switzer and Williams, 1967, p. 253).

Deaf Leadership Power

In recent years, an invigorating force has made itself felt in the national deaf community, gradually arousing the habitually passive "silent minority" to positive action. The force is embodied in deaf leadership, both individual and organizational.

Organizations per se are no new thing in the field of the deaf. The first and most influential were established in this country in the nineteenth century. These were organizations *for* the deaf. They were founded and administered by nondeaf persons and were mainly concerned with the education of deaf children. The principal national organizations of the period were: The Volta Bureau and its controlling organization, the American Association to Promote the Teaching of Speech to the Deaf, both founded by Alexander Graham Bell; the Convention of American Instructors of the Deaf and Dumb (now the Convention of American Instructors of the Deaf); and the Conference of Principals of American Schools for the Deaf (now the Conference of Executives of American Schools for the Deaf). In addition, there were numbers of parent associations, also *for* the deaf and similarly concerned with the education of deaf children.

In this kind of *for*-the-deaf organizational network, leadership was in the hands of the nondeaf. The adult deaf remained a more or less outside group whose welfare was relegated mainly to religious organizations and church missions. Deaf spokesmen for deaf citizenry were few and far between.

Organizations composed *of* deaf persons had difficult beginnings. Their founding was met with sharp disfavor by educators of the deaf, on the grounds that such organizations would increase the likelihood of intermarriages among deaf members, with a resultant increase in the deaf population. "Clannishness" was another source of objection. Not only were there objections, there was active opposition. But objections were also raised to the acceptance of deaf members into nondeaf clubs and national associations and organizations. This left deaf adults in a state of enforced ostracism from the organizational network on both deaf and hearing fronts.

The deaf, however, found a way in. They formed alumni associations. There could be no open objection to this move, simply subtle discouragement. Among the earliest alumni associations were: the Alumni Association of the High Class of the New York School, founded in 1859; the Ohio Alumni Association, founded in 1870; and the Alumni Association of the Wisconsin School, founded in 1876. Another of these early organizational moves was the establishment of the New England Association *of* the Deaf in 1853 to raise funds for a monument to Thomas Hopkins Gallaudet.

At the same time, deaf persons at the local community level were forming clubs and small societies of the deaf, mostly for social purposes but with some extending fraternal benefits to members in need. From these scattered beginnings, it was only a step to the next phase of organization, the consolidation of various groups, without loss of their own identity, into state associations of the deaf. One of the earliest was the Empire State Association of Deaf-Mutes (now the Empire State Association of the Deaf), founded in 1865 in New York State.

The climax of all these moves came in 1880 with the founding of the first national organization of deaf persons: the National Association of the Deaf. Its stated purpose was to promote the welfare of the deaf in educational measures, in employment, in legislation, and in any other field pertaining to or affecting the deaf of America in their pursuit of economic security, social equality, and all their just rights and privileges as citizens. With the founding of this organization, the deaf population could add a voice of its own to the national organizational scene.

In the beginning, the voice was a comparatively weak one, owing mainly to the scarcity of deaf leaders, the overwhelming reforms that had to be made, and the ingrained passivity of the silent minority. But with the passage of Public Law 565 in 1956, help came from a powerful friend of the deaf, Mary Switzer, then head of the U.S. Office of Vocational Rehabilitation; Boyce R. Williams, a major deaf figure, served the Office as chief consultant on deaf affairs and needs. The encouragement and funding supplied at this government level sparked a nationwide era of projects in behalf of the deaf, beginning with the first Mental Health Center for the Deaf, a project initiated in 1955 by Boyce Williams and myself (Adler, 1978) and situated at the New York State Psychiatric Institute in New York City (Levine, 1956, 1960, 1963; Rainer, Altshuler, and Kallman, 1963).

The opportunities provided by the Office of Vocational Rehabilitation required that the accumulation of unmet needs be carefully analyzed and assigned priority rankings for orderly management. Accordingly, a Workshop was conducted in 1960 on Research Needs in the Vocational Rehabilitation of the Deaf (Rogers and Quigley, 1960), at which specialists listed research proposals in order of priority in the areas of psychological assessment, language, the subculture of the deaf, vocational development, education, and family genetics and institutionalization. The scarcity of deaf professional persons led to a heavily nondeaf steering committee for this workshop. Perhaps for this reason, no great emphasis was placed on establishing programs for training deaf leaders. Or perhaps this unprecedented opportunity to get research under way at long last overshadowed all else. In any event, deaf leadership training played a minor role at the meeting. Awareness of the need came later.

By 1969, Mary Switzer sounded the training alert: "In view of the present shortage of professional personnel capable of meeting needs generated by the complex problems of deafness, training programs assume an importance equaling that of research" (1969, p. v). At the same time, a review of government-funded long-term professional training programs in the area of deafness stated that, "Annually, 15 persons, five of whom may be deaf persons, are selected for participation in a special leadership training program" (Adler, 1969, p. 43). The importance of deaf leadership in the service of deaf persons was thus "officially" recognized (Petersen, 1972).

A general picture of deaf leadership at about this time may be drawn from an address by Williams:

> deaf leadership is beginning to stir. It may be that the maturation of the large ratio of deaf leadership has only recently reached a point that it may effectively attack the reasons for the undereducation of deaf persons. . . . However, much outstanding deaf leadership talent and much time are absorbed in important recreational and social activities that are essential for group and often for individual emotional health. So much manpower is absorbed in this area that less is left for development of the socio-education front. . . . However, the deaf leader is now beginning to speak up to public officials and is encouraged by the warm reception he usually receives. (1970, pp. 6, 7, 9)

Even more striking evidence of the growing impact of deaf leadership was its arousal of the silent minority from its traditional passivity. "Deaf Power" slogans began to appear in local clubs; and in certain cities, street demonstrations were held to give public visibility to the deaf members of society and their demands for recognition as first-class citizens.

In all these advances, an outstanding role was played by the most influential organization *of* the deaf, the National Association of the Deaf. As described by Williams:

> When . . . [the National Association of the Deaf] established a staffed headquarters in Washington, it provided a solid base to which public services, State associations of the deaf, deaf individuals, parents of deaf children, interested persons, organizations, or agencies could relate. . . . As the NAD acquired skill, government was able to request more and more services. Several important workshops have been staged by the NAD, such as the San Francisco Workshop for Interpreters, the Salt Lake City Leadership Workshop, the International Seminar on Research in Vocational Rehabilitation of the Deaf, and others, all of which strengthened the NAD and helped government carry out its responsibilities. . . . The NAD quickly organized to establish the Registry of Interpreters for the Deaf so that growing government need for qualified interpreters could be met. . . . The most ambitious and important service that this organization is now providing is the national census of the deaf, a long-standing need which will provide the firm base that is required for program projection. (1970, pp. 10–11)

Many hundreds of projects have been conducted in behalf of the deaf in training, research, and rehabilitation by organizations, agencies, universities, colleges, and individuals throughout the country, both before and since these remarks by Williams. Information on government-funded projects can be found in the inclusive listings in *Deafness Annual,* published by the Professional Rehabilitation Workers with the Adult Deaf, Inc. (now the American Deafness and Rehabilitation Association, Inc.). Of particular concern to deaf leaders, over and above rehabilitation in the inclusive sense, are educational reforms, adult education, law and the deaf, deaf driving and insurance problems, abridgments of legal and civil rights, problems of the aging deaf population, and the expansion of interpreter services. And worthy of note is the increasing prominence of deaf participants in all these activities.

This discussion would not be complete without a special bow to the generally unsung heroes of many of these advances in deaf leadership. They are the presidents, directors, or executive directors of associations *of* the deaf. Theirs is the kind of job that demands the utmost in endurance, perseverance, and frustration-tolerance. A behind-the-scenes look at what is involved is provided by John B. Davis, President of a state association of the deaf:

> As President of the IAD for eight years I have had to live with the inertia of people inside and outside the association. I have had to learn to withstand disappointments in the failure to bring about needed advances for the deaf. I have

also had to deal with the condescension of professionals who claim to know everything about deafness.

I have been unable to delegate many of my duties, which is highly unusual for the president of a large organization. The reason for this is the very low educational level of the majority of deaf people. Few deaf persons are knowledgeable enough about general community affairs to make contributions to their associations. In addition, few have the language skills necessary for effective verbal presentation of issues. . . .

The most difficult obstacle I have had to deal with and which all of the deaf face is that of communication. . . . True, the typewriter-telephone is a new and God-sent media for the deaf but how many deaf people can use the typewriter? How many of them have the money to pay for the service? More often than not the handwritten letter is the only means of communication available. The most frustrating part is after the letters have been written they often remain unanswered because many deaf people shy away from any situation that would reveal their low educational level. There are many times when I have had to travel long distances just to communicate an important message. . . .

Not being a college graduate, I have often met with condescension from professionals at meetings. Sometimes such meetings do not have qualified interpreters who could give me enough information for me to be fully involved in the meeting. Many times I remain silent because I have not been able to keep up with the proceedings and I feel that my presence is a token gesture. (1972, pp. 35, 36)

Davis's experiences are far from unique. It is safe to say they are the universal burden of all deaf professional persons and leaders. However, Davis sees the involvement of deaf individuals in professional activities as one way of broadening the base of awareness of the needs of the deaf. He concludes, "If improvements are to be expected, they will have to come from deaf leaders taking part in all programs involving deafness" (1972, p. 37). Davis and all who serve in similar capacities in associations of the deaf deserve special commendation for their too often unrecognized contributions to deaf leadership.

To paraphrase Best (1943), deaf leaders are indeed the gamest of them all. As a result of their perseverance and stamina, there are now deaf leaders, participants, and/or members in all national organizations serving the deaf and in a great many local ones, current listings of which are found in the Directory issue of the *American Annals of the Deaf.* The interests and advocacies of these bodies do not always coincide, as witness the divisive issue of oral versus total communication. But then neither do the opinions of all deaf persons.

There are some who feel that there are too many organizations in the field of the deaf, and this may be so. But insofar as these organizations provide a base for further development of deaf leaders, they have justified their existence.

Summary Comment

The exceptional range and combinations of variables that characterize the "deaf" environment are reflected in the exceptional range and combinations that characterize the deaf population. Similarly, the many deficits in the developmental and educational environments of deaf persons are mirrored in matching deficits in the majority members of the population. The "environmental microcosm" postulate of the eco-behavioral and culture-pattern theorists appears as valid for the deaf as the nondeaf. Both are largely "products" of the fashioning environment.

This being so, an extraordinary highlight in these sketches from life is the remarkable resiliency of the deaf as a group, and the equally remarkable progress made after the school years, progress which would not be expected from the depressed levels of school achievements. How does this come about? What are the responsible propelling factors? How does the phenomenon fit into environmental theory? These and many other questions are part of the search, which still has far to go in solving the psychological riddles presented by the deaf.

But one thing at least is true. As Best has said of the deaf, "They face life courageous and intrepid, knowing that the odds are against them in the race which they must run, and in the struggle in which they must engage" (1943, p. 637). The sketches from life suggest that the deaf do not give up despite the odds, not even such as Roberto. Among the most intrepid of the propelling forces is deaf leadership; and among the most courageous are the deaf leaders.

References

Adler, E., Ed. 1969. Long-term professional training programs in the area of deafness, Rehabilitation Services Administration. *Deafness,* Monograph No. 1, p. 43.

Adler, E. 1978. Mental health services to deaf people: an historical review. *Gallaudet Today,* Fall, 5–6.

Best, H. 1943. *Deafness and the Deaf in the United States.* New York: Macmillan Co.

Carpenter, A. A., Comp. 1967. Catalog of Captioned Films for the Deaf. Washington, D.C.: Bureau of Education for the Handicapped, Office of Education, HEW.

Castle, D. L. 1977. Telephone and distance communication devices for the hearing impaired. *Deaf American,* 29: 15–16.

Community Organization with the Deaf: Proceedings of a Community Resources Institute. 1967. Project no. RD-2088-6. Tucson, Arizona: University of Arizona Rehabilitation Center.

Community Responsibilities for Meeting the Needs of Deaf Persons. 1964. Project no. VRA 64-3. Washington, D.C.: Office of Vocational Rehabilitation, HEW, and San Francisco Hearing Society.

Craig, W. N., and Craig, H. B., Eds. 1978. U.S. Office of Education for the Handicapped, Division of Media Services. *American Annals of the Deaf*, 123: 338–41.

Crammatte, A. B. 1968. *Deaf Persons in Professional Employment*. Springfield, Ill.: Charles C. Thomas.

Crammatte, A. B., and Schreiber, L. F. 1961. *Proceedings of the Workshop on Community Development through Organization of and for the Deaf*. Washington, D.C.: Office of Vocational Rehabilitation, HEW.

Davis, J. B. 1972. The frustrations of being a president of a state association for the deaf. *Deafness Annual*, 2: 35–38.

Du Bow, S. 1979. Federal action on interpreters and telecommunications. *American Annals of the Deaf*, 124: 93–96.

Freebairn, T. 1974. *Television for Deaf People*. New York: Deafness Research and Training Center.

Friedman, M. 1964a. No longer just a dream: The deaf now use telephones. *Empire State News*, 26 (April): 2, 5.

Friedman, M. 1964b. NAD convention sees telephonic marvels. *Empire State News*, 26 (July): 1.

Furfey, P. H., and Harte, T. J. 1968. *Interaction of Deaf and Hearing in Baltimore City, Maryland*. Washington, D.C.: Catholic University of America.

Fusfeld, I. S. 1955. Suggestions on causes and cures for failures in written language. Paper presented at the 37th Regular Meeting of the Convention of American Instructors of the Deaf, West Hartford, Connecticut, June 27, 1955. Mimeographed.

Gendel, J. M. 1974. List of devices to help the hearing impaired in everyday living. *Highlights*, 53 (Fall): 16–18.

Hairston, E. E. 1974. Captioned films and telecommunication/learning resources branches, Division of Media Services. *Deafness Annual*, 4: 275–89.

Higgins, E. 1973. Television for deaf viewers. *Gallaudet Today*, 4: 6–7.

Jackson, W., and Perkins, R. 1974. Television for deaf learners: A utilization quandary. *American Annals of the Deaf*, 119: 537–48.

Jacobs, L. 1974. The community of the adult deaf. *American Annals of the Deaf*, 119: 41–46.

Jamison, S. I., and Crandall, J. T. 1974. Telephonic assistance devices for deaf people. *Deafness Annual*, 4: 143–58.

Keller, E. C. 1978. Quoted in *APSD Newsletter*, 1: 4.

Lawrence, G. 1979. Amy's a hearing-ear dog. *Shreveport Times*, Sunday, January 28, p. 3F.

Leon, V. 1977. TV at Gallaudet College. *Gallaudet Today*, 8: 25–29.

Levine, E. S. 1956. The mental health clinic for the deaf. *Silent Worker*, 9: 7–8.

Levine, E. S. 1960. Psychiatric-preventive and sociogenetic study of the adjustive capacities, optimum work potentials, and total family problems of literate deaf adolescents and adults. *American Annals of the Deaf*, 105: 272–74.

Levine, E. S. 1963. Historical review of special education and mental health services. In J. D. Rainer, K. Z. Altshuler, and F. J. Kallmann, Eds., *Family and Mental Health Problems in a Deaf Population*. New York: Department of Medical Genetics, New York State Psychiatric Institute, Columbia University. Pp. xvii–xxvi.

Lloyd, G. T., Ed. 1972. *Planning for Deaf Community Development*. New York: Deafness Research and Training Center, New York University.

Petersen, E. W., Ed. 1972. *Deaf Leadership Training for Community Interaction: A Manual for "Grassroots" Leadership*. Washington, D.C.: Social and Rehabilitation Service, Rehabilitation Service Administration, HEW.

Rainer, J. D., Altshuler, K. Z., and Kallmann, F. J., Eds. 1963. *Family and Mental Health Problems in a Deaf Population*. New York: Department of Medical Genetics, New York State Psychiatric Institute, Columbia University.

Rogers, M., and Quigley, S. P., Eds. 1960. Research needs in the vocational rehabilitation of the deaf. *American Annals of the Deaf*, 105: 335–70.

Sanderson, R. G. 1969. The gallants. In R. L. Jones, Ed., *The Deaf Man and the World*. National Forum II. Washington, D.C.: Council of Organizations Serving the Deaf. Pp. 9–17.

Schein, J. D. 1964. *The Deaf Community Study of Metropolitan Washington, D.C.: Methodological Report*. Washington, D.C.: Gallaudet College.

Schein, J. D., and Delk, M. T., Jr. 1974. *The Deaf Population of the United States*. Silver Spring, Md.: National Association of the Deaf.

Sendelbaugh, J. W. 1978. Television viewing habits of hearing-impaired teenagers in the Chicago metropolitan area. *American Annals of the Deaf*, 123: 536–41.

Stewart, L. G. 1972. A truly silent minority. *Deafness Annual*, 2: 1–2.

Switzer, M. E. 1969. Introduction. *Deafness*, Monograph No. I, pp. iv–v.

Switzer, M. E., and Williams, B. R. 1967. Life problems of deaf people. *Archives of Environmental Health*, 15: 249–56.

Television and Deaf Persons: An Update. 1978. *Gallaudet Today*, Spring 1978 issue.

Williams, B. R. 1970. Community development for deaf people. Erwin Kugel Lecture, January 16, 1970, New York Society for the Deaf, pp. 1–17.

Workshop II: Video Technology and Programs for the Deaf: Current Developments and Plans for the Future. 1969. Washington, D.C.: Office of Education, Bureau of Education for the Handicapped, HEW.

7 Sketches from Research

As a complement to the preceding sketches of the deaf as obtained from life, we turn to sketches of the deaf as obtained from research and interpreted through theory. The focus is on personality, the normal mental potential of the deaf having long since been established (Levine, 1960, 1963; Mindel and Vernon, 1971). We ask: What have personality tests to say about the deaf? How does personality theory interpret their behaviors? And finally, how do the findings obtained from research compare with those obtained from life?

Personality Studies

This section summarizes the findings of selected personality studies of the deaf. The ones that follow are arranged in rough chronological order for historical overview; and are presented under the names of the tests used so that the reader can easily scan for type and variety and compare results from test to test. Unless otherwise stated, the tests were neither designed nor standardized for a deaf population, the reason being the lack of psychological instruments so treated.

Thurstone Personality Schedule

Among the earliest personality studies of the deaf was that conducted by Lyon (1934), using the Thurstone Personality Schedule with 87 deaf high-school pupils of a state residential school. Lyon found that "the percentage of deaf pupils classified in Groups D and E (Emotionally Maladjusted, Should Have Psychiatric Advice) is more than twice that of college freshmen of approximately the same age" (1934, p. 3).

Brunschwig Personality Inventory for Deaf Children

Lyon's findings were broadly confirmed in a study conducted by Lily Brunschwig (1936). The Brunschwig study is of particular interest in that the Inventory had been standardized by the investigator on a deaf pupil population. It was used in a comparison of 182 deaf students of a state residential school and 348 hearing public school students. Brunschwig found that in all comparisons, "the deaf averaged poorer adjustment scores than the hearing, differences between the means of the deaf and hearing being statistically significant in six out of twelve comparisons" (1936, p. 132).

Bernreuter Personality Inventory

Still further evidence of differences between deaf and hearing persons was derived from an investigation conducted by Pintner, Fusfeld, and Brunschwig (1937), in which the Bernreuter Personality Inventory was used to ascertain the adjustment status of 50 deaf students of Gallaudet College, and 126 deaf adults. Revisions were made in the wording of those test items that seemed likely to present language difficulties for deaf subjects, and special care was taken in administration. The results showed that the deaf subjects were "only slightly more emotionally unstable, only a little more introverted, and not quite so dominant as the normal hearing" (1937, p. 326).

Fears-and-Wishes Checklist

A checklist of 39 possible fears was devised and a list of 7 pairs of wishes was put together by Pintner and Brunschwig (1937) in order to compare the fears and wishes of deaf and hearing children. Although the groups, consisting of 159 deaf and 345 hearing children, were in similar school grades, the deaf children were 2–3 years older chronologically. The investigators found that on the whole there was great similarity between the fears of the deaf and of the hearing subjects. As to wishes, a statistically reliable difference was found in the direction of greater preference for immediate gratification on the part of the deaf, which the investigators interpreted as indicating a less mature attitude toward life.

Vineland Social Maturity Scale

The social maturity of the deaf was the topic of three early studies, conducted by Bradway (1937), Burchard and Myklebust (1942), and Streng and Kirk (1938).

The subjects of the Bradway study were 92 pupils of a state residential school, all of whom were deaf before the age of 2 years, plus 11 pupils of the same school who became deaf after age 5. Bradway found this combined deaf group "to be 20 percent inferior to hearing subjects in social competence throughout all age levels examined" (1937, p. 138) when compared with the test norms of the nondeaf standardization group.

These findings were confirmed by the Burchard and Myklebust study, in which 104 deaf pupils of a state residential school were the subjects.

However, contrary results were obtained by Streng and Kirk, whose subjects were 97 deaf and hard-of-hearing pupils of a day school. The investigators found the subjects to be average in social maturity.

Haggerty-Olson-Wickman Behavior-Rating Schedule

Studies using this Schedule were conducted by Burchard and Myklebust (1942), Kirk (1938), and Springer (1938a). In Kirk's study, 112 deaf and hard-of-hearing pupils of a day school were used as subjects. The results showed a significantly greater number of problem tendencies among the deaf and hard-of-hearing group than among normally hearing children. These findings were confirmed by Burchard and Myklebust, using the same instrument in a study of 187 deaf pupils of a state residential school. However, Springer, in a comparison of 377 deaf and 415 hearing pupils, found very little difference between the groups and, in fact, found that the deaf rated more favorably than the hearing on certain items of the Schedule.

Brown Personality Inventory for Children

Studies using the Brown Inventory were conducted by Springer (1938b) and Springer and Roslow (1938). In the Springer study, the Inventory was used with 400 deaf pupils of day and state residential schools, and 327 hearing pupils of the regular public schools. The results showed that all the groups of deaf children received much higher neurotic scores than the hearing control children. These findings were confirmed in the Springer and Roslow study, in which a comparison of responses to the Inventory was made for equated groups of 59 deaf and 59 hearing pupils.

Free Association Test

The word-responses of deaf subjects aged 11–17 years to printed stimulus words were compared by Kline (1945) to those of hearing children of the same ages. The words used were familiar to the deaf subjects. Even so, Kline found differences in response between the deaf and hearing groups, with more failure of response among the deaf as well as a larger percentage of commonest responses. Personality interpretation was not carried out.

Rorschach Projective Technique

The use of the Rorschach Technique with deaf subjects marks the first major departure from inventory and rating types of studies. The earliest Rorschach studies were conducted by Altable (1947) in Mexico, Levine (1948, 1956) and McAndrew (1948) in this country, and Beizman (1950) in France.

Altable's subjects were 45 mostly illiterate, congenital "deaf-mutes" of both sexes, ranging in age from "under 10" to 20 years. McAndrew's were

25 deaf residential-school pupils, also of both sexes, of ages 10–15 years; Levine's subjects were 31 adolescent deaf girls of a residential school who had been carefully screened as typical, well-adjusted deaf teenagers. Beizman's were 27 "deaf-mutes" ranging in age from 11 to 21 years.

Despite the sharp differences in the subjects of these studies, certain common personality findings emerged: (1) conceptual deficiencies; (2) emotional immaturity; (3) rigidity and egocentricity; (4) deficient social adaptability; and (5) constricted interests and motivations.

Interpretation of these findings differed from investigator to investigator. Altable stressed the maladjustive and neurotic features of "deaf" Rorschach patterns. McAndrew noted the similarities between the patterns of her deaf subjects and those of somewhat younger hearing children. Beizman emphasized the poverty of response on the part of the deaf subjects, and likened their response patterns to those of very young hearing children or in some respects to those of the mentally deficient.

Levine, however, viewed the patterns from a somewhat different angle. The aim of the Levine study was to obtain a personality picture of a "normal" group of deaf subjects, hence the careful screening of subjects for typicality and adjustment. In these circumstances, the subjects could not logically be considered "maladjusted" simply on the basis of deviant-from-hearing Rorschach patterns. Rather, the patterns of the deaf subjects were interpreted as representing a particular mode of adaptation to a deviant fashioning environment. It was further hypothesized that the pattern is by no means a fixed concomitant of deafness but is subject to change with changes in the influencing environment. It was recognized that if similar Rorschach patterns were found in persons reared in "hearing" environments, they might well suggest abnormality. But in the case of deaf subjects, the patterns suggest the manner in which normal psychological potentials can be shaped by an abnormal fashioning environment. This is not to imply that the patterns are strong enough to withstand the pressures of life outside the protective environment of a residential school. To strengthen the patterns would require improvement and reform in the influencing environment. This view was in essence supported by Bindon (1957b) in a later Rorschach study conducted in England using the Monroe Inspection Technique.

A still later Rorschach study was conducted by Goetzinger et al. (1966), using the Structured Objective Rorschach Test (SORT) modification of the original technique. This investigation compared 24 deaf and 24 hearing control adolescents on various personality attributes. On a number there were significant group differences: "the deaf manifested higher aggression, less cooperation, above average tendencies in Consistency of Behavior, less than average Anxiety, and higher degree of Non-conformity" (1966, p. 521). The investigators report further that "the deaf did not differ from the controls of this study in range of interests, in tact, in confidence, in moodiness, in impulsiveness, and in flexibility" (1966, p. 520). However, the gulf in terminology, procedure, and interpretation between this test and the Rorschach is so wide that the investigators recommend that further study of the SORT with hearing as well as deaf subjects be conducted.

Lowenfeld Mosaic Test

The Lowenfeld Mosaic Test of personality was used in three unpublished but related investigations by Schonberger (1952) using deaf male subjects, Healey (1952) using deaf female subjects, and Gelbmann (1952) comparing male and female subjects. In his male subjects, Schonberger found implications of constrictive, withdrawal tendencies together with an overemphasis on emotional control. For the female subjects, Healey found indications of greater immaturity than with the hearing controls, together with more neurotic traits and greater tendencies toward constriction and withdrawal. On comparing male and female deaf subjects, Gelbmann found greater insecurity, anxiety, and emotional repression among the males than among the females, while the females showed more maladjustment than the males in other personality areas and also a greater tendency toward a schizoid type of adjustment.

Rohde-Hildreth Sentence Completion Test

Using the insufficiently exploited sentence completion technique, Ayers (1950) administered the Rohde-Hildreth test to a group of deaf adolescents. She found less self-justification needs among her subjects as compared with the hearing, but stronger need for aid, protection, and sympathy as well as greater needs to please, follow, and admire, and to relate facts, explain, interpret, and judge.

Make-a-Picture Story (MAPS)

Investigations using the MAPS technique were conducted by Bindon (1957a) and by Hess (1960, 1969). In the Bindon study, two groups of deaf adolescents and a matched hearing group were used. One of the deaf groups was composed of children who had become deaf as a result of maternal rubella, and the other of children who became deaf from other causes and before the age of 2 years. Bindon's results showed significantly fewer normal and significantly more schizophrenic signs in the deaf groups than in the matched hearing group. Also noted were the impoverished fantasy productions of the deaf, which, the investigator remarks, are generally suggestive of the social isolation and illogical, unrealistic thinking of the subjects.

In the Hess study, the investigator used his own nonverbal modification of the MAPS in comparing a group of deaf subjects with two hearing groups:

one emotionally adjusted and the other emotionally disturbed. All subjects were in the age range of 8–10 years. The findings showed that the deaf differed from the hearing in exhibiting greater impulsivity, increased fantasy, superficial interpersonal contacts, shallow emotional investments, selective sensitivity for minority groups, and depressive qualities. Hess found further that certain group differences show behaviors characteristic of the deaf, such as the preceding, while others show similarities between the deaf group and the maladjusted hearing group. Particularly noted was the finding of an expansive fantasy life, in direct disagreement with Bindon. Hess interprets this finding as signifying "that the restrictions met by the deaf in their interpersonal relationships might be compensated for by increased fantasy gratification of their needs" (1969, p. 17).

California Test of Personality

In response to increasing doubts about whether the personality of the deaf can be soundly assessed with tests standardized on the hearing, Vegely and Elliott (1968) launched their own inquiry into the subject using the California Test of Personality, an inventory type of measure. They found the responses of their deaf subjects to be inferior to those of the hearing. The question this raised in the minds of the investigators was whether this inferiority was a real deviation on the part of the deaf subjects or whether it was an artifact of the test. In an interesting approach to the problem, they found that the inferior performance of the deaf subjects could not be adequately explained as an artifact of the test but was real deviation. They concluded that the California test can be used as it stands in evaluating the adjustment of a given deaf child to the norms and standards of hearing society.

IES (Impulse, Ego, Superego) Test

The IES Test is an interesting instrument constructed for clinical and research purposes within the frame of psychoanalytic theory. It is designed to assess the relative strengths of impulses, ego, and superego, and to estimate the effects of impulse and superego forces upon ego functioning. The instrument was used by Zivkovic (1971) with a group of deaf subjects that numbered 29 boys and 25 girls with a mean age of 18 years, and a control group of hearing subjects that included 37 boys and 15 girls with a mean age of 17 years. The hypotheses tested were that "impulsivity will be more prominent in the deaf than in the hearing subjects, and ego and superego forces will be more outstanding in the hearing than in the deaf subjects. The increase of impulsivity and decrease of ego and superego forces in the deaf will be manifested in their overt behavior, in their way of perceiving the outside world, in their fantasy life and in their ego integration" (1971, p. 863). Of 36 comparisons made between the scores of the deaf and the hearing,

Zivkovic found 15 statistically significant differences agreeing with the hypotheses, and 8 opposite to expectations. He concluded that the deaf subjects tended to perceive the world subjectively rather than realistically, and as a place where impulses are freely expressed. He also noted that behavior in accord with superego values was seldom found, and remarked on the presence of a great deal more rigidity and restriction in the behavior of the deaf than in that of the hearing.

Missouri Children's Picture Series (MCPS)

This is a different type of test designed for use with children in the age range of 5 to 16 years. It is a nonverbal test consisting of 3-by-5 cards on which are line drawings of children engaged in various activities: 238 in all. The subject's task is to group the cards into "fun" and "not fun" categories. Vegely (1971) used the test in a study of 160 deaf children distributed evenly by sex and number for the age groups 10, 12, 14, and 16 years. Attributes measured by the test include conformity, masculinity/femininity, maturity, aggressivity, inhibition, hyperactivity, sleep disturbances, psychosomatization. The findings indicated that as a group, the deaf subjects obtained scores associated with normal adjustment, with a tendency for low scores among the male subjects on the masculinity/femininity scale.

Hand Test

Using the Hand Test (Bricklin, Piotrowski, and Wagner, 1962; Wagner, 1962), a study conducted by Levine and Wagner (1974) marks the first explicit effort to break away from the traditional "the"-personality-of-"the"- deaf research design, by taking cognizance of the great heterogeneity that characterizes the deaf population. To accomplish this, the investigators selected as subjects three groups of young deaf adults representing the exceptional, average, and below-average groupings previously described. The outstanding difference among the groups was in level of linguistic ability, with the exceptional group at advanced high school and college reading achievement levels, the average at about 6th-grade level, and the below-average at little more than 2nd-grade level. In other respects there was substantial conformity among the subjects. The large majority had profound, congenital deafness; all had begun school at about the same age and had attended for a minimum of 10 years preceding the study, were of at least average intelligence, and had no health problems or other physical disabilities.

The test used in the investigation seemed uniquely suited to deaf subjects. The projective stimuli of the Hand Test are nine simple line drawings of hands in ambiguous poses, each on a separate card. The subject "projects" by telling the examiner what the hands appear to be doing. On a tenth blank card, the subject is asked to imagine a hand and tell what it is doing. The fact that most deaf adults habitually communicate with their hands gave the test a comfortable touch. Further, the test was administered in whatever communicative mode the subject habitually used.

The results of the investigation demonstrated wide divergence in personality patterns among the groups, with 20 out of 24 Hand Test variables significantly discriminating among them. Briefly: the personality patterns of members of the exceptional group proved to be remarkably similar to the patterns of their hearing high-school and college peers; the patterns of the average group, while not showing any unusual amount of deviance, did exhibit various evidences of psychological weakness consistent with communicative restrictions; and the pattern of the below-normal group was characterized by high pathological signs together with rigid attachment to the simple routinized aspects of behavior, inability to cope with and a general unresponsiveness to the complexities of reality, yet a clear awareness of a "difference" from other people, with accompanying feelings of inferiority. Obviously, this study successfully challenges the myth of "the" personality of "the" deaf.

To sum up, this sampling of personality studies includes the large majority of psychological instruments used in such research with deaf subjects. The general research theme is one of deviance and maladjustment. Whether this is real deviance on the part of the subjects, an "artifact" of the test instruments, as Vegely and Elliott ask, or an expression of environmental more than individual deviance is explored in the discussion at the end of this chapter.

Personality Theorizing

The challenge facing personality theorists concerned with the deaf is to interpret the known facts in the light of a given theory. Personality research has obviously provided only descriptive information. We turn, therefore, to the theorists for underlying explanations. Fitting theory to fact (or fact to theory) is no mean task, particularly in light of the enormous number of personality theories in the psychological marketplace (Hall and Lindzey, 1978; Ruitenbeek, 1964).

The summaries that follow are of necessity highly abridged and are grouped by major theory applied.

Psychoanalytic Theory

Expressed in the 1920s was Freud's belief that the ego wears an auditory lobe (Freud, 1947). By this he meant that the reality inputs provided by hearing, particularly in the form of spoken language, are of central importance in differentiating the ego or "I" from the unconscious, instinctual drives that dominate the original composition of the psyche. As explained by Blum, "in being able to tie together words and ideas, the ego is better equipped to handle the external world as well as impulses from within" (1953, p. 64). Applying this view to prelinguistically deaf persons leads to the Freudian conclusion that an inability to acquire language in consonance with psychic need registers in retarded or impaired ego formation.

Isakower ascribes the same central importance to hearing and verbal language in the formation of the superego:

> It is self-evident that experiences and impressions of the environment are necessary in order that a super-ego be built up. It is just as self-evident that these experiences and impressions are acquired by way of sense-perception. But can one imagine that purely optical sense-impressions, for example, by themselves and without showing any linguistically ordered structure could possibly lead to the building up of a function of logical and ethical judgement? Without further discussion, this question can certainly be answered in the negative. But the claim of the auditory sphere to the primary place in the building up of the super-ego would be thereby established. (1939, p. 345)

Isakower concludes with the statement, "The following formula then suggests itself: Just as the nucleus of the ego is the body-ego, so the human auditory sphere as modified in the direction of a capacity for language is to be regarded as the nucleus of the super-ego" (1939, pp. 345–46).

In effect, psychoanalytic theory as applied by Freud and Isakower rests on the central importance of verbal language in ego and superego formation. The "auditory sphere" and hearing are repeatedly mentioned simply because they are the major vehicle for language input. Where verbal language cannot be acquired in tune with psychic need, notably through hearing, the theory holds that there will be deficiencies in the formation of both ego and superego.

On the basis of his clinical experiences with deaf persons, Finkelstein (1968) finds confirmation for the Freudian view. He bases the justification for his view on the personality pictures of the deaf as derived from research: preference for immediate gratification; a tendency toward impulsivity; deficient social adaptability, egocentric motives, shallow emotional investments, and impoverished fantasy productions. Findings such as these point to underdevelopment of ego-functioning. As possible causes, Finkelstein points to the difficulties experienced by a young deaf child in identifying with hearing parents. He also notes the tensions and ambivalence that hamper many such parents in giving the child the loving security needed for ego strength. In effect, Finkelstein sees the deaf child as making contact "with the real world with an Ego weakened by his sensory defect, weakened by a defect in the ability to identify himself, and weakened by a defect in the amount of love he receives" (1968, p. 6).

Taking issue with the central importance of verbal, heard language in ego and superego development are Wile (1933) and Knapp (1953). Wile, one of the earliest psychoanalytically oriented workers with the deaf says, "I do not agree that all ideas are dependent upon the tongue. All signs, movements, and actions are ideas regardless of whether there is a linguistic equivalent or not" (1933, p. 472). Of the deaf he says, "Their visual contacts with the world enable them to set up their ego structure firmly and give it sound foundations" (1933, pp. 466–67). Basing his judgments on close clinical relations with deaf persons, Wile finds that the vigorous herd forces among the deaf promote an active social life which, in turn, serves to release the ego from negative pressures. He also notes a tremendous ego pressure for self-expansion among deaf persons, and interprets this as arising from a sense of isolation if not outright social rejection, which is compensated for "by gaining the maximum capacity to live within one's own peer group with a sense of rising values" (1933, p. 471). Wile's sensitive and insightful interpretations are summed up in his statement that for the deaf "the greatest struggle involves the attainment of an ability to live in harmony with one's self, to overcome one's inner feelings of ineptness, one's sense of solitariness in the dark, one's sense of isolation from the social life of those capable of speech, and to develop a socialized ego without sacrificing individuality and independence" (1933, p. 471). The strong conviction of this eminent psychiatric pioneer in work with the deaf was that there should be greater emphasis on the language of symbols in the early development of a deaf child than on the language of "alphabet and sounds." Wile's belief is echoed today in the rising tide of total communication.

Like Wile, Knapp calls attention to the nonheard and nonverbal modes of language in human communication, and observes that the congenitally deaf whose "auditory spheres" lack the capacity for verbal language do not thereby "have a congenital atrophy of conscience" (1953, p. 682). He notes, however, that listening does contribute to superego and ego formation and functions (1953, p. 685).

Nass (1964) takes a closer look at superego functioning in the deaf; he studied the development of conscience in deaf as compared with hearing children, based on the responses of the subjects to Piaget stories involving moral judgments. He found that in situations involving peer reciprocity and independence from adults, deaf children as represented by his subjects mature earlier than hearing ones, or at a comparable level. However, significantly higher scores were earned by the hearing subjects in situations involving a more subtle recognition of the distinction between motivation for and results of an action. However, differences appeared to level off by age 12, at which time no measurable differences in conscience development were found between the deaf and hearing subjects. Nass wisely modifies the finding with the caution, "The relations among conscience, morality, and superego are not clear . . . and a study of the responses of children to stories involving moral judgments cannot permit a direct test of this broader problem of differences in superego development" (1964, p. 1074).

Other psychoanalytically oriented investigations have been conducted through studies of the dreams of deaf persons. In the study by Mendelson, Siger, and Solomon (1960), the postulate employed was "that an individual deprived of the normal auditory and verbal processes of perception and communication in his social and cultural environment, will uniquely incorporate necessary modifications of such perception and communication into his fantasy behavior and dreams" (1960, p. 883). Three groups of deaf college students served as subjects; in the first group deafness was present since birth; in the second, before age 3; and in the third, after age 5. The investigators found that the dreams of the deaf subjects, regardless of age of onset of deafness, were markedly different from dreams of hearing persons. The difference was most marked among the congenitally deaf, whose dreams were characterized by greater vividness, more brilliant color, and greater frequency of dream recall, suggesting the greater frequency of dream occurrence. A number of interesting but inconclusive speculations are proposed by the investigators to account for the differences. Like Wile and Knapp, these investigators also express disagreement with the Isakower formula: "we have seen abundant evidence of superego structuring in our deaf populations" (1960, p. 887). They recommend continued investigation of the nonverbal aspects of superego formation and function.

In the dream study conducted by Sherman (1970), a 51-item questionnaire based on psychoanalytic theory was the instrument-of-inquiry in a comparison of the dreams of 50 deaf and 51 hearing college students. Sherman found no distinct differences between the groups in dream colors, vividness, spatial dimension, or frequency of recall. Significant differences were found in the occurrence of sound and the experiencing of emotions dreamt. Sound would not be expected to play as prominent a role in the dreams of the deaf as in those of the hearing. Concerning experienced dream-emotions, the investigator found that "the emotions in the deaf subjects' dreams were significantly not as lifelike as those of hearing students. Even in the specific emotion of fear the majority of the deaf group could not feel the emotion as they were dreaming it" (1970, p. 62). Sherman interprets this as signifying an "overcontrol of the primary process by the superego" and concludes that "this superego domination casts dubious light on the Isakower theory" (1970, p. 62).

As with many other provocative but inconclusive investigations, so with studies of dreams of the deaf—the challenge is for continued inquiry. For example, it would be interesting to test Isakower's statement that *"speech elements in dreams are a direct contribution from the superego to the manifest content of the dream''* (1954, p. 3, italics in original), by applying the postulate to sign language in dreams of the deaf. Also, the emotional flatness of dreams of the deaf as reported by Sherman warrants further study, particularly in view of the emotional flatness of the responses of deaf subjects as reported in projective personality research. For all dream studies, however, Knapp cautions that it is ''unwise to assign dream sensations, such as color, any universal connection with one or another 'compartment' of personality such as superego'' (1956, p. 332), since there is much in dream interpretation that is more speculative than definitive.

Existential Theory

In existential theory, man is regarded as the central force in his own development, continually striving for change and growth through involvement, commitment, and personal choice. In applying this theory to deaf individuals, Krippner and Easton stress the importance of finding a personal meaning to life. Lack of involvement and inability to find such meaning ''produces many individuals who behave in a mechanical manner, typically characterized by passivity, isolation, dependency, and emotional flatness'' (1972, p. 440). This picture, the investigators point out, is ''a strikingly appropriate description of many deaf children and adults'' (1972, p. 440). They maintain further that the pervasive existential problem of deafness ''is the hesitancy and fear of becoming involved in the life process'' (1972, p. 441). The investigators consider this to be largely an outcome of communicative mismanagement since early childhood and suggest corrective measures along total communication lines.

Eriksonian Theory

Eriksonian theory maintains that the whole human life cycle can be seen as progressing in a sequence of eight integrated critical phases, each of which has its own specific maturational task that must be successfully achieved in order to serve as effective preparation and foundation for the subsequent critical phase (Erikson, 1959). Erikson describes his eight critical phases in terms of extremes of successful and unsuccessful solution: (1) basic trust versus mistrust; (2) autonomy versus shame and doubt; (3) initiative versus guilt; (4) industry versus inferiority; (5) identity versus identity diffusion; (6) intimacy versus isolation; (7) generativity versus stagnation; (8) integrity versus despair.

Schlesinger and Meadow (1972) interpret the excessive amount of emotional disturbance they found among deaf pupil-populations in the light of Eriksonian theory, and ask whether communicative factors are significant in blocking satisfactory solutions to Erikson's early critical phases. They conclude that the main obstructing factors result from ineffective communicative exchange between a deaf child and important life figures from infancy onward, and express the conviction that many of the developmental handicaps so imposed can be lessened if not eliminated through early manual communicative intervention.

Clinical Psychiatry

Deaf persons with mental illnesses often provide significant theory-leads in the search for the elusive determinants of personality patterns. The most intensive work with mentally ill deaf persons has been that conducted at the Department of Medical Genetics of the New York State Psychiatric Institute, Columbia University. Some of the theory-leads coming from this source are summarized as follows:

> As a result of his hearing loss, the deaf child suffers both in the cognitive aspects of learning and thinking and the emotional correlates of communication with his parents in his early years. It was observed in the course of the project that certain unique personality features were present among deaf persons. They often showed a poorly developed ability to understand and care about the feelings of others; and they had inadequate insight into the impact on others of their own behavior and its consequences. With a generally egocentric view of the world and with demands unfettered by excessive control machinery (conscience), their adaptive approach may be characterized as gross coercive dependence. Their preferred defensive reactions to tension and anxiety are typified by a kind of primitive riddance through action. Even in the presence of more sophistication, defensive reactions remain at the level of simple projection. This mode of handling tension is reflected in impulsive behavior and the absence of much thoughtful introspection. (Rainer and Altshuler, 1966, pp. 141–42)

A number of interesting observations are made by Altshuler (1971) concerning symptoms of psychosis among the deaf patients of the mental health project. Alleged auditory hallucinations are reported by deaf patients about as often as by hearing schizophrenics. Altshuler interprets this phenomenon as either serving a wish-fulfilling function for the deaf patient or as a specific demand of the disease process, with audition cast in the form the subject imagines. Altshuler also remarks on the rare occurrence of obsessional character problems and psychotic depressions in his population. However, impulsive behavior was marked. He speculates that the various perceptual modes play broadly enabling roles in human adaptations, and the absence of a particular mode may prevent the normal development of certain adaptive options. Audition, for example, may be "somehow necessary to the internalized control of rage" (1971, p. 1525). In its absence, rage is externalized and impulsive.

Another source of information derived from mentally ill deaf patients was the project conducted by the Psychosomatic and Psychiatric Institute of Michael Reese Hospital in Chicago (Grinker, 1969). Two of the project's staff, Mindel and Vernon, report that "one of the most disturbing findings of the study was the pervasive underachievement of the outpatient population" (1971, p. 100). Despite average mental ability, many of the teenagers had an educational achievement level of 2nd or 3rd grade, with related impoverishment in general knowledge of social codes as well as lack of sex information. The investigators succinctly remark that "the failure of the educational system undermined efforts at psychotherapy and rehabilitation" (1971, p. 100). An interesting disagreement between this project and the New York State Psychiatric project concerned depressive illness among the patients. Depressive illness (as a primary diagnosis) as well as depressive affect were prominent in the Chicago project but rare in the New York State project. The Chicago staff interprets depressive signs as an internalization of thoughts of failure; the New York staff interprets its lack of depressive findings as due in part to the tendency of the patients to attribute failure to outside environmental causes rather than to personal ones. A strong underlying theme of the Chicago report is the critical need of deaf children for the communicative skills with which to establish the environmental relationships and interplay that are essential for healthy development and maturation. The Chicago staff expresses a strong indictment of education for failing to meet this need.

To sum up, the implications from personality theories and from clinical psychiatry suggest a picture of personality inadequacies, if not outright maladjustment, much along the lines of the test findings. The root cause is seen as lack of sufficient communicative input and individual–environment interplay from infancy onward. The corrective measure favored by most theorists is early manual communicative intervention.

Discussion

The inference from personality studies of the deaf is that beneath the buoyant life-behavior of most deaf persons lurks a pattern of emotional disturbance and maladjustment. With few exceptions, study after study confirms the view. So deeply ingrained is the concept that the mere mention of the term "personality of the deaf" flashes a stereotypic image to the professional community, an image of emotional immaturity, rigidity, social ineptness, and other such maladaptive traits (Donoghue, 1968).

The trouble with the image is that it is not a picture of personality; it is simply a list of traits. In themselves, traits do not answer the key question: What constellation of interlocking and counterbalancing psychic and cognitive forces constitutes the personality patterns of deaf persons? Despite decades of "personality" testing, we still do not have the answer. The full story has been obscured by numbers of beclouding factors, not the least of which are the tests themselves.

Growing disenchantment with traditional personality tests is spreading through contemporary psychology (Cronbach, 1970). As Buros remarks:

> In this era of remarkable progress in science and technology, it is sobering to think that our most widely used instruments for personality assessment were published 20, 30, 40, and even more years ago. Despite the tremendous amount of research devoted to these old, widely used tests, they have not been replaced by instruments more acceptable to the profession. Nor has the research resulted in a consensus among psychologists concerning the validities of a particular test. . . . In fact, all personality instruments may be described as controversial, each with its own following of devotees. (1970, pp. xxv–xxvi)

Thoughtful reviews of particularly troublesome issues in personality testing are presented by Mischel (1977) and Hogan, DeSoto, and Solano (1977). These include the trait concept in measurement, the role of environment, the multiple determinism of behavior, and what Hogan and associates call the "mindless research" resulting from the ease with which test data can be collected.

Of particular relevance to personality assessment of the deaf is Mischel's "norm-centered" versus "person-centered" issue. Mischel describes the difference: "A norm-centered approach compares people against each other, usually on a trait or attribute continuum—for example, amount of introversion-extroversion" (1977, p. 248). In contrast, the person-centered approach aims to describe a given individual in relation to the particular psychological foundations and conditions of his life.

Most of the "personality" tests used with the deaf are of the norm-and-trait-centered type. Further, the norms and traits are derived from data collected on hearing standardization groups, and the tests were originally used as clinical aids in psychiatric diagnosis. As such, most of them are heavily weighted with trait-items specifically selected to "snapshot" evidences of personality deviance among the hearing. There is no argument against their clinical use for this purpose. But neither can their findings be considered a balanced picture of total personality, and particularly not of personality patterns of deaf persons.

The use of such tests with the deaf is a matter of sheer necessity. Some time ago, I conducted an informal search for mental and personality tests specifically standardized for deaf populations. The search included the United States, through the more than 2,000 tests cited in Buros's *Tests in Print* (1961), and numbers of foreign countries through direct communication. The result was a grand total of 11 such tests standardized on the deaf, of which 9 were intelligence tests and 2 were personality tests—one an inventory devised by Brunschwig (1936) for deaf children, the other a non-verbal adaptation of the Make-a-Picture Story by Hess (1960), also for deaf children. This extreme paucity forces testers of the deaf to supplement these slim resources by dipping into the pool of measures standardized on the hearing. And thereby arises a debate.

Some claim that because the deaf live in the same world as the hearing, they should be tested with the same psychological measures. And others protest the unfairness of assessing deaf subjects with tests and norms based on hearing life experiences. One of the earliest protestors was Welles, who believed that personality inventories "are not probing the underlying drives which are the causal factors in any individual's emotional behavior, but are merely making a sampling of symptomatic material" (1932, p. 23). Another was Habbe, who said with irony that "that investigator is courageous who obtains a list of 'yes' and 'no' responses from several hundred personality inventories and proceeds therefrom to deduce conclusions relating to various individuals in the group thus studied" (1936, p. 11). Both of these investigators based their observations on their work with hearing-impaired subjects.

That the deaf and hearing live in the same physical world is obvious. But psychological test items are not based on the physical but on the psychological attributes of the "worlds" inhabited by test subjects. The question is: Do the deaf live in the same *psychological* world as the hearing? Do the items of hearing-standardized personality tests mean the same thing to the deaf conceptually or indicate the same psychological condition for the deaf adaptively as for hearing subjects? Can deaf and hearing subjects be validly compared on items which may carry different connotations for each? An illustration is the following item from the Minnesota Multiphasic Personality Inventory: "While in trains, busses, etc. I often talk to strangers." For most deaf persons there will be two opposite but equally correct answers to the statement. One is "No"; the other, "Yes." The ensuing scoring dilemma stems from the fact that the usual answer would be "no" if the stranger were a hearing person, but "yes" if the stranger were deaf. Examples of other inappropriate items in tests used with the deaf are: "My hearing is apparently as good as that of most people," also taken from the Minnesota Inventory; and "Do you prefer traveling with someone who will make all the necessary arrangements to the adventure of traveling alone?" from the Bernreuter Personality Inventory.

These few somewhat extreme examples give an idea of what it means to test deaf persons with measures based on hearing life experiences and reactions. When deaf persons answer items in such tests from their own life experiences (providing they understand the test language), they run the risk of "deviating from the norm," and so being scored "maladjusted." Even when a conscientious examiner carefully pores over the test, weeds out the grossly inappropriate items and simplifies the test language, the principles on which the remaining items were selected and standardized are not thereby altered. They are still based on hearing life experiences and hearing pathological signs, hence are just as inappropriate for the deaf as are the eliminated items, albeit less obviously so. The same holds true, in principle, for projective as well as inventory tests.

To one familiar with the life behavior of deaf children and adults, with their ability to cope, with their remarkable tolerance for frustration, and with their social energies and enthusiasms, the test-derived personality picture is singularly noninformative, flat, and lifeless. The most conspicuous omissions are the psychic dynamisms that act to maintain individual integrity. What emerges is "emotional immaturity, rigidity, social ineptness" and other such test-derived signs that are more indicative of sociocultural deprivation than of personality. What we need to know is the interplay of counterbalancing psychic forces that enable deaf persons to cope, survive, and even advance. That we lack this knowledge is the expected outcome when our personality picture of an individual, whether deaf or hearing, is derived from tests that emphasize simple, quantifiable responses, that are constructed to follow single lines of trait inquiry, and that are based on comparisons with norms—in the case of the deaf, inapplicable norms.

The conviction in contemporary psychology is that new approaches in personality testing and research are long overdue. As Mischel observes: "The future of personality measurement will be brighter if we can move beyond our favorite pencil-and-paper and laboratory measures to include direct observations as well as unobtrusive nonreactive measures to study lives where they are really lived and not merely where the researcher finds it convenient to look at them" (1977, p. 248). The statement calls to mind the rationale of Barker's eco-psychological research, discussed in chapter 1, and exemplifies the growing trend in personality psychology to reach out into real-life environments and study personality and behavior in terms of real-life encounters.

Various techniques for accomplishing this kind of assessment are cited by Bersoff (1973), who calls his own technique "psychosituational assessment." The major aim is to describe an individual as he interacts with and is affected by the environment and its occupants. For example, in the environment of a classroom, Bersoff's approach would include the behaviors of both the child and the teacher; they "co-constitute" the behavior setting, and careful observations and notations are made of the flow of behaviors evoked by their interactions and confrontations.

It will take some time before such complex changes in personality assessment are perfected, and even more before they are applied to the deaf. In the meanwhile, judgments about the "personality of the deaf" must reach beyond the static results of conventional tests and testing; and even beyond conventional concepts of "mental health." There is something more to the personality patterns of deaf persons than the tests reveal, something that enables them to meet the demands and tensions of life with more spirit than passivity, with more energy than inertia, more humor than anger, more hope than despair; and that impels even someone like Roberto to reach to the stars. It is time to look beyond the test-elicited stereotype of "the" deaf personality, derived, it must be pointed out, largely from studies of deaf schoolagers and clinical cases, and to balance the picture with studies of the real-life coping mechanisms and survival strategies of deaf adults, such as seen in the sketches from life.

References

Altable, J. P. 1947. The Rorschach psychodiagnostic as applied to deaf-mutes. *Rorschach Research Exchange and Journal of Projective Techniques,* 11: 74–79.

Altshuler, K. Z. 1971. Studies of the deaf: Relevance to psychiatric theory. *American Journal of Psychiatry,* 127: 1521–26.

Ayers, P. 1950. Some aspects of personality in deaf adolescents. Ph.D. dissertation, University of California.

Beizman, C. 1950. Quelques considerations sur le Rorschach des sourd-muets. *Enfance* 3: 33–48.

Bersoff, D. N. 1973. Silk purses into sow's ears: The decline of psychological testing and a suggestion for its redemption. *American Psychologist,* 28: 892–99.

Bindon, D. M. 1957a. Make-A-Picture Story (MAPS) test findings for rubella-deaf children. *Journal of Abnormal and Social Psychology,* 55: 38–42.

Bindon, D. M. 1957b. Rubella-deaf children: A Rorschach study employing Monroe Inspection Technique. *British Journal of Psychology,* 48: 249–58.

Blum, G. S. 1953. *Psychoanalytic Theories of Personality.* New York: McGraw-Hill.

Bradway, K. P. 1937. The social competence of deaf children. *American Annals of the Deaf,* 82: 122–40.

Bricklin, B., Piotrowski, Z. A., and Wagner, E. E. 1962. *The Hand Test: A New Projective Test with Special Reference to the Prediction of Overt Aggressive Behavior.* Springfield, Ill.: Charles C. Thomas.

Brunschwig, L. 1936. *A Study of Personality Aspects of Deaf Children.* Teachers College Contributions to Education, No. 687. New York: Teachers College, Columbia University.

Burchard, E., and Myklebust, H. R. 1942. A comparison of congenital and adventitious deafness with respect to its effect on intelligence, personality, and social maturity. *American Annals of the Deaf,* 87: 140–54.

Buros, O. K. 1961. *Tests in Print.* Highland Park, N.J.: Gryphon Press.

Buros, O. K. 1970. *Personality: Tests and Reviews.* Highland Park, N.J.: Gryphon Press.

Cronbach, L. J. 1970. *Essentials of Psychological Testing.* 3d ed. New York: Harper and Row.

Donoghue, R. J. 1968. The deaf personality—a study in contrasts. *Journal of Rehabilitation of the Deaf,* 2: 37–52.

Erikson, E. H. 1959. *Identity and the Life Cycle.* New York: International University Press.

Finkelstein, J. 1968. Ego aspects of deafness. Paper presented at the Workshop for Psychiatrists on Deafness and the Deaf, New York University, May, 1968.

Freud, S. 1947. *The Ego and the Id.* London: Hogarth Press.

Gelbmann, F. 1952. A study of sex differences in personality characteristics of the deaf as determined by the Mosaic Test. Master's thesis, Catholic University of America.

Goetzinger, C. P., Ortiz, J. D., Bellerose, B., and Buchan, L. G. 1966. A study of the S. O. Rorschach with deaf and hearing adolescents. *American Annals of the Deaf,* 3: 510–22.

Grinker, R. G. 1969. Psychiatric diagnosis, therapy, and research of the psychotic deaf. Final report. (Available from Dr. Grinker, Michael Reese Hospital, Chicago, Illinois.)

Habbe, S. 1936. *Personality Adjustments of Adolescent Boys with Impaired Hearing.* Teachers College Contributions to Education, no. 697. New York: Teachers College, Columbia University.

Hall, C. S., and Lindzey, G. 1978. *Theories of personality.* 3d ed. New York: Wiley.

Healey, R. E. 1952. A study of personality differences between hearing and non-hearing girls as determined by the Mosaic Test. Master's thesis, Catholic University of America.

Hess, D. W. 1960. A study of personality and adjustment in deaf and hearing children using a non-verbal modification of the Make-A-Picture Story (MAPS) Test. Ph.D. dissertation, University of Rochester.

Hess, D. W. 1969. Evaluation of the young deaf adult. *Journal of Rehabilitation of the Deaf,* 3: 6–22.

Hogan, R., DeSoto, C. B., and Solano, C. 1977. Traits, tests, and personality research. *American Psychologist,* 32: 255–64.

Isakower, O. 1939. On the exceptional position of the auditory sphere. *International Journal of Psychoanalysis,* 20: 340–48.

Isakower, O. 1954. Spoken words in dreams. *Psychoanalytic Quarterly,* 23: 1–6.

Kirk, S. A. 1938. Behavior problem tendencies in deaf and hard of hearing children. *American Annals of the Deaf,* 83: 131–37.

Kline, T. K. 1945. A study of the free association test with deaf children. *American Annals of the Deaf,* 90: 237–58.

Knapp, P. H. 1953. The ear, listening and hearing. *Journal of the American Psychoanalytic Association,* 1: 672–89.

Knapp, P. H. 1956. Sensory impressions in dreams. *Psychoanalytic Quarterly,* 25: 325.

Krippner, S., and Easton, H. 1972. Deafness: An existential interpretation. *American Annals of the Deaf*, 117: 440–46.

Levine, E. S. 1948. An investigation into the personality of normal deaf adolescent girls. Ph.D. dissertation, New York University.

Levine, E. S. 1956. *Youth in a Soundless World*. New York: New York University Press.

Levine, E. S. 1960. *The Psychology of Deafness*. New York: Columbia University Press.

Levine, E. S. 1963. Studies in the psychological evaluation of the deaf. *Volta Review*, 65 (Special Research Issue): 496–512.

Levine, E. S., and Wagner, E. E. 1974. *Personality Patterns of Deaf Persons: An Interpretation Based on Research with the Hand Test*, Monograph Supplement 4-V39, *Perceptual and Motor Skills*.

Lyon, V. W. 1934. Personality tests with the deaf. *American Annals of the Deaf*, 79: 1–4.

McAndrew, H. 1948. Rigidity and isolation: A study of the deaf and blind. *Journal of Abnormal and Social Psychology*, 43: 474–94.

Mendelson, J. H., Siger, L., and Solomon, P. 1960. Psychiatric observations on congenital and acquired deafness: Symbolic and perceptual processes in dreams. *American Journal of Psychiatry*, 116: 883–88.

Mindel, E. D., and Vernon, M. 1971. *They Grow in Silence*. Silver Spring, Md.: National Association of the Deaf.

Mischel, W. 1977. On the future of personality measurement. *American Psychologist*, 32: 246–54.

Myklebust, H. 1960. *The Psychology of Deafness*. New York: Grune and Stratton.

Nass, M. I. 1964. Development of conscience: A comparison of the moral judgment of deaf and hearing children. *Child Development*, 35: 1073–80.

Norris, A. G., Ed. 1972. *Deafness*, vol. 2. Silver Spring, Md.: Professional Rehabilitation Workers with the Adult Deaf.

Pintner, R., and Brunschwig, L. 1937. A study of certain fears and wishes among deaf and hearing children. *Journal of Educational Psychology*, 28: 259–70.

Pintner, R., Fusfeld, I. S., and Brunschwig, L. 1937. Personality tests of deaf adults. *Journal of Genetic Psychology*, 51: 305–27.

Rainer, J. D., and Altshuler, K. Z. 1966. *Comprehensive Mental Health Services for the Deaf*. New York: New York State Psychiatric Institute, Columbia University.

Rainer, J. D., Altshuler, K. Z., Kallmann, F. J., and Deming, R., Eds. 1963. *Family and Mental Health Problems in a Deaf Population*. New York: New York State Psychiatric Institute, Columbia University.

Ruitenbeek, H. M. 1964. *Varieties of Personality Theory*. New York: Dutton.

Schlesinger, H. S., and Meadow, K. P. 1972. *Sound and Sign*. Berkeley: University of California Press.

Schonberger, W. J. 1952. A study of the personality characteristics of the deaf and the nondeaf as determined by the Mosaic Test. Master's thesis, Catholic University of America.

Sherman, W. A. 1970. A comparative assessment of hearing and deaf dream characteristics. *Journal of Rehabilitation of the Deaf*, 4: 54–64.

Springer, N. N. 1938a. A comparative study of the behavior traits of deaf and hearing children of New York City. *American Annals of the Deaf*, 83: 255–73.

Springer, N. N. 1938b. A comparative study of psychoneurotic responses of deaf
and hearing subjects. *Journal of Educational Psychology*, 29: 459–66.

Springer, N. N., and Roslow, S. 1938. A further study of the psychoneurotic responses of deaf and hearing children. *Journal of Educational Psychology*, 29:
590–96.

Streng, A., and Kirk, S. A. 1938. The social competence of deaf and hard of hearing
children in a public day school. *American Annals of the Deaf*, 83: 244–54.

Vegely, A. B. 1971. Performance of hearing-impaired children on a nonverbal personality test. *American Annals of the Deaf*, 116: 427–34.

Vegely, A. B., and Elliott, I. I. 1968. Applicability of a standardized personality test
to a hearing-impaired population. *American Annals of the Deaf*, 113: 858–69.

Wagner, E. E. 1962. *Hand Test: Manual for Administration, Scoring and Interpretation*. Los Angeles: Western Psychological Services.

Welles, H. H. 1932. *The Measurement of Certain Aspects of Personality among
Hard of Hearing Adults*. Teachers College Contributions to Education, no. 545.
New York: Teachers College, Columbia University.

Wile, I. S. 1933. Some mental hygiene problems of the deaf. In *Proceedings of the
International Congress on the Education of the Deaf*. West Trenton, N.J.: New
Jersey School for the Deaf.

Zivkovic, M. 1971. Influence of deafness on the structure of personality. *Perceptual
and Motor Skills*, 33: 863–66.

Part Four
THE
PSYCHOLOGICAL
EXAMINATION

8 Psychology and the I Background

ONE MIGHT suppose that the unique situation presented by humans reared in a "silent world" would have drawn psychologists to the field of the deaf as if by a magnet. However, a glance at the historical facts indicates otherwise. Indeed, the countless problems associated with prelinguistic deafness have discouraged all but the most intrepid from entering the field.

The way in is barred by a number of stubborn obstacles. To overcome them demands competencies of an unusual order, as reviewed in chapter 9. All in all, they present formidable challenges to psychological practice with a deaf clientele. Yet despite the barriers, psychologists have managed to survive a sometimes interrupted and often disheartening journey through the field of the deaf and, what is more, to bring the journey to its present optimistic state. How this came about provides both background and context for later discussion. The following historical sketch traces some of the trends and highlights.

The Pioneers

With the opening of the first public schools for the deaf in the early nineteenth century, educators found themselves faced with a mass of illiterate human enigmas whose minds were trapped in silence and ignorance, but who nevertheless had to be taught. The question was: How? What kind of minds did these enigmas possess? How much of the world's culture and custom could they assimilate; how much of society's standards, obligations, and values? In short, what could be done to bring life to these minds as yet unborn?

Ordinarily, psychology would have been called upon to help find the answers. But these were the early days. Psychology was still in the throes of its own evolutionary struggles. No help could be expected from this quarter.

Educators of the deaf had perforce to struggle with their problems alone.

They did their own observing, experimenting, and interpreting. Their schools resembled psychological laboratories as well as educational workshops. As pioneer investigators of the dynamics of human behavior in a context of deafness, these early educators can truly be said to have been the first psychologists in the field of the deaf. Poring over their publications, the reader is struck by the range of their interests and observations and by the keenness of their perceptions. Unhampered by rules of objectivity, their curiosity and speculations were free to explore any enticing path of psychological inquiry.

One such path led to a momentous achievement, albeit unrecognized as such in the small, isolated field of the deaf. In 1889, David Greenberger, then principal of the Institution for the Improved Instruction of Deaf Mutes, now the Lexington School for the Deaf, published his procedures for "testing" the intelligence of deaf children (Greenberger, 1889). The "test-tasks" and evaluative concepts were not too dissimilar from those used today. However, this was some two decades before the father of all psychological tests—the Binet-Simon scale—appeared on the scene.

Greenberger himself seems not to have recognized the psychological importance of his singular achievement. He considered his procedures more an educational than a psychological contribution, a possible solution to a common educational dilemma of the times. This was the problem of estimating the intelligence of applicants for school admission whose mental abilities could not be readily discerned. Some of the children were noncommunicative but not necessarily deaf; many belonged in institutions for the mentally retarded; and others had fine minds behind the dull façades, minds only waiting to be activated. Greenberger called such children the "doubtful cases" and complained that to differentiate among them "is one of the most difficult tasks that devolved upon the head of an institution for deaf-mutes" (1889, p. 93). Interestingly enough, it was the same type of problem in the regular schools that led to the later construction of the Binet-Simon intelligence test, which in turn led to the development of the whole psychological testing movement as we know it today. It was an educator of the deaf who anticipated this solution, but its full significance was not perceived. There was no follow-up at the time. But psychology was in the air, and the need to "understand" children was considered essential to educational success. Among the firm believers was Taylor, who, like Greenberger, was an educator of the deaf. As early as 1894, Taylor deplored the fact that although children are the most important creatures on earth, they are the least understood. He pushed for greater recognition of the values of psychology to the education of the deaf, and urged a closer study of deaf pupils. In this he was joined by other forward-looking educators of the deaf, and it was largely through their insistence that pioneer psychological investigations were begun.

A compelling interest of these early studies was how deaf pupils compared with hearing ones in regard to various mental and physical attributes. The instruments used in these investigations reflect the tests of the period, and include such tasks as spelling, memory, strength of grip, tapping, sensory acuity, and perception of size and weight (Mott, 1899, 1900; Taylor, 1897, 1898). The studies generally showed the deaf to be as good as and in certain instances superior to the hearing.

It remained for the most thoroughgoing investigation of the time to come up with less favorable findings. This was a study conducted by MacMillan and Bruner (1906), which showed the deaf to be considerably poorer than the hearing in a prime intelligence measure of the day—the cancellation of A's. In their wisdom, the investigators did not leap to conclusions. They reasoned that this inferiority could possibly mean no more than delayed rather than retarded development; that if the deaf child's education were begun considerably earlier than the customary 6 years, this inferiority might well be reduced if not altogether eliminated. (This possibility had not escaped others in the field. As early as 1893 a "Union of Kindergartners for the Deaf" was organized for the purpose of introducing preschool programs in all schools for the deaf [Hudson, 1893, 1894].)

A highly important outcome of the MacMillan-Bruner study was that it demonstrated the practical value of the psychological examination. Educators were ripe for such demonstrations and eager for help. Thus, when the first English translation of the Binet-Simon test appeared in 1910, it was greeted with enthusiastic interest by many educators in the field of the deaf. Greenberger's proposal had not been entirely forgotten. The Binet-Simon intelligence test was looked upon as a possible means toward that end.

Era of Search for the I.Q.

The appearance of the Binet-Simon test and its objective frame of reference stimulated a new era in psychological involvement with the deaf, one devoted largely to establishing the mental status of the population. Inaugurating the era was Rudolf Pintner, himself a psychologist. From the time of his first publication on the deaf in 1915 until his untimely death in 1942, Pintner was directly or indirectly responsible for much of the psychological research in the field, and for the introduction of professional psychologists.

The first important effort in the search for the I.Q. was an attempt by Pintner and Paterson to use the Binet-Simon test with the deaf (Pintner and Paterson, 1915). The Goddard revision was tried with 22 deaf pupils whose average chronological age was 12.5 years. The test was administered in whatever methods of communication the subjects preferred, but even so, 4 were completely unable to take the test. Of the remaining 18, the results showed an average mental age of 7.9 years and an average mental retardation of 4.58 years. However, the investigators were by no means satisfied with their findings. They complained of countless difficulties in test administration and deplored the complete unsuitability of many of the test questions to the life situation of the deaf. In short, they concluded that verbal measures of the Binet type could not be used with the deaf and recommended the use of performance tests instead.

The construction of the Pintner-Paterson Performance Scale in 1917 was the direct outcome of their recommendation. The Binet Scale suggested the theoretical frame of reference; but on the performance scale, intelligence was measured through manipulative rather than verbal tasks. The appearance of this objective scale which could be administered nonverbally opened a new test avenue for the study of the mental abilities of the deaf.

The next quarter-century witnessed a tremendous surge of psychological activity. The stress was on investigation rather than service. Studies were conducted on personality (as already reviewed), on scholastic achievement, special skills, and on other attributes and aptitudes (Pintner, Eisenson, and Stanton, 1941); but the major focus was on establishing the mental status of the deaf.

In the early years of this search for the elusive "deaf" I.Q., the principal tests used were paper and pencil nonlanguage group tests, and the popular performance scales. Among the former were studies using the Pintner Nonlanguage Mental Test (Day, Fusfeld, and Pintner, 1928; MacKane, 1933; Reamer, 1921; Shirley and Goodenough, 1932) and the Goodenough "Draw-a-Man" test (Petersen and Williams, 1930; Shirley and Goodenough, 1932; Springer, 1938). Performance scale studies were conducted using the Drever-Collins Performance Scale, one of the earliest tests standardized on deaf children (Drever and Collins, 1928), the Grace Arthur Point Performance Scale (Bishop, 1936; Burchard and Myklebust, 1942; Lyon, 1933), the Randall's Island Performance Series (Schick, 1933), and the Advanced Performance Series (Lane and Schneider, 1941). Studies were also conducted with the Kohs Block Design (Petersen, 1936) and with the Porteus Maze test (Zeckel and van der Kolk, 1939). The findings of the studies were in sharp conflict, with retardation ranging from minor to substantial being reported by more than half the investigators and "average range I.Q." reported by the others.

The influx of conflicting estimates of the mental abilities of the deaf from these and other studies proved pretty disconcerting to educators of the deaf.

They were at a loss concerning which mental level to gear their educational programs to. In an effort to break the deadlock, MacKane (1933) used a battery of performance scales—the Drever-Collins, the Pintner-Paterson, and the Grace Arthur—plus the Pintner Nonlanguage Mental Test with 130 deaf children ranging in age from 10 to 12 years, each of whom was paired with a matched hearing subject. But here too the findings were at odds, with about a 1-year retardation reported for performance test results and as much as 2 years on the Pintner Nonlanguage Mental Test.

Understandably, the enthusiasm with which educators had welcomed psychology into the fold was considerably shaken by these returns. The hope had been that psychology would open the door to a clearer view of deaf persons and the needs of deaf pupils. But the hope was dashed by the conflicting picture that emerged. In their disappointment, educators held psychologists largely to blame, claiming with Aurell that "the ordinary students of psychology are not fully qualified to deal with the psychology of the deaf. They lack the empiric knowledge of the deaf which can be gained only by teaching them and living with them in everyday life. . . . Their lack of familiarity with the deaf is too obvious to inspire a teacher of the deaf with confidence" (1934, p. 230).

Psychologists, on the other hand, held the psychological tests largely to blame. By this time it was recognized that traditional performance tests were not the ideal investigative instruments. Deaf children had become so accustomed to taking them that they could "do them in their sleep," as one disgruntled worker put it. The time had come to try other tests and techniques. Educators might indeed have soured on psychology, but psychology did not give up the search.

Reviews of efforts to break away from traditional text instruments can be found elsewhere in the literature (Levine, 1960a, 1963, 1971, 1976). In brief, these efforts focused on three lines of investigation: (1) the search for other types of intelligence tests that showed promise for use with deaf subjects even though they had been standardized on the nondeaf; (2) the construction and standardization of intelligence tests designed specifically for the deaf; and (3) efforts to identify "valid" tests by establishing the concurrent validity of various intelligence tests used with the deaf.

Examples of the other types of intelligence tests tried out in this breakaway period include: the full-scale Wechsler-Bellevue Scale for the Measurement of the Intelligence of Adolescents and Adults, Form I (Levine, 1956a); the nonverbal Raven's Progressive Matrices, 1938 edition (Oléron, 1950); the Long and Welsh Test of Causal Reasoning, Brody Nonverbal Abstract Reasoning Test, Deutsche questions (Templin, 1950); the full-scale Wechsler Intelligence Scale for Children (Smith, 1962); the performance portions of various Wechsler scales (Goetzinger and Rousey, 1957; Lavos, 1962); and the verbal and nonverbal portions of the Federal Service Examination (Stunkel, 1957).

The findings obtained from these and other nontraditional test approaches indicated that the deaf are of normal mental potential, with average range I.Q.'s on nonverbal and nonlanguage measures but with considerably less than average I.Q. scores on verbal tests. Of the verbal test retardation, Templin commented, "Since this retardation persists even when intelligence is controlled, a heavy share of the burden for this deficiency must be attributed to the specific training of these deaf subjects" (1950, p. 269).

Certain psychologists saw a way out of the test dilemma through the construction of intelligence tests specifically designed for the deaf and standardized on a deaf population. Among the tests so designed both in this country and abroad are the following: the previously cited Drever and Collins Performance Scale (Drever and Collins, 1928); the Ontario School Ability Examination (Amoss, 1936); the Nebraska Test of Learning Aptitude for Young Deaf Children (Hiskey, 1941); the DuToit Group Test (DuToit, 1954); the Borelli and Oléron Performance Scale (Borelli and Oléron, 1954); the Baar Nonlanguage Scale for Children (Baar, 1957); the Hayashi Intelligence Test for Deaf Children, modeled after the Nebraska Test (Hayashi, 1959); the Snijders-Oomen Non-Verbal Intelligence Tests (Snijders and Snijders-Oomen, 1959); and the Smith-Johnson Non-verbal Performance Scale (Smith and Johnson, 1978). Several of these tests were standardized on hearing as well as deaf children, namely the Nebraska, the Snijders-Oomen, and the Smith-Johnson Scale.

In view of the small number and overlapping applicability of intelligence tests standardized on deaf children, nondeaf-standardized tests maintained their important position in test practices with such children. In consequence, a number of studies addressed the question of whether these as well as tests standardized on the deaf were actually measuring what they purported to measure. The approach was through an examination of concurrent validity. Kirk and Perry (1948) compared the Ontario and Nebraska tests, using as criterion test the Terman 1937 revision of the Stanford-Binet Scale, and found the Ontario scores closer to Binet results than were the Nebraska scores. Another study of the Nebraska Test was conducted by MacPherson and Lane (1948), using as criteria tests the Advanced Performance Scale for their older deaf subjects, and the Randall's Island Series for the younger ones. High correlations among the tests were found, thereby implying the validity of the Nebraska Test as a measure of intelligence for deaf children. Other tests studied along concurrent validity lines included: the various Wechsler performance scales (Brill, 1962; Graham and Shapiro, 1953; Larr and Cain, 1959); Raven's Progressive Matrices (Harris, 1959; Levine and

Iscoe, 1955; Seifert, 1960); the Chicago Nonverbal Examination (Johnson, 1947; Lavos, 1950); the Leiter International Performance Scale (Birch and Birch, 1951; Mira, 1962); and the Columbia Mental Maturity Scale (Kodman, Waters, and Whipple, 1962). Lavos (1954) studied the interrelationship among three nonlanguage intelligence tests used with the deaf—the Chicago Nonverbal, the Pintner General Ability, and the Revised Beta—and found good correlations among them, with validity assumed from the correlations. However, despite conscientious inquiry, no "best test" emerged from the search.

Other aspects of test attributes were also examined by inquiring psychologists. Such studies include: the predictive ability of the Hiskey Test for academic achievement, with equivocal results (Giangreco, 1966); the test-retest reliability of the Chicago Non-Verbal, the 1938 Raven's Matrices, and the Terman Nonlanguage Multi-Mental tests, with a finding of significant increase in retest scores on all the tests (Goetzinger, Wills, and Dekker, 1967); construction of a scale of "cognitive capacity" for the deaf, consisting of such familiar performance tasks as the Knox Cube, Alexander Passalong Binet Beads adaptation, a form-assembly task, and a block design task (Kearney, 1969); a deaf–hearing group comparison using Raven's 1947 Colored Matrices, which showed no significant difference between the groups (Goetzinger and Houchins, 1969); and a comparison of teachers' ranking of intelligence with the test results obtained from the Leiter International Performance Scale and the Raven's Colored Matrices, with the finding of no difference between teacher evaluations and test results for each test used (Musgrove and Counts, 1975). Of special interest to me was a study by Ross (1970), which followed the lines of my investigation (Levine, 1956) in which the full Wechsler Adult Intelligence Scale was used for a comparison of verbal I.Q.'s and performance I.Q.'s of the deaf subjects. The Ross study found a 34-I.Q.-point difference between the two in favor of the Wechsler Performance Scale I.Q., and points out the sharper predictive value of the verbal I.Q. in various life-achievement areas as opposed to the performance I.Q.

Although the normal mental potentials of the deaf were firmly established by the cumulative results of these studies, there still remained the question of how to account for the poor showing in learning-related accomplishments. The I.Q. score could not provide the answer. Investigation branched out into other areas. One group of studies concentrated on digging beneath the I.Q. with Piaget test-tasks in order to get at the information-processing patterns of the deaf. The assumption was that such tasks would provide a more refined means for ascertaining if there were any malfunction with the information-processing system to account for problems in the acquisition and application of knowledge. Heading the move was psychologist Hans

Furth (1964, 1966; Levine, 1976). The conclusion reached by Furth, his associates and followers was that there are no basic malfunctions in the cognitive capacities of the deaf, and that whatever inferiority may be found in cognitive competence can be attributed to experiential and linguistic deficits and communication handicaps. This was more or less how the old I.Q. investigators saw the picture. The key inquiry that initiated the Furth studies still needs answering, namely, What is the *nature* of the cognitive processes and imagery that sustain thinking and reasoning in a context of deafness? Obviously psychologists have decades of work ahead of them in the field of the deaf before answers are found to the many unresolved questions that haunt inquiry.

The Flowering of Psychological Services

Although psychological investigations of the deaf flourished and spread during the post–World War II decades, psychology as a service profession had harder going. Attitudes toward psychologists remained strongly influenced by Aurell's judgment. That the difficulties experienced by these workers stemmed mainly from a lack of training opportunities went unnoticed. However, the post-war years brought a pressing need for rehabilitation services (Office of Vocational Rehabilitation, 1956, 1957a,b, 1958), and it was largely through advances in vocational rehabilitation legislation that psychology as a service profession gradually found its way into the field of the deaf.

In the course of legislative advance, it was recognized that there is a psychological component to rehabilitation that requires at least as much attention as the physical or vocational. It was at this time that the terms "total rehabilitation," "helping the whole man," and "helping the person to help himself" appeared in rehabilitation literature and thinking. Psychology was in the air again, and this time its focus was on the human aspects of physical disability, including deafness.

Among the first to perceive the possible value of psychological services to deaf children was the Bureau for Handicapped Children of the New York State Department of Education. As early as 1954, the Bureau conducted a round-table conference in collaboration with the Lexington School for the Deaf on such services. This was probably the first such meeting held on the subject, certainly the first in New York State. The questions considered are as timely now as they were then. They included: (1) What general categories of services fall under the heading "psychological services for hearing-impaired children"? (2) What specific services are presently being rendered by psychologists in the field? (3) What psychological services are being rendered by nonpsychologists? (4) What are the outstanding problems in psychological evaluation of the deaf and the hard of hearing? (5) What are the outstanding needs? (6) Which psychological tests and measures are presently found useful with the deaf, the hard of hearing? (7) For what kinds of recommendations should the psychologist be responsible, how should they be formulated, how communicated? (8) Which outstanding problems might be solved or helped through a psychological service program and how should such a program be organized? (9) What background of training and experiences are considered necessary for the person engaged in rendering psychological services to the hearing-impaired? Serving as base of reference for discussion was the psychological service program newly initiated at the Lexington School for the Deaf (Levine, 1948). The proceedings of this prophetic conference were not published, simply mimeographed, and so the impact remained on a narrow, local level.

Considerably broader notice was accorded psychology when the first federal grant under PL 565 was made to the field of the deaf in 1956 (Office of Vocational Rehabilitation, 1956). The award went to the now celebrated Mental Health Center for the Deaf at the New York State Psychiatric Institute (Levine, 1960b; Rainer et al., 1963). In view of psychology's deep involvement in mental health, the grant served a singular advocacy function for psychological service to the deaf.

Further recognition of the profession came with the first national conference on psychological assessment of the deaf in 1959, sponsored by the U.S. Office of Vocational Rehabilitation and conducted by the Department of Psychology and Psychiatry of The Catholic University of America in collaboration with Gallaudet College. Here, too, there were no published proceedings. Another of the "firsts" in which psychology was involved was a national conference on research needs in the vocational rehabilitation of the deaf (Rogers and Quigley, 1960), also sponsored by the Office of Vocational Rehabilitation. From these beginnings there eventually emerged an exceptional flow of research, demonstration, and training projects in the service of the deaf, excellently listed and annotated in the *Deafness Annual* publications of the Professional Rehabilitation Workers with the Deaf (later the American Deafness and Rehabilitation Association).

The decade that followed witnessed a gradual increase in the number of psychologists entering the field, some of whom were themselves deaf. Activities branched in many directions and included not only research but also psychological assessment, advocacy and outreach, counseling, psychotherapy, publications, in-service training, and more (Levine, 1976).

However, this flowering of activities brought psychology under close scrutiny, especially in view of the mandated psychological assessment responsibilities under the education of All Handicapped Children Act. The feedback was not favorable. Yet it is clearly irrational to expect psychologists who lacked the necessary training, to cope effectively with the complex problems of assessment presented by the deaf; but the equally irrational feeling still persists in many lay and professional circles, that psychologists are magically prepared for any assignment involving human behavior. When this proved not to be the case in work with the deaf, a general undercurrent of dissatisfaction threatened a lack of confidence in the profession similar to that expressed in the past.

To forestall this eventuality, a national survey was conducted to get the psychologists' side of the story (Levine, 1974). Work on the survey was begun in 1971 with an initial plan and an immediate handicap. The plan was to develop and mail-distribute as comprehensive a questionnaire as feasible (Appendix H) to psychological service providers to the deaf, in order to obtain first-hand information about their backgrounds, experiences with the deaf, their psychological practices, problems, and recommendations. The handicap was the lack of a mailing list, registry, or other reference material for identifying and locating such personnel. Fortunately, the Alexander Graham Bell Association for the Deaf and the National Association of the Deaf made available their general mailing lists. Through their good offices, 178 usable returns were received from respondents in 48 states; of these returns, 76 represented special schools for the deaf; 62, special classes for the deaf; 24, wholly or partially integrated situations; and 16, nonschool facilities. The combined total of deaf individuals served in all these facilities was over 24,000.

Responses to the questionnaire were unusually detailed, thoughtful, and frank, almost as if the respondents were grateful for the interest shown. The general theme indicated the respondents were, if anything, even more unhappy with their professional lot in the field of the deaf than were the consumers with their services. The large majority were practicing without any substantive knowledge of deafness or the deaf, without having been afforded an opportunity for specialized training, and without the ability to communicate manually or to establish productive interpersonal relations with manual deaf clients. Most had never even met a deaf person prior to assuming professional practice with such individuals. Their problems were compounded by exceptional difficulties in the use and interpretation of psychological tests with the deaf. A considerable number of respondents commented that their employers had only vague notions of what to expect from psychologists: some assumed they were experts in all aspects of practice; others, that their principal ability and function was to test. Among the recommendations made was universal support for a closer look at the picture by way of a national conference.

The recommendation was carried out in 1974 when a three-day national conference on The Preparation of Psychological Service Providers to the Deaf was convened at Spartanburg, South Carolina, hosted by the South Carolina School for the Deaf and the Blind and supported in part by the Rehabilitation Services Administration of the Department of Health, Education, and Welfare (Levine, 1977). The conference objectives were to: (1) review the functions that qualified service-psychologists are normally expected to carry out in line with their professional training and responsibilities; (2) analyze and determine the functions expected of psychological service providers to the deaf in the various settings in which they practice; (3) analyze and determine the special bodies of knowledge, skills, and competencies required to carry out these functions effectively; (4) recommend courses of study and various types of training programs through which these competencies could be acquired; and (5) propose ideas concerning such issues as program accreditation and worker certification.

At this first such national conference, informally called the Spartanburg Conference, the aim was to reach out for input not only to service providers but also to other major figures and professional disciplines that were directly or indirectly involved in the psychological frame. Experiences and reactions were obtained from the more than 100 participants from every state of the continental United States who represented special schools and classes for the deaf, rehabilitation agencies and centers, special services in hearing and speech and in mental health, college- and university-based programs on the deaf, national organizations and agencies of and for the deaf, parent organizations, and denominational services. The disciplines represented included psychology, education, rehabilitation, counseling, administration, denominations, audiology, speech and hearing therapy, interpreting, and parentage. Among the participants 12 were hearing impaired, of whom 7 designated themselves as "deaf."

Despite the short duration of the conference, the contributions covered much ground, including psychological service functions, special competencies, training, and tentative suggestions regarding certification and accreditation (Levine, 1977). A detailed account cannot be given here, but some of the recommendations are included in later discussions. In brief, after decades of underrecognized importance, a start was made at the Spartanburg Conference to establish psychological practice with the deaf as a professional specialty in its own right.

Follow-up to the conference was almost immediate. Projects in line with the Spartanburg recommendations were begun all over the country, with the development of training programs at a number of facilities. It appears that service psychology is well on the way to doing justice to itself in this highly complex area of human behavior and, more importantly, doing justice to its deaf clientele. It now remains for some innovative thinking to be given to new kinds of psychological instrumentation that will do justice to both.

References

Amoss, H. 1936. *Ontario School Ability Examination*. Toronto: Ryerson Press.

Aurell, E. 1934. A new era in the history of the education of the deaf. *American Annals of the Deaf*, 79: 223–30.

Baar, E. 1957. *Sprachfreie entwicklungsteste (nach Buhler-Hetzer und Schenk-Danzinger)*. Basel and New York: S. Karger.

Birch, J. R., and Birch, J. W. 1951. The Leiter International Performances Scale as an aid in the psychological study of deaf children. *American Annals of the Deaf*, 96: 502–11.

Bishop, H. M. 1936. Performance scale tests applied to deaf and hard of hearing children. *Volta Review*, 38: 447, 484–85.

Borelli, M., and Oléron, P. 1954. *Une Nouvelle echelle de performance*. Paris: Centre de Psychologie Appliquée.

Brill, R. G. 1962. The relationship of Wechsler I.Q.'s to academic achievement among deaf students. *Exceptional Children*, 28: 315–21.

Burchard, E., and Myklebust, H. R. 1942. A comparison of congenital and adventitious deafness with respect to its effect on intelligence, personality, and social maturity. *American Annals of the Deaf*, 87: 140–55, 241–51, 342–60.

Day, H. E., Fusfield, I. S., and Pintner, R. 1928. *A Survey of American Schools for the Deaf*. Washington, D.C.: National Research Council.

Drever, J., and Collins, M. 1928. *Performance Tests of Intelligence*. Edinburgh: Oliver and Boyd.

DuToit, J. W. 1954. Measuring the intelligence of deaf children: A new group test. *American Annals of the Deaf*, 99: 237–52.

Furth, H. G. 1964. Research with the deaf: Implications for language and cognition. *Psychological Bulletin*, 62: 145–64.

Furth, H. G. 1966. *Thinking without Language*. New York: Free Press.

Giangreco, C. J. 1966. The Hiskey-Nebraska Test of Learning Aptitude (Rev.) compared to several achievement tests. *American Annals of the Deaf*, 111: 566–77.

Goetzinger, C. P., and Houchins, R. R. 1969. The 1947 Colored Raven's Progressive Matrices with deaf and hearing subjects. *American Annals of the Deaf*, 114: 95–101.

Goetzinger, C. P., and Rousey, C. L. 1957. A study of the Wechsler Performance Scale and the Knox Cube Test with deaf adolescents. *American Annals of the Deaf*, 102: 388–99.

Graham, E., and Shapiro, E. 1953. Use of the performance scale of the Wechsler Intelligence Scale for Children with the deaf. *Journal of Consulting Psychology*, 17: 396–98.

Greenberger, D. 1889. Doubtful cases. *American Annals of the Deaf*, 34: 93–99.

Harris, D. B. 1959. A note on some of the ability correlates of the Raven Progressive Matrices 1947 in the kindergarten. *Journal of Educational Psychology*, 50: 228–29.

Hayashi, S. 1959. Intelligence test for the deaf children. *Japanese Journal of Educational Psychology*, 5: 96–101; and *Psychological Abstracts*, no. 6804.

Hiskey, M. S. 1941. *Nebraska Test of Learning Aptitude for Young Deaf Children.* Lincoln: University of Nebraska.

Hudson, A. F. 1893, 1894. The union of kindergartners for the deaf. *American Annals of the Deaf*, 38: 277–78; 39, 25–27.

Johnson, E. H. 1947. The effect of academic level on scores from the Chicago Non-Verbal Examination for primary pupils. *American Annals of the Deaf*, 92: 227–34.

Kearney, J. E. 1969. A new performance scale of cognitive capacity for use with deaf subjects. *American Annals of the Deaf*, 114: 2–14.

Kirk, S. A., and Perry, J. 1948. A comparative study of the Ontario and Nebraska tests for the deaf. *American Annals of the Deaf*, 93: 315–24.

Kodman, F., Jr., Waters, J. E., and Whipple, C. I. 1962. Psychometric appraisal of deaf children using the Columbia Mental Maturity Scale. *Journal of Speech and Hearing Disorders*, 27: 275–79.

Lane, H. S., and Schneider, J. L. 1941. A performance test for school-age deaf children. *American Annals of the Deaf*, 86: 441–47.

Larr, A. L., and Cain, E. 1959. Measurement of native learning abilities of deaf children. *Volta Review*, 61: 160–62.

Lavos, G. 1950. The Chicago Non-Verbal Examination. *American Annals of the Deaf*, 95: 379–87.

Lavos, G. 1954. Interrelationship among three tests of non-language intelligence administered to the deaf. *American Annals of the Deaf*, 99: 303–14.

Lavos, G. 1962. W.I.S.C. psychometric patterns among deaf children. *Volta Review*, 64: 547–52.

Levine, B., and Iscoe, I. 1955. The Progressive Matrices (1938), the Chicago Non-Verbal and Wechsler Bellevue on an adolescent deaf population. *Journal of Clinical Psychology*, 11: 307–8.

Levine, E. S. 1948a. An investigation into the personality of normal deaf adolescent girls. Ph.D. dissertation, New York University. University Microfilms.

Levine, E. S. 1948b. The psychological service program of the Lexington School for the Deaf. *American Annals of the Deaf*, 93: 149–64.

Levine, E. S. 1956a. *Youth in a Soundless World.* New York: New York University Press.

Levine, E. S. 1956b. The mental health clinic for the deaf. *Silent Worker*, 9: 7–8.

Levine, E. S. 1960a. *Psychology of Deafness: Techniques of Appraisal for Rehabilitation.* New York: Columbia University Press.

Levine, E. S. 1960b. Psychiatric-preventive and sociogenetic study of the adjustive capacities, optimum work potentials, and total family problems of literate deaf adolescents and adults. *American Annals of the Deaf*, 105: 272–74.

Levine, E. S. 1963. Studies in psychological evaluation of the deaf. *Volta Review*, 65: 496–512.

Levine, E. S. 1971. Mental assessment of the deaf child. *Volta Review*, 73: 80–104.

Levine, E. S. 1974. Psychological tests and practices with the deaf: A survey of the state of the art. *Volta Review,* 76: 298–319.

Levine, E. S. 1976. Psychological contributions. In R. Frisina, Ed., *A Bicentennial Monograph on Hearing Impairment,* Washington, D.C.: Alexander Graham Bell Association for the Deaf.

Levine, E. S., Ed. 1977. *The Preparation of Psychological Service Providers to the Deaf.* PRWAD Monograph no. 4. Silver Spring, Md.: Professional Rehabilitation Workers with the Deaf.

Lyon, V. W. 1934. Personality tests with the deaf. *American Annals of the Deaf,* 79: 1–4.

MacKane, K. 1933. *A Comparison of the Intelligence of Deaf and Hearing Children.* Contributions to Education, No. 585. New York: Teachers College, Columbia University.

MacMillan, D. P., and Bruner, F. G. 1906. *Children Attending the Public Day Schools for the Deaf in Chicago.* Special Report of the Department of Child Study and Pedagogic Investigation, Chicago Public Schools, May 1906. Chicago.

MacPherson, J. G., and Lane, H. S. 1948. A comparison of the deaf and hearing on the Hiskey Test and on performance sales. *American Annals of the Deaf,* 93: 178–84.

Mira, M. P. 1962. The use of the Arthur Adaptation of the Leiter International Performance Scale and the Nebraska Test of Learning Aptitude with preschool deaf children. *American Annals of the Deaf,* 107: 224–28.

Mott, A. J. 1899, 1900. A comparison of deaf and hearing children in their ninth year. *American Annals of the Deaf,* 44: 401–12; 45; 33–39.

Musgrove, W. J., and Counts, L. 1975. Leiter and Raven performance and teacher ranking: A correlation study with deaf children. *Journal of Rehabilitation of the Deaf,* 8: 18–22.

Oléron, P. 1950. A study of the intelligence of the deaf. *American Annals of the Deaf,* 95: 179–95.

Petersen, E. G. 1936. Testing deaf children with the Kohs Block Designs. *American Annals of the Deaf,* 81: 242–54.

Petersen, E. G., and Williams, J. M. 1930. Intelligence of deaf children as measured by drawings. *American Annals of the Deaf,* 75: 273–90.

Pintner, R., and Paterson, D. G. 1915. The Binet Scale and the deaf child. *Journal of Educational Psychology,* 6: 201–10.

Pintner, R., Eisenson, J., and Stanton, M. 1941. *The Psychology of the Physically Handicapped.* New York: F. S. Crofts & Co.

Rainer, J. D., Altshuler, K. Z., Kallmann, F. J., and Deming, R., Eds. 1963. *Family and Mental Health Problems in a Deaf Population.* New York: Department of Medical Genetics, New York State Psychiatric Institute, Columbia University.

Reamer, J. C. 1921. Mental and educational measurements of the deaf. *Psychological Monographs,* 29, no. 132.

Rogers, M., and Quigley, S. P., Eds. 1960. Research needs in the vocational rehabilitation of the deaf. *American Annals of the Deaf,* 105: 335–70.

Ross, D. R. 1970. A technique of verbal ability assessment of deaf adults. *Journal of Rehabilitation of the Deaf*, 3: 7–15.

Schick, H. F. 1933. The use of a standardized performance test for pre-school age children with a language handicap. *Proceedings of the International Congress on the Education of the Deaf*, June, 1933. West Trenton, N. J.: New Jersey School for the Deaf. Pp. 526–32.

Seifert, K. H. 1960. The Progressive Matrices and its application to deaf-mute children. *Neue Blätter für Taubstummenbildung*, 14: 16–22.

Shirley, M., and Goodenough, F. L. 1932. A survey of deaf children in Minnesota schools. *American Annals of the Deaf*, 77: 238–47.

Smith, A. J., and Johnson, R. E. 1978. *Smith-Johnson Nonverbal Performance Scale*. Los Angeles: Western Psychological Services.

Smith, C. S. 1962. The assessment of mental ability in partially deaf children. *Teacher of the Deaf*, 60: 216–24.

Snijders, J. Th., and Snijders-Oomen, N. 1959. *Non-verbal Intelligence Tests for Deaf and Hearing Subjects*. Groningen, Netherlands: J. B. Wolters.

Springer, N. N. 1938. A comparative study of the intelligence of a group of deaf and hearing children. *American Annals of the Deaf*, 83: 138–52.

Stunkel, E. R. 1957. The performance of deaf and hearing college students on verbal and non-verbal intelligence tests. *American Annals of the Deaf*, 102: 342–55.

Taylor, H. 1894. The mind of the child. *American Annals of the Deaf*, 39: 244–48.

Taylor, H. 1897, 1898. A spelling test, *American Annals of the Deaf*, 42: 364–369; 43, 41–45.

Templin, M. 1950. *The Development of Reasoning in Children with Normal and Defective Hearing*. Minneapolis: The University of Minnesota Press.

Office of Vocational Rehabilitation. 1956. *New Hope for the Disabled: Public Law 565*. Washington, D.C.: Government Printing Office.

Office of Vocational Rehabilitation. 1957a. *Announcement: Rehabilitation Research Fellowships*. Washington, D.C.: Government Printing Office.

Office of Vocational Rehabilitation. 1957b. Announcement: Research and Demonstration Grants in Vocational Rehabilitation. Washington, D.C.: Government Printing Office.

Office of Vocational Rehabilitation. 1958. *Training Grant Programs of the Office of Vocational Rehabilitation*. Washington, D.C.: Government Printing Office.

Zeckel, A., and van der Kolk, J. J. 1939. A comparative intelligence test of groups of children born deaf and of good hearing by means of the Porteus Test. *American Annals of the Deaf*, 84: 114–23.

9 Psychological Examiners: Special Qualifications

IN ORDINARY PRACTICE, psychology's main operational tool is communication—linguistic, conceptual, and behavioral. When communication ceases to function effectively, psychological practice suffers a crippling handicap. Such is the situation for which psychologists to the deaf must be prepared. But this is not the only handicap. Others are created by psychology's powerful patterns in rehabilitation: education and society. Helping deaf persons take their place in society is only a part of psychological service. The other part involves getting society to accept its deaf members so that they can complete the rehabilitation process in the mainstream of real life. This can be the most obstructive problem of all. In the case of the deaf, society's traditional aversion to disability is compounded by problems of communication and undereducation. These interlocking difficulties add up to weighty responsibilities for psychologists to the deaf, and require exceptional competencies.

Problems of communication pose the need for psychologists to master the language forms used by deaf persons, to be able to "think deaf" conceptually, and distinguish customary from deviant behaviors in a context of deafness. Problems involving educational inadequacies and societal indifference pose the need for psychologists to engage in educational reform, public education, outreach, and advocacy.

To accomplish these multiple tasks requires unusual personal qualifications and technical skills, and encompasses an extraordinary range of functions. These are briefly outlined in this chapter as a prelude to subsequent discussion of psychological examination procedures.

Services

In 1977, the American Psychological Association published annotated standards "to improve the quality, effectiveness, and accessibility of psychological services to all who require them" (1977a, p. 1). The services covered by current standards as broadly delineated by a special Task Force (APA Task Force, 1975, p. 687) include the following:

A. Evaluation, diagnosis, and assessment of individuals, groups, and programs.
B. Interventions for the remediation and facilitation of the functioning of individuals and groups, such as psychotherapy, counseling and behavior therapy.
C. Program development services, including those relating to client habilitation and rehabilitation; training of staff in personnel development and management procedures; community participation and development; or company, institutional, and organizational policies regarding human resources.
D. Consultation relating to the following: (a) clients (individuals, families, organizations, agencies, or educational institutions); (b) the administration and operation of facilities or organizations; (c) the community served by the individual, the facility, or organization; (d) the training and education of psychology staff; and (e) the conduct of research, research design, and dissemination of psychological research findings.
E. The teaching of psychology in accredited academic institutions, per se, is not considered a psychological service that would require a state license, or certificate, or endorsement by the state psychological association by voluntary certification.

From this broad base of customary services, there emerged a more detailed analysis of psychological functions expected of service providers to the deaf, as submitted by participants at the national conference on The Preparation of Psychological Service Providers to the Deaf (the Spartanburg Conference). The following summary was excerpted from the conference report (Levine, 1977, pp. 19–21) and represents a *resource pool* of functions from which specific services suited to a particular setting and situation can be abstracted.

Summary of Functions

I. *Services to the Individual*
  A. Evaluation (assessment, diagnosis, differential diagnosis, intake, developmental profiles, eligibility, etc.)
  B. Integration of psychological and team findings
  C. Interpretation of integrated findings
  D. Recommendations
  E. Recording
  F. Reporting (written and/or person to person)

G. Treatment
H. Follow-up
I. Case-finding

II. *Services to the Facility*
   A. In-service training of facility personnel.
   B. Foster preventive mental health philosophy and methods
   C. Assist administration in decision-making
   D. Assist administration in program evaluations and the development of new programs
   E. Provide consultive service to facility personnel
   F. Assist in personnel screening and problems
   G. Publicize programs and services
   H. Promote inter-agency contacts and collaboration
   I. Provide consultive services to "outside" agencies and professionals
   J. Recruit other specialties into the field

III. *Services to the Community* (Deaf and Hearing)
   A. Interpret the implications of deafness to public, community, parents, and professional groups
   B. Serve as advocate for the deaf in community actions such as mental health, legislative, educational
   C. Act as friend to the deaf community: interpret hearing world; input current happenings; stress and interpret mental health to deaf individuals and families
   D. Outreach to every available forum including mass media for public relations and education
   E. Recruit quality workers for the field
   F. Foster programs of preparation for such workers
   G. Serve as community consultant on problems and issues involving the deaf

IV. *Research*
   A. Keep up with current research
   B. Identify significant problems that need researching
   C. Conduct research when feasible
   D. Maintain records that can be used by researchers
   E. Cooperate with selected researchers
   F. Stimulate spirit of inquiry in staff personnel
   G. Review and analyze significant research with administration and staff, and consider utilizing where feasible
   H. Disseminate own research publications

V. *Administration and Supervision*
   A. Supervise staff psychological workers
   B. Program in-service training for staff psychologists and psychological aides
   C. Provide orientation training for interpreters working with psychologists
   D. Supervise psychological interns and apprentices
   E. Evaluate psychological workers and psychological program
   F. Self-study program to improve services
   G. Maintain psychological equipment, test file, publishers' catalogues, etc.
   H. Maintain psychological report file
   I. Develop psychological reference library

VI. *Continuing Professional Development*
   A. Maintain professional and personal integrity
   B. Observe ethical standards of psychologists (American Psychological Association, 1977b) and ethical principles in research with human participants (American Psychological Association, 1973)
   C. Maintain membership and participate in activities of professional organizations
   D. Keep current with related literature
   E. Initiate and participate in professional institutes, workshops, conferences, continuing education courses, etc.
   F. Cooperate with and serve as resource person to other professionals

At first glance, this formidable listing of services appears overwhelming; but surprisingly enough, numbers of full-time psychologists to the deaf routinely perform most of them as need dictates, without consciously perceiving them as specific "functions." A situation arises that calls for a particular kind of management and they respond. The problem is that there are too few such workers to satisfy the need. The problem grows more pressing as mandated accountability under PL 94–142 imposes its requirements for sound psychological assessment of all handicapped children.

Competencies

To carry out the preceding services—or at least a basic minimum—and to effectively assess deaf persons calls for unusual personal and professional competencies. What these skills involve is summarized in the detailed Spartanburg Conference report. Excerpted from the report is the following listing of "minimum standard" competencies involved in serving a deaf population.

Basic Competencies

1. The ability to express and receive messages in whatever communicative modes and concept levels are habitually used by a deaf subject; or, until this point is reached.

2. The ability to understand the art and skills of interpreting for the deaf, and to work effectively through interpreted communication.

3. The ability to recognize significant leads in testing, the case history, and in interview and observation, and to understand their psychological implications.

4. For lack of psychological tests standardized on deaf youth and adults, the ability to select from a pool of hearing-standardized tests those best suited to a particular deaf subject, and to make whatever adaptations are required in language and administration that will elicit best-performance yet preserve test objectivity.

5. The ability to interpret test findings not only in relation to the behaviors elicited by the test but more particularly in relation to the subject's special background of experiences and deprivations.

6. The ability to understand the concepts of the severely undereducated, for whom reality is often a jigsaw of unconnected pieces, and whose concepts simply represent their efforts to put the pieces together to make some sense.

7. The ability to recognize deviant or psychopathic behavior in a context of deafness and to conduct differential diagnosis.

8. The ability to work effectively with multidisciplinary team members including parents, and to understand the psychological implications of their respective contributions.

9. The ability to formulate psychological reports in a way that gives a living picture of a human being, noting strengths and not only weaknesses, for it is mainly on the too often unrecognized strengths that remediations rest.

10. The ability to work comfortably with deaf subjects and inspire trust and confidence by projecting warmth, caring, and patience.

11. The ability to put all these together into sound recommendations, guided, in the words of one conference participant, by "where the subject was, where he is, where he should be, and how to get him there."

Underlying these abilities are a number of basic knowledge-imperatives, among them: (1) to "know" the deaf in terms of heterogeneity, culture, community, and persons; (2) to know the impact of deafness on family and child; (3) to know the diverse educational practices to which the deaf are exposed, for these represent major influences in their fashioning, adjustments, and problems; (4) to know the educational reform movements and their rationale, because educational reforms represent the best preventive mental health moves undertaken in behalf of the deaf; and (5) above all, to know—as Allen Sussman, the eminent deaf psychologist, often and rightly advises—how to "think deaf" and "talk deaf" when such is required.

This sounds like an overwhelming roster of special competencies, and in a sense it is. But it has its rewards, not only in providing quality services to a deserving but psychologically neglected population, but also in heightening the professional expertise of psychologists willing to brave the difficulties to profit from the challenge.

Points of Special Emphasis

Highlighting the special competencies were a number of points that were particularly stressed at the Spartanburg Conference. The following are a few of them.

1. *The Psychologist as a Person.* Psychologists to the deaf need to possess certain personal qualifications and attributes that "fit" into the frame of operations required with this population. These qualities include patience, warmth, flexibility, humor, and basic human-interactive skills involving empathy, rapport, and insights. Persons in whom deafness arouses aversion, tensions, or anxieties have no place in work with the deaf, least of all as psychologists.

2. *The Team Role.* To serve the multiple psychologically related problems raised by deafness requires a wide array or team of professional specialists, each of whom has a particular contribution to make to a psychologist's understanding of the person under examination. It is therefore essential that psychologists understand the "languages" of the various specialists and the significance of the information conveyed.

3. *Reporting.* On their part, psychologists must make every effort to communicate with team specialists in terms they can understand. This means avoiding technical jargon and esoteric theory references. A special complaint voiced by conference participants was that many psychological reports are simply summaries of test scores with mechanical interpretations that dwell on the scores and tell little about the individual. Such reports have little usefulness in planning for habilitation or rehabilitation.

4. *Confidentiality.* A recurring theme of the conference was the need for confidentiality in work with a deaf clientele. The deaf world is a closely knit community in which everyone more or less knows everyone else. The temptation is strong to pass on the "latest news" about a community member, with the usual embellishments as the word gets around, and sometimes with

dire results. Deaf subjects of psychological examination or treatment are well aware of this state of affairs and need to be assured that confidentiality will be observed and honored.

5. *The Tester Image.* The image of psychologists as testers has long been ingrained in the thinking of both the lay and professional public. As one conference participant stated, "This image is perpetuated by schools, employers, state departments, and by psychologists themselves, particularly those who do not feel secure enough with the deaf to do other than test. There needs to be broader outreach and public education in the field in behalf of psychologists: what they are and how they function" (Levine, 1977, p. 22). The conference participants overwhelmingly rejected the tester image.

6. *Professional Qualifications.* It was the strong consensus of all conference participants that in order to qualify for psychological practice with a deaf clientele, psychologists must first meet the requirements and standards of their own accredited psychological organizations, such as those formulated by the American Psychological Association. As expressed by a hearing-impaired conference participant, "The deaf deserve no less."

This statement is the best possible argument for the establishment of training programs to produce high-quality providers of psychological service for the deaf.

References

American Psychological Association. 1977a. *Standards for Providers of Psychological Services.* Washington, D.C.

American Psychological Association. 1977b. *Ethical Standards of Psychologists.* Rev. ed. Washington, D.C.

American Psychological Association. 1973. *Ethical Principles in the Conduct of Research with Human Participants.* Washington, D.C.

APA Task Force on Standards for Service Facilities. 1975. Standards for providers of psychological services. *American Psychologist,* 30: 685–94.

Levine, E. S., Ed. 1977. *The Preparation of Psychological Service Providers to the Deaf.* (Report of the Spartanburg Conference.) Monograph No. 4, *Journal of Rehabilitation of the Deaf.*

10 Methods of Psychological Examining: A Review

THE HIGH-QUALITY psychological services the deaf deserve call for examiners who not only "know" the deaf but who also know the basic techniques of psychological examination, namely tests and testing, observation, interview, and the case history. No one of these techniques professes to yield a full psychological picture, but each in its own way helps fill the gaps that deafness can create in the others.

The common misconception is that the techniques in themselves perform psychological assessments. They do not. They are strictly information-gathering strategies. Psychological assessments, on the other hand, lie not in collecting information—although this too requires special skills—but in the identification and interpretation of significant facts. The only "instrument" designed for this purpose is the examiner. It is the examiner who tells what the information *means* in a given case. No instrument or technique can replace an examiner's interpretive competence and wisdom. This is where knowing the deaf plays a critical role.

The amount of information needed to "know" a particular individual and understand his needs and problems varies from case to case. Extensive information is not always necessary. For example, a well-adjusted young high-school graduate seeking help with educational planning would not be expected to require the same type of examination as a young adult with a history of chronic vocational failure, or a child with bizarre behavior, or a deaf pupil on the verge of mainstreaming. In some cases, a complete work-up is called for; in others, only selected lines of inquiry are needed. Again, the situation and the examiner's perceptions determine the amount of information required.

When a situation calls for intensive study, delicate decision-making, and extra caution, maximum information-input is desirable, and all four data-gathering methods are called into service. The special advantage of using all four approaches is that each taps a different kind of information from a different source, thus providing an examiner with broader coverage than would be possible from a single method. Psychological testing provides objective information about an individual's present status and level of function in regard to important behaviors and various abilities. The case history tells about the experiences and events that have gone into the fashioning of the individual, as obtained from a variety of informants and perspectives. Interview gives facts supplied by the individual himself or herself, thus enabling an examiner to get a glimpse of the world through the eyes of the subject; while observation enables an examiner to see, among other things, how the individual fares in a variety of interpersonal and social encounters.

Through this battery of approaches, subjective, objective, and reported information is obtained covering both past and present. It is from the pool of data so assembled that psychological interpretations and assessments are made, and predictive inferences are drawn. A closer look at each of these approaches serves as introduction for discussing their use with deaf subjects.

Psychological Tests and Testing

Traditionally, the most popular approach used by psychologists for information-gathering is the test-and-measure method. The overwhelming appeal of psychological tests lies in the fact that instruments falling under the "test" umbrella are available to cover a broader and more varied range of measurement purposes (see the Buros *Mental Measurements Yearbooks*) in less time and with relatively fewer errors and bias (at least in theory) than any other psychological technique. For mass consumers such as schools, industry, and government, there can be no more compelling qualifications.

However, serious questions are being raised in contemporary psychology concerning the use and abuse of the test-and-measurement concept, in particular the overdependence on tests for individual evaluation (Buros, 1970; Cleary, et al., 1975; Cronbach, 1970; Green, 1978; Hogan et al., 1977; Jensen, 1980; Testing report released, 1978; L. Wright, 1970). It would be a simple matter if human behavior could be mirrored in a string of test scores. All that would be needed would be to link an I.Q. with a personality test score, add on an achievement score plus the scores of whatever other tests had been administered, and so arrive at a picture of a behaving person. But human nature is not so obliging; nor, for that matter, are the tests.

Human behavior resists compartmentalization, and resents quantification. Tests, on the other hand, are rooted in compartmentalization and quantification. As Heim remarks, "the term 'personality test' by tacit consent means a test which cuts out the cognitive elements (as though this were possible)" (1970, p. 19); and in a similar vein, the term "intelligence test" by tacit consent cuts out personality, "aptitude test" would cut out both intelligence and personality, and so forth—again, as though this were possible. Heim calls this "an affront to psychology, to common sense, and to semantics" (1970, p. 19). Such is the growing mood in contemporary psychology.

Furthermore, the increasing influence of ecological theory and mandated accountability has multiplied the objections to overdependence on tests and scores. In the spirit of ecology, the shift is from a focus on scores to a focus on experiences; from a view of the individual as depicted by tests to a review of the influences that went into his making (Bersoff, 1973). As to mandated accountability, for a psychologist this rests not only on knowing a person's test scores, but more particularly on knowing the person. The two are not necessarily compatible, as can be inferred from the earlier "sketches from life" and "sketches from research." Nevertheless, when psychological tests are properly understood and wisely used, they can serve an important information function.

In individual appraisal, the most generally favored targets for information are intelligence and personality. Not that anyone has yet succeeded in arriving at a satisfactory definition of either—as easily define such abstractions as truth and beauty as the abstractions intelligence and personality. Nonetheless, ingenious test constructors have succeeded in entrapping samplings of these elusive qualities in quantifiable tests and measures. How this is done provides basic insights into test utilization and evaluation. A classic example of the accomplishment can be found in David Wechsler's *The Measurement of Adult Intelligence* (1944).

The procedures and statistics used by Wechsler and other meticulous test constructors represent strategies for getting around the barrier of measuring behaviors that do not exist in quantitative form nor function in isolation from one another. To illustrate: the constructor of, let us say, an intelligence test begins the job by selecting or evolving the theory of intelligence on which to base his operations; thinks out the types of behaviors and test tasks that seem to fit the theory; and postulates how intelligence will show itself in task performance in the particular population for whom the test is designed— whether child, adult, disadvantaged, or whatever. He then sets about trying out and refining his concepts in numbers of trials, using actual task-items with actual populations. But since working with totals of either items or populations is out of the question, the constructor works with samples. The imperative here is that the samples must be exact replicas of the totals they stand for, albeit in mini-form; in other words they must be *representative* samples.

At the same time certain yardstick units must be built into the test to make behavior measurement possible. The units are represented by the test's score and norm systems; they are analogous to the inches, pounds, and other standard units of physical measurement. Scores codify an individual's test performance into easily handled numerical credits, while norms represent the usual performance of the population sample used in the final stage of test construction, commonly termed the standardization population. Both the scores and norms of a given test are restricted to this sample and to the population it represents. This is an extremely important point for examiners of the deaf to bear in mind, since a subject's standing on a given test is a *relative* measure derived by *comparing* the scores earned by the individual with the norms derived from the representative population. In the case of deaf subjects, this generally means comparing scores with norms derived from a nondeaf population.

A major aim of these complex procedures is to produce an instrument that is capable of objective measurement; but tests being instruments of intricate design, there is plenty of room for bias and error in both test structure and test usage unless special precautions are exercised to guard against them.

In respect to test structure, the main precautions are subsumed in the concepts *validity* and *reliability*. Validity is concerned with the fundamental question that haunts all conscientious test constructors and users: Does the instrument actually measure the behavior or ability that it purports to measure? There are a number of different ways of examining and using validity. These may be summarized in the following questions: (1) Is each of the individual test items a true example of the behavior or ability being measured, and do the collective items constitute a proper *proportional* distribution of that which is being measured? (*content validity*); (2) To what degree are the individual test items examples of the specific behavior being measured as defined by the underlying theory or construct on which the test is based, and to what degree are the collective items a representative sample of that behavior? (*construct validity*); (3) How close is the correspondence between a test's scores and dependable outside criteria concerning the individual's *current* status in respect to the behavior measured? (*criterion-oriented concurrent validity*); (4) How close is the correspondence between a test's scores and dependable outside criteria concerning the individual's *future* performance in the behavior being measured? (*criterion-oriented predictive validity*). These broad questions illustrate the main concerns in studies involving validity. For details, see Cronbach (1970) and the *Standards for Educational and Psychological Tests,* published by the American Psychological Association (1974)

The concept *reliability* refers mainly to the internal consistency of a test and to its temporal consistency from use to use. There are a number of ways of examining reliability, each of which deals with a different question: (1) How close is the correspondence between test scores when the same test is given again after a reasonable period of time? (*stability*); (2) How close is the correspondence of scores obtained from split parts of the test such as split-half, odd-even, or other parallel splits? (*internal consistency*); (3) How close is the correspondence of scores from alternate or parallel forms of the test when administered in the *same* time frame? (*stability*); (4) How close is the correspondence of scores when alternate forms of the test are given at *different* times? (*stability* and *equivalence*). A good illustration of the determination of reliability coefficients can be found in Wechsler's WAIS manual (1955) for each test of the WAIS as well as for the various scales.

In addition to these structural controls there are the controls involved in a test's usage. An important part of a test's objectivity depends on using precisely the same manner of administration and scoring with a subject as was used with the original standardization population. The intent here is to guard against biasing influences either on the part of the tester or in the test environment by spelling out procedures in such a way as to assure that everyone taking the test does so under uniform conditions and is subject to uniform scoring practices. Specifications for test administration and scoring are therefore included in every manual of dependable instruments, together with a table of adequately determined norms of performance.

Possibly the greatest subjective latitude allowed a psychologist in a test situation lies in the interpretation of a subject's performance, as distinct from pure measurement. As Freeman states:

> The data and indexes derived from psychological tests are, for the most part, objectively determined; but their clinical use involves judgment, subjective assessment, and interpretation based upon a variety of data from several sources. The experienced clinical examiner will supplement the test's numerical results with his observations of the testee's attitudes during the examination and the manner in which he attacks the problems of the test: his degree of confidence or dependence, his cooperativeness or apathy, his negativism or resentment, the richness or paucity of his responses. The individual test situation thus can be, in effect, an occasion for general psychological observations—really a penetrating psychological interview. (1962, p. 119)

Freeman emphasizes that the ability to perform such interpretive analyses comes "from working with persons rather than with tests alone" (1962, p. 139).

To sum up, a psychological test that has weathered the procedures involved in creating a responsible instrument is customarily termed "standardized," and exposes its key structural data by way of a test manual that includes:

1. Specific and unequivocal directions for test administration.
2. Specific and unequivocal directions for scoring.
3. A table of adequately determined norms of performance.
4. Data concerning validity.

5. Data concerning reliability.

6. Data concerning the nature and selection of the population sample on whom the test was standardized.

A "qualified" subject for a particular test is one whose background, condition, and experiential exposures fit in with those of the standardization population.

A key problem in psychological testing is that consumers are apt to expect more of tests than the instruments were originally designed to accomplish. In this, consumers are abetted by competitive practices among test publishers. Buros complains that "at present, no matter how poor a test may be, if it is nicely packaged and if it promises to do all sorts of things which no test can do, the test will find many gullible buyers" (1965, p. xxiv). An experienced examiner is not so easily taken in.

For the foreseeable future, psychological testing as we know it today will continue to serve a useful function in countless areas of inquiry (See Buros' *Mental Measurements Yearbooks*), with the added understanding that in individual assessment "the significance of test scores is greatest when they are combined with a full study of the person by means of interview, case history records, application blanks and other methods" (Cronbach, 1970, p. 8).

Observation

Of all the information-gathering procedures summarized here, observation appears to be most in tune with the movement toward real-life behavioral evaluation. Propelled by the ecological viewpoint as well as by mandates for the "least restrictive" educational environment, observation is taking significant strides from the test-room into the classroom for information about behaving children (Boehm and Weinberg, 1977; Ekanger and Westervelt, 1967; Hunter, 1977; Kent and Foster, 1977; Lynch, 1977; Sitko, Fink, and Gillespie, 1977). Sitko and associates explain:

Programs that attempt to measure the strengths and weaknesses of children in various areas are being criticized because typically they involved the development of instructional decisions based upon normative or standardized testing that occurs outside the environment or curriculum found in the classroom and are therefore not situationally specific. Education is also faced currently with a host of norm referential global measures of school aptitudes that have modest predictive validity and virtually no individual diagnostic validity. Moreover there exists a very limited range of diagnostic instruments, many based on doctrinaire, poorly researched theories of learning disabilities and behavior disorders. Hence, it is extremely difficult to establish precise and valid relationships between the specific diagnoses and prescribed remediations inherent in current test related programs. (1977, p. 25)

Simply expressed, people do not perform in life as on formboards; nor behave in life as on personality inventories; nor achieve in life as on achievement tests. Therefore it is rarely if ever possible to decide on the basis of test scores alone which is the least restrictive educational environment for a given child without also observing the child in action and interaction with peers, teachers, instructional methods, the curriculum, and many other real-life variables. And in real life as on tests, it is essential to know the nature of behavior-evoking stimuli in order to judge the relevancy of the elicited behaviors. Hence, classroom observation includes not only the child but also such behavior-evoking stimuli as teacher, peers, and a host of other observable events.

In situ observation requires special skills and special instruments. The skills are acquired through training and practice. The instruments for classroom observation are designed so that systematic recordings can be made of selected aspects of the targeted behavior as well as relevant and observable features of the classroom setting. Lynch estimates that there are several hundred such instruments in use, with over a hundred in published form; he describes them as typically consisting of ''several printed sheets on which the observer marks or writes while selectively attending to certain classroom events during their occurrence'' (1977, p. 2). The format of the particular recording sheets selected for use depends on the focus of observation, the nature of the behavior sample being observed, and on the type of recording to be made. The following types of observation systems and instruments are summarized from Hunter (1977).

1. *Category systems* include instruments that permit a record of each event under observation in accordance with predetermined categories (coded in numbers or symbols) to which the event belongs. Some of the categories focus on events involving cognitive behaviors; others, on affective behaviors; and still others, on events involving teacher feedback and interaction with students. The observer writes down the category number or symbol of the events as heard or seen, thus permitting a final count by categories of all events that transpire. These can ultimately be presented as a profile.

2. *Rating systems* require observation and simultaneous rating-recordings of selected behaviors on the part of teachers or students in a specified time-frame. Ratings are generally in terms of presence, quality, and frequency of the behaviors under observation.

3. *Time and Sign systems*. Record forms used in these systems resemble checklists or tally sheets in which all the behaviors selected for observation are listed, and the observer simply checks off specific behaviors as they occur during the same time-frame.

4. *Specimen Description and Free Observation systems*. These systems

refer to detailed recordings of all that transpires in a given situation within more or less extended periods of time. Continuous note-taking is required of the observer, or audio- or videotape recordings may be made. Scoring or coding is imposed on the record after it is completed.

5. *Event sampling*. This method involves recording the descriptions of specific behavioral events of a predetermined type as they occur. Examples are: fighting, spitting, crying, and temper tantrums. The meaning of the behavior is studied in relation to the provoking agent and the situation in which it occurs.

As may be inferred from the nature of the methods and instruments involved in naturalistic observation, there is plenty of room for bias and error in the collection of data. These are matters of special concern to researchers, in particular investigators of the validity and reliability of the observation instruments and the dependability of the observers. Reviews of such research can be found in the cited references, with excellent summaries in Hunter (1977) and Kent and Foster (1977).

Important by-products of observation's invasion of classrooms are striking disclosures of inadequacies in teacher performance and in teacher-training programs. The result has been a growing move to rate teacher performance for operational competence (Rosner, 1972) and to stress the related skills in teacher-training. Included among them are: providing a classroom climate of acceptance; the exercise of democratic controls; clarity and organization in the presentation of lessons; teacher enthusiasm and humor; respect for the learner; and constructive feedback to pupils. Another important by-product is the broadened role of the school psychologist in educational evaluations and in the decision-making process.

Although the observation technique has advanced to a position of unprecedented prominence, owing largely to the mandates for educational accountability, it has long been used as an information-gathering method in settings other than classrooms. Ekanger and Westervelt (1967) tell of the value to a day-care-center staff when observation was extended to include the child's home-and-family setting. When the practice was first proposed to the staff, it met with resistance; but, as the authors comment, such resistance is the expected initial response to new and time-consuming procedures. As the values of the procedure became apparent, resistance faded. It is my conviction that no child-observation procedure is complete without home-and-family observation data.

McGowan and Porter (1967) describe the use of observation in prevocational evaluation procedures with individuals, such as certain disabled persons, whose capabilities cannot be assessed by traditional techniques. Evaluation takes place in a prevocational "unit" which is described as "a vocational diagnostic laboratory in which patients try out various job samples taken directly from industry" (1967, p. 102). This evaluation method is known as the Work Sample Method; the evaluator observes the performance of a given client on various work-tasks and evaluates it by comparison with the known performance of successful employees in similar work situations.

The use of observation in studies of psychopathological states has a long clinical history. In more recent times, outstanding contributions have been made by Ruesch (1957) and by Ekman and Friesen (1974). Ruesch bases his clinical approach on observations of a patient's communicative behavior and has devised a comprehensive guide for obtaining and recording such data (1957, pp. 192–313) as gleaned from observation and interview in various settings. Ekman and Friesen are conducting highly ingenious investigations of observed nonverbal behavior as diagnostic indicators in psychopathology. In both instances, the ability to obtain, organize, record, and interpret the data demands high clinical competence as well as special competence in the use of observation and related instruments. But the same can be said of all conscientious applications of psychological methodology.

Interview

The basic aim of interview in psychological assessment is to obtain a wide-angled view of a subject's perceptions of the world in which he lives, of his place in it, and of his hopes, problems, and coping mechanisms. Compared with psychological testing and with observation, interview offers the individual considerably more latitude for self-expression. In psychological testing, the flow of information is hemmed in by test-tasks; in observation, by the behaviors under scrutiny. But in a well-conducted interview, information-flow proceeds through seemingly free interpersonal communication—"seemingly" because the proceedings are at all times under the strict though unobtrusive control of the interviewer. Gordon describes the basic functions of the interviewer as follows:

> The basic tasks of the interviewer include accurately communicating the question to the respondent; maximizing the respondent's ability and willingness to answer the question; listening actively to determine what is relevant; and probing to increase the validity, clarity, and completeness of the responses. All of the strategies, techniques, and tactics of interviewing must contribute in some way to accomplishing these central tasks. (1969, p. 355)

Among the inhibitors of information-flow, Gordon notes such factors as ego threat, trauma, forgetting, chronological confusion, and unconscious behavior; among the facilitators he notes such factors as giving recognition, supplying sympathetic understanding, providing altruistic appeals, facilitating catharsis, and fulfilling the need for meaning.

For an interviewer to successfully accomplish his mission demands exquisite skills and craftsmanship. The interviewer must not only know where he is leading a subject and why but also how best to elicit and channel self-revelation. This demands the ability to exercise a wide assortment of apparently opposite behaviors. The interviewer must be empathetic yet objective, flexible yet organized, a participant and also an observer, a follower yet a leader, relaxed yet alert, nonjudgmental yet a critical analyst.

Essential to all initial interviews is establishing a relationship of mutual trust and empathy between the two participants. The person being interviewed must be made to feel free to tell his story as if to a friend; the interviewer must feel and project a sincere interest in and nonjudgmental acceptance of what he is being told. A good way to start the proceedings is by explaining the purpose of the interview and the confidentiality of the procedure. At the same time, the interviewer must enter the situation with some flexible pre-plan in mind concerning the kinds of information to be sought and the areas to be explored, a tentative sequence of topics to be covered, the interview language, the kinds of question forms and probing strategies that can be used for eliciting further information or for shifting a flow of repetitive discourse to another topic, and alternative strategies for dealing with inhibition and resistance. These are among the major controls involved in assembling an organized body of information through interview.

The interviewer must also be prepared to deal with persons who enter the interview situation with reluctance or with a chip on the shoulder. Reluctance is met with empathetic encouragement; a chip-on-the-shoulder attitude is often best met by permitting the person to let off steam until he has cooled sufficiently to perceive the interviewer's sincere and nonjudgmental interest in him as a person whom he desires to help.

It is not possible in this brief summary to explore the full range of possible events with which interviewers must be prepared to cope, nor the range of coping methods employed. Excellent discussions can be found in Gordon (1969), in Kahn and Cannell (1957) and in Meyer, Liddell, and Lyons (1977). Basically, the key to coping lies in the individual's perceptions of the interviewer's attitudes as projected in verbal and nonverbal behavior. The following recommendations along these lines are excerpted from Hadley (1958).

1. Get the interview off to a good start by conveying to the person a sincere and nonjudgmental interest in him, and by clearly explaining that the purpose of the interview is to ascertain how best to provide assistance.

2. Frame questions clearly, economically, naturally.

3. Adjust the sequence of topics to be discussed to the anxiety level of the informant.

4. Move rapidly through the interview, but without pushing.

5. Record information at the time of interviewing.

6. Ask "ticklish" questions straightforwardly.

7. Exert skill and tact in handling pauses and silences.

8. Attempt to get beneath superficial answers.

9. Note discrepancies in the interviewee's discourse, and check as unobtrusively as possible.

10. Handle emotional scenes tactfully but firmly.

11. Be prepared for questions.

Note-taking can be one of the great inhibitors in interview situations. Some interviewers have developed the skill of unobtrusive note-taking by lap-recording, that is, resting the recording form on a lapboard which is more or less concealed from the interviewee by the desk or tabletop, and by devising various short-cut codifications for the rapid recording of certain kinds of data.

The degree of validity and reliability of the interview rests on the accuracy and completeness of the data collected. These in turn depend on a number of factors summarized by Gordon as: (1) the type of information sought; (2) the nature or state of the interviewer; (3) the concepts which guide the interview; and (4) the methods used by the interviewer. Gordon emphasizes that "no refinement in data analysis can counteract the effects of faulty data-collection methods that provide raw information which is false, distorted, or incomplete" (1969, p. 2). And again, the basic imperative for accurate data in establishing validity and reliability holds for interview as for all psychological data-gathering methods concerned with human assessments.

Case History

The basic purpose of a comprehensive case history is to obtain as complete a picture as possible of the interplay of events, experiences, and attributes that have gone into the making of an individual, the better to understand how he came to be as he is, and to identify the causes and appropriate interventions for whatever behavioral handicaps may be present. While it is true, as H. F. Wright observes, that the behavior of a person is "in the nature of a stream that can never be seen in its entirety" (1960, p. 73), a comprehensive history aims to approach the "entirety." However, in drawing inferences from history data, the individual items of information have little meaning in themselves. As discrete data, they may be likened to the unassembled pieces of a jigsaw puzzle. It is only when the relationship of the pieces to one another and to the whole is perceived that they fall into logical place and a personality picture emerges. To an experienced worker, a full history provides most of the leads needed for understanding the nature and problems of an individual.

The content of case records varies with the kinds of data sought and the use to be made of the information. For example, in vocational rehabilitation settings, McGowan and Porter (1969) list the following as topics that should be reported in a client's case record.

1. Determining eligibility for vocational rehabilitation services.
2. Client's perception of his problems.
3. Counselor–client relationships.
4. New information (medical, vocational, psychological, personal, financial, etc.) as it comes in during the life of the case.
5. Discussion of alternative vocational goals.
6. Case evaluation.
7. Justification of rehabilitation plans.
8. Changes in rehabilitation plan.
9. Case supervision during beginning period of vocational training or employment.
10. Case-service interruptions.
11. Case re-evaluation.
12. Loss of contact with client.
13. Readiness for employment.
14. Job placement plan.
15. Case closure.

The focus in this list is obviously on vocational planning. In case histories dealing with emotionally disturbed individuals, the focus would be on the onset, nature, and description of disturbance, treatment interventions, and other relevant details in the patient's life and experiences; and in the case histories of children, the focus is mainly on developmental data, fashioning environments (both family and school), on learning abilities and progress, and on manifest behaviors and behavior problems. For settings serving deaf children or adults, a detailed history inventory form that spans the chronological range from infancy through adulthood is included in Appendix F.

It cannot be stressed strongly enough that in assembling a history the purpose is not to accumulate a mass of facts, dates, and names but to reconstruct a life story that has a beginning and a chronological sequence of events, reactions, and consequences leading up to the present. In the process of reconstruction, there will be gaps in the story to fill, facts to check, conflicting reports to reconcile, and areas of inquiry to be brought up to date. History does not end with the present. It is part of a continuing story that will be referred to and added to by future workers.

Therefore case history must be recorded with an awareness of future as well as present usability. Significant information should be annotated in regard to: (1) the name and address of a particular informant; (2) the age of the person at the time the information about him was reported; (3) the date the information was received; and (4) the reliability of the informant and his relationship to the subject. In this latter connection, a fairly safe procedure is to build interpretation on data obtained from responsible primary sources, i.e., those with authentic, firsthand experiences with both the subject and with the lines of inquiry on which they report, uncontaminated by personal biases or emotional overtones. For example, specialists who have actually examined the individual can be considered primary sources for their respective findings. However, parents, friends, or relatives who are simply reporting the results of professional examinations cannot be considered primary sources for such information. As a rule, professional reports are too technically expressed for precise understanding not only by laypersons but often by professional colleagues from other disciplines. Psychologists who find themselves the recipients of cryptic professional reports should not hesitate to request explanation and clarification.

Reliable information can sometimes be surprisingly difficult to obtain from parents. Even in the brief histories of young children, uncertainty is not uncommon concerning the course and chronology of events and reactions. With older school-agers, it is the usual occurrence. The past is clouded by present problems, lapse of time, and emotional rather than factual recall. Where this is the case, a more objective account of events must be sought from knowledgeable but less deeply involved informants.

Recording must also reflect an awareness of the importance of significant written reports and documents provided by informants, particularly professional reports. Photocopies should be attached to or included in appropriate sections of the history, both to preserve chronological continuity and to safeguard the information against possible loss of the original documents. Above all, recording should not be so abbreviated and cryptic as to be meaningless to other readers. In effect, a good history is a concise but understandably written sequential record of pertinent facts in a life story, chronologically complete and cross-checked for accuracy.

References

American Psychological Association. 1974. *Standards for Educational and Psychological Tests*. Washington, D.C.
American Psychological Association. 1977. *Standards for Providers of Psychological Services*. Washington, D.C.

Bersoff, D. N. 1973. Silk purses into sow's ears: The decline of psychological testing and a suggestion for its redemption. *American Psychologist,* 28: 892–99.

Boehm, A. B., and Weinberg, R. A. 1977. *The Classroom Observer: A Guide for Developing Observation Skills.* New York: Teachers College Press.

Buros, O. K. 1965. *The Sixth Mental Measurements Yearbook.* Highland Park, N.J.: Gryphon Press.

Buros, O. K. 1970, *Personality Tests and Reviews.* Highland Park, N.J.: Gryphon Press.

Cleary, T. A., Humphreys, L. G., Kendrick, S. A., and Wesman, A. 1975. Educational uses of tests with disadvantaged students, *American Psychologist,* 30: 15–41.

Cronbach, L. J. 1970. *Essentials of Psychological Testing.* 3rd Ed. New York: Harper & Row.

Ekanger, C. A., and Westervelt, G. 1967. Contributions of observation in naturalistic settings to clinical and educational practice. *Journal of Special Education,* 1: 207–13.

Ekman, P., and Friesen, W. V. 1974. Nonverbal behavior and psychopathology. In R. J. Friedman and M. M. Katz, Eds., *The Psychology of Depression: Contemporary Theory and Research.* Washington, D.C.: Winston & Sons. Pp. 203–32.

Freeman, F. S. 1962. *Theory and Practice of Psychological Testing.* 3rd Ed. New York: Holt, Rinehart and Winston.

Gordon, R. L. 1969. *Interviewing: Strategy, Techniques, and Tactics.* Homewood, Ill.: Dorsey Press.

Green, B. P. 1978. In defense of measurement. *American Psychologist,* 33: 663–79.

Hadley, J. M. 1958. *Clinical and Counseling Psychology.* New York: Alfred A. Knopf.

Heim, A. 1970. *Intelligence and Personality: Their Assessment and Relationship.* Baltimore: Penguin Books.

Hogan, R., DeSoto, C. B., and Solano, C. 1977. Traits, tests, and personality research. *American Psychologist,* 32: 255–64.

Hunter, C. P. 1977. Classroom observation instruments and teacher inservice training by school psychologists. *School Psychology Monograph,* 3: 45–88.

Jensen, A. R. 1980. *Bias in Mental Testing.* New York: Free Press.

Kahn, R. L. and Cannell, C. F. 1957. *The Dynamics of Interviewing.* New York: John Wiley & Sons.

Kent, R. N., and Foster, S. L. 1977. Direct observational procedures: Methodological issues. In A. R. Ciminero, K. S. Calhoun, and H. E. Adams, Eds., *Handbook of Behavioral Assessment.* New York: John Wiley & Sons. Pp. 279–328.

Korman, M. 1971. *Levels and Patterns of Professional Training in Psychology: Conference Proceedings, Vail, Colorado.* Washington, D.C.: American Psychological Association.

Levine, E. S. 1977. *The Preparation of Psychological Service Providers to the Deaf,* PRWAD Monograph no. 4. Silver Spring, Md.: *Journal of Rehabilitation of the Deaf.*

Lynch, W. W. 1977. Guidelines to the use of classroom observation instruments by school psychologists. *School Psychology Monograph,* 3: 1–22.

McGowan, J. P., and Porter, T. L. 1967. *An Introduction to the Vocational Rehabilitation Process.* Rev. Washington, D.C.: Government Printing Office.

Meyer, V., Liddell, A., and Lyons, M. 1977. Behavioral interviews. In A. R. Ciminero, K. S. Calhoun, and H. E. Adams, Eds., *Handbook of Behavioral Assessment.* New York: John Wiley & Sons. Pp. 117–52.

Roch, J. 1968. *Interviewing Children and Adolescents.* New York: St. Martin's Press.

Rosner, B. 1972. *The Power of Competency-based Teacher Education: Report of the Committee on National Program Priorities in Teacher Education.* Boston: Allyn and Bacon.

Ruesch, J. 1957. *Disturbed Communication.* New York: W. W. Norton.

Sitko, M. C., Fink, A. H., and Gillespie, P. H. 1977. Utilizing systematic observation for decision making in school psychology. *School Psychology Monograph,* 3: 23–44.

Testing report released; Research unit created at NIE, Washington, D.C. 1978. *APA Monitor,* 9 (1): 6–9.

Wechsler, D. 1944. *The Measurement of Adult Intelligence.* 3rd. Ed. Baltimore: Williams & Wilkins Co.

Wechsler, D. 1955. *WAIS Manual: Wechsler Adult Intelligence Scale.* New York: The Psychological Corporation.

Wright, H. F. 1960. Observational child study. In P. H. Mussen, Ed., *Handbook of Research Methods in Child Development.* New York: John Wiley & Sons. Pp. 71–139.

Wright, L. 1970. The meaning of I.Q. scores among professional groups. *Professional Psychology,* 1: 265–69.

Part Five
EXAMINATION GUIDES

INTRODUCTION

PROBLEMS ASSOCIATED with prelinguistic deafness spill over into psychological examination procedures and practices. Even granted an examiner's special competence, interpretation of the results of a psychological examination requires special insights, perceptions, and knowledge. How vulnerable, for example, are mental, scholastic, social, and emotional development to lack of hearing ability; how vulnerable the fashioning environment, parent–child relations, community acceptance, personal fulfillment? What attributes constitute psychological assets and liabilities in the life of one who cannot hear? What attainments represent the average, the exceptional, the failing? What personality traits characterize the normative, the unusual, the deviant? What compensatory imperatives are required to fill the voids created by prelinguistic deafness? How can a psychological examination distinguish between individual potentials and the handicaps inflicted by failures in the fashioning environment? To what extent may the deaf be assessed by hearing standards?

These are among the questions that crowd the minds of conscientious examiners bent on realistic interpretation of examination findings. Added to the difficulties are problems arising from the lack of psychological instruments designed for use with the deaf, plus the enormous range of individual differences encountered among deaf subjects of examination.

To cover the total range of problems likely to arise in psychological practice with the deaf is well beyond the scope of this volume. The principal aim of the guides that follow is to provide suggestions and cautions where difficulties in examination are most apt to occur, and to clarify the rationale of special procedures and lines of inquiry.

The procedures to be reviewed focus on three target age levels—infancy, school age, and adult. Each age group is separately discussed, with emphasis on how various special considerations arising out of deafness apply to the basic methods of psychological examining: case history, interview, observation, and psychological testing. Related guides are included in the Appendices of this volume.

A look at one such guide—the inventory for case history information, Appendix F—highlights the exceptional range of information and the wide variety of informants involved in the behavioral evaluation and interpretation of hearing-impaired individuals. Commonly included are parents, teachers, otologists and other medical personnel, audiologists, speech and hearing therapists, social workers, intake personnel, rehabilitation counselors, and other specialists as required. The whole evaluation process is a collaborative operation, with the psychologist functioning as a member of an evaluation team. A highly important factor in sound psychological assessments is a psychologist's capacity to function as an *effective* team member, able to receive and impart information smoothly and knowledgeably. This skill is as deeply involved in psychological assessment as is the psychological examination itself.

Finally, the psychological examination of deaf children has only recently acquired a commanding position in special education, due largely to the assessment requirements of PL 94-142. Similarly, the need for infant assessment assumes increasing importance with the growing trend toward infant programs and the early fitting of hearing aids. The guides that follow are offered in response to such practical considerations, and not as examples of standard procedure. On the contrary, it is my aim and hope that this book will stimulate more intensive studies of psychological examination approaches that can profitably be used with deaf subjects so that more effective procedures and instruments than now exist will eventually be developed.

11 Infant Assessment

WITH THE flowering of parent–infant programs for hearing-impaired children and the early fitting of hearing aids—sometimes in the first weeks of life—the assessment of infant development becomes an important component of habilitative evaluation. Assessment at the infant level is a comparatively new function for most psychologists to the hearing-impaired. Traditionally, the major focus has been on school populations. Descending the age-scale to infancy involves a different theory base and different techniques from those customarily used in psychological testing.

The reason for these differences stems from the fact that infancy represents a state of rapid bio-physiological change. Although growth occurs in an ordered and systematic manner, the various systems involved are in a condition of ongoing metamorphosis, not yet stabilized into firm patterns of integration and reinforcement. Therefore, assessment is preferably based on *developmental* behaviors rather than on such traditional measures as the I.Q.

Especially disappointing to examiners is the fact that "test scores earned in the first year or so have relatively little predictive validity" (Bayley, 1970, p. 174). An interesting review of research at the infant level discloses the following predictive possibilities: (1) until the second year of life, prediction from infant tests to later-determined I.Q.'s is relatively poor; and (2) before the age of 1 year, the best single predictor of the I.Q. appears to be the socioeconomic status of the parents (McCall, Hogarty, and Hurlburt, 1972, pp. 745–46). Not until the age of about 2 years do I.Q.'s become fairly stable and so acquire a degree of predictive validity. This chapter focuses on the chronological range preceding this point of stability.

Although prediction is eminently desirable, it is not the major aim of infant assessment. The fundamental purpose is to find out if the basic developmental equipment of the tiny being is in good working order for the tasks of environmental exploration, interplay, and incorporation that underlie enculturation; and if the developmental environment is conducive to productive input, stimulation, and exploration. For related details, the reader is referred to the abundant literature on child development. The guides that follow

sketch the use of the basic psychological techniques in gathering information
of special importance in infant assessment.

Case History

A psychological examiner looks to the case history for leads that help in
understanding what an infant is telling through its patterns of behavior.
Among the leads are details concerning: (1) the experiences, exposures, and
hazards that have gone into the making of the behaviors; (2) the developmental levels of manifest behaviors as compared with a central average; (3)
the presence of suspicious deviations from normal expectations; and (4)
remedial interventions, if any, that have been used and to what effect. Items
of information that warrant special attention include the following.

1. *Parental attitudes toward pregnancy.* A psychological environment
awaits an infant even before it is born, as determined by the attitudes of
parents in wanting or not wanting the baby. Where attitudes are unfavorable,
an infant is handicapped from the start. The presence of a disability worsens
the picture. Because the need for acceptance is a critical factor in child adjustment, information concerning parents' attitudes toward having the child
provides important leads to the child's psychological environment and later
problems of adjustment.

2. *Maternal condition during pregnancy.* Where there is a maternal history involving illnesses and incidents during pregnancy such as those noted
in Appendix F, the history inventory, there is grave danger of permanent
damage to the nervous system of the developing fetus. This etiological possibility may lead to a variety of disabilities, persistent behavior deviations,
retardations, and exceptional learning difficulties, especially in language
mastery. Detailed information of the mother's condition during pregnancy is
therefore an important component of infant biographies.

3. *Perinatal events.* Permanent damage to brain tissue may also be
caused by the physical trauma and events of birth, with results similar to
those noted in section 2. Listed in Appendix F are a number of conditions
commonly associated with brain damage at birth.

4. *Medical and health information.* Even after the hazards of birth have
been successfully weathered, "the list of infections, traumas, and toxic
agents that may injure [an infant] is almost endless" (Gesell and Amatruda,
1947, p. 110). A number are listed in Appendix F. Often the presence of
disabling sequelae to such hazards is not or cannot be detected in routine pe-
diatric examination but may be picked up in the course of the developmental
examination. Where there is a history of illness in infancy, the examiner is
alerted to watch out for behavior signs of various postinfection disabilities.

5. *Auditory status of family.* As previously discussed, whether a hearing-impaired infant's parents are deaf or hearing provides leads to the infant's developmental, psychosocial, and rearing environment. Involved in these determinations are the parents' educational and socioeconomic status, their perception of the parent role in child rearing, the practices employed, and their attitudes toward a hearing-impaired offspring.

6. *Auditory-diagnostic history and status of infant.* Another index of a deaf infant's adjustive environment is the nature of the family's diagnostic experiences preceding the discovery of deafness. Where these experiences have been prolonged and frustrating, they may leave a permanent psychological scar on parent–child relations. Therefore, the examiner should have detailed information about the diagnostic experiences of parent and child, together with whatever audiological procedures and findings have been reported. Among other things, this can orient the examiner to the possible responses of the baby to developmental examination tests involving hearing ability.

The infant's auditory history needs to include details concerning the age of onset of impaired hearing, pre- and post-disability behaviors including vocalizations, remedial interventions used, at what age they were begun and with what results both behaviorally and auditorially.

7. *Communication patterns.* Information concerning parent–child communication patterns provides good leads to the nature of the infant's interplay with the human environment and possibly to the amount of message-input and exchange likely to take place. Toward this end, information needs to be obtained concerning details of parent–child communication habits—oral, purely auditory, manual, gestural, pantomime, etc.—and of the infant's facility in the expressive and receptive aspects of the method or combination of methods habitually used.

8. *Developmental status.* Determination of an infant's developmental status is discussed in a following section dealing with the developmental examination. Of prime importance are pronounced deviations from normal expectation as disclosed in previous as well as current examination.

Interview

Interview at the infant level naturally takes place with parents. A customary procedure is for an initial and comprehensive interview to be conducted by intake personnel with both parents. Sometime later the examiner conducts a briefer interview with the mother, immediately preceding the developmental examination.

The main purpose of the pre-examination interview with the mother is to obtain information about the infant's highest levels of attainment in everyday behavior, particularly in the significant behavior zones, classified by

Gesell and Amatruda (1947, p. 100) as: motor behavior (including handedness and manner of manipulation of objects); language behavior (including gestures); play behavior (including toys); domestic behavior (including feeding, dressing, toilet, cooperation); emotional behavior (including dependency, management, playmates, specific behavior deviations); and health history (including teething). An associated purpose is to enable the examiner to get the feel of the mother's insights and reactions to the baby's disability, and to see the infant through the mother's eyes. This seems a tall order for a brief interview, but the more skilled the interviewer, the less the time required.

Interview Preparation

Basic information. In situations where an examiner is not provided with full intake information before the interview with the mother, certain basic items should be obtained ahead of time, such as:

1. *Age of infant.* Knowing the infant's age, which may range anywhere from a few weeks to 2 years, prepares an examiner for the chronological focus of the interview, the kinds of equipment needed for the examination, and the probable range of test-tasks to be used.

2. *Auditory status of baby.* The examiner should also have information about the probable amount of hearing loss in order to have a base of reference for the baby's general reactions to ordinary sound as well as to later administered test-tasks based on response to sound.

3. *Auditory status of interviewee.* Whether the person being interviewed is deaf or hearing alerts the examiner to the methods of communication that may be required and to the possible need for an interpreter.

Unestablished disability. Where intake information indicates that "something is wrong with the infant" but no determination has been made of what it is, the examiner faces the tricky assignment of differential diagnosis and is thereby alerted to be on the watch for soft signs of behavioral deviation observed during the course of parent interview, which will be checked later during the formal developmental examination.

Emotional confrontation. Examiners of hearing-impaired and disability-suspect infants must be especially sensitive to the probability that many of the parents and babies have already weathered a long, frustrating variety of doctor-shopping experiences and conflicting diagnoses and recommendations. Examiners should therefore be prepared for infants who are frightened of strangers and suspicious of their intentions, and for parents who are at the end of their tether and mistrustful of yet another "authority" figure.

Pre-examination Interview Procedures

The pre-examination interview is conducted after all preliminary matters have been attended to. The mother is the usual inteviewee.

Where emotional tensions are apparent or suspected, the major initial goal is to reduce these to a minimum by creating a relaxed atmosphere of calm confidence. Examiners familiar with the diagnostic travails of so many parents of hearing-impaired infants are able to take emotional reactions, even hostility, in stride with unruffled personal feelings. They meet the tensions with understanding and gentle management until both mother and infant come to feel at ease. To accomplish this requires special interpersonal skills; but it must be done since the infant's examination cannot begin until a measure of confidence has settled over mother and baby, and the examiner is ''accepted.''

Information is elicited from the mother in an informal, conversational way that is, above all, neither judgmental nor inquisitorial. Where a mother is overcharged with a need to tell her story, the examiner lets her take the lead while unobtrusively steering the conversation into desired channels. Where a mother is inhibited, the examiner begins the interview with neutral observations that are not likely to arouse tensions.

Many mothers tell their stories by way of anecdotes. These should not be lightly dismissed. They often contain significant behavior-facts or leads that are apt to be overlooked in direct questioning.

Interview time is also used to establish trustful feelings on the part of the baby toward the examiner. A frightened, nonfriendly baby is nonchalantly ignored as the interview with its mother gets under way. When the baby calms down a bit, an occasional smile is cast in its direction by the examiner, and a nontest toy casually offered. If the toy is not accepted, so be it; it is simply offered again later on. When the toy is accepted, this is a sign that the examiner is also being accepted. The baby is then gently exposed to the regular-examination toys and procedures.

The amount of time allotted for a pre-examination interview is especially important if examination of the infant has been scheduled to follow the interview. If the interview is prolonged and exhausts the baby's patience or extends into feeding and nap times, examination must be put off for another day. At this next session, it is best to proceed with the examination at once, if the infant is willing; and if the interview with the mother has not been completed, it should follow examination.

Finally, the incredible perceptivity of very young children, even infants, to emotional climates cannot be lightly dismissed. When information is being relayed by the mother about problems, the child feels the tensions generated and can be observed to stare with round-eyed dismay at the unhappy facial expressions of the mother and the worried looks cast in its direction. An emotionally charged interview about a perceptive child should not be conducted in its presence. If this cannot be avoided, some distracting nontest toys should be on hand, and both mother and interviewer should maintain guarded control over their facial expressions and the direction of their glances.

The Developmental Examination

The major targets of a developmental examination are the behavior zones previously mentioned, i.e., motor behavior, coordination, and skills; sensorimotor coordinations and sensory-perceptual acuities and function; language behavior; emotional behavior; adaptive and interpersonal behaviors, including play and domestic behaviors. Where a behavior deviation is detected or suspected, it is advisable not to leap to a diagnostic conclusion on a first examination. Wide physiological deviations are not uncommon from infant to infant, and the behavior deviations detected may be due to this circumstance. Repeated examinations need to be made and differential diagnostic clues followed until a definitive diagnostic picture emerges. For example, lack of response to sound may be due to any one or combination of such conditions as deafness, mental retardation, cerebral dysfunction, complete emotional neglect, and more. Sometimes it is necessary to wait until the infant is older before the real situation can be pinned down. During this time, it is good policy to see that all the inputs and environmental advantages necessary for healthy development are afforded the baby, plus whatever remedial supports seem indicated until eventually a diagnosis based on the outcome of treatment is derived. Where differential diagnostic leads seem to point to hearing difficulties, the developmental examination needs to be supplemented by special medical (neurological, otological, etc.) and audiological examinations.

Special Considerations

The following special considerations characterize infant-behavior evaluations as compared with regular psychological test practices.

1. *Examiner qualifications.* Professional competence in infant examination requires certain personal attributes on the part of examiners, over and above technical skill. A number have been indicated in passing. In addition, of even more fundamental importance than technical expertise "is the requirement that the examiner be able to interact effectively with infants at various levels of development in order to motivate relevant responses to the test stimuli within the short span of time that small children's interest can be

held'' (Bayley, 1969, p. 27). The examiner must neither be frightened of nor maudlin about babies. He or she must simply feel comfortable with babies and able to adapt to their rhythm of operations without stress or strain.

2. *Equipment*. Equipment for infant-level examinations must be such as to accommodate postural maturity: nonsitting babies, sitting with support, sitting alone, and chair sitting. Such equipment includes: (a) a flat surface such as the top of an ordinary examining table, on which the infant can display postural and other motor behaviors; (b) a bed tray placed on the examining table for the presentation of test materials; (c) a crib in which the infant can be placed during the interview with the parent, or a highchair in which a sitting infant can be placed for certain tests; and (d) at later stages, a nursery table and chairs for baby and examiner. There should, of course, also be chairs for the adults who may be present. Another useful item is a playpen in which older babies can be placed during the parent interview, and their play-behavior with non-test toys observed. Obviously, all this equipment plus space for moving about requires a room of generous size (or, in fact, two rooms), which should be furnished in a comfortable but unostentatious way.

3. *Flexibility of examination*. In contrast to the fixed procedures standardized for the administration of psychological tests, the administration of developmental scales, particularly at the early infant levels, is characterized by great flexibility. The examiner may well have been ''accepted'' by the infant, but even so remains subject to the fluctuating moods, wishes, and interests of the baby. In order to maintain rapport and secure best performance, the mother is present during the examination both to assure the infant with her presence and to assist in the examination when it seems that best performance can be elicited when a task is presented by the mother rather than the examiner. Further, if the examiner's presence distracts the infant from the task in hand, the examiner moves to a position away from the direct gaze of the baby. When the baby looks to an examiner for approval, nods and smiles are in order. If the baby grows tired or bored, proceedings are halted for a time, and mother-comfort is given if this seems called for. Finally, the order of presentation of test items is also generally flexible, depending on the directions specified in the test manual. With babies happily disposed to interpersonal relations, the examiner can relax his guard somewhat, and enjoy in wonder the remarkable abilities of these small beings who are scarcely at the threshold of life.

Instruments of Examination

The terms ''developmental schedule'' and ''developmental scale'' are preferred to the term ''test'' for the psychological instruments used in infant examination. "Test" implies something definitive and stable in the form of a quantitative score. In my opinion, this is not an appropriate concept for the rapid growth changes that characterize infancy. But opinions differ, as illustrated by the popular *Cattell Infant Intelligence Scale* (Cattell, 1940), which is largely a downward extension of the 1937 Stanford-Binet, Form L for the age range 3 months to 30 months, and which employs mental age and intelligence quotient concepts in evaluation.

Of the infant evaluation scales available (see current psychological test catalogues of leading publishers and the latest Buros *Mental Measurements Yearbook*), two are of special merit particularly in the examination of disability-suspect and hearing-impaired infants.

1. *Gesell Developmental Schedules* (Gesell and Amatruda, 1947). Developed under Gesell's direction at the Yale Clinic of Child Development, this is probably the earliest, best known, and most comprehensive approach to infant behavior evaluation. The age range covered is from 4 weeks to 6 years, and at the early infant level, the behavior zones examined include: motor behavior, adaptive behavior, language behavior, and personal-social behavior. Each behavior zone is tapped by a comprehensive array of test tasks.

2. *Bayley Scales of Infant Development* (Bayley, 1969). This is an excellently conceived and constructed approach to the assessment of children in the age range from 2 through 30 months. The Scales are designed to evaluate developmental status on a tripartite basis: (1) the Mental Scale, which focuses on such behaviors as sensory-perceptual acuities, memory, learning, problem-solving ability, vocalizations and beginning verbal communication, and early evidences of abstract thinking ability; (2) the Motor Scale, which deals mainly with behaviors reflecting motor coordination and skills; and (3) the Infant Behavior Record, which assesses the nature of the child's social and objective orientation toward his environment.

In addition to information available in psychological test catalogues and the test reviews to be found in the Buros *Mental Measurements* publications, a good guide for new infant-examiners is actual observation of examination procedures as conducted by experts. The examination of infants can be difficult and demanding, and new examiners can profit greatly from watching the experts in action.

Observation

Infant behavior assessment is based on trained observation. This encompasses a great deal more than simply response to test items. In themselves, the items present a special kind of stimulus designed to elicit certain kinds of information. Ideally, the full scope of a given infant's behavior is best evoked and observed in a real-life context. But granting the unfeasibility of this ideal for busy practitioners, quite a variety of revelatory behaviors are manifested and can be assessed during the course of examination, beyond responses to test items. These include: interaction with the mother, reaction to strangers, to new surroundings; cooperative interaction; comfort/discomfort behaviors; play. Such "incidental" behaviors are as much a part of the assessment picture as are responses to test items.

Certain developmental schedules have special forms for recording these behaviors. For example, in the Bayley Infant Behavior Record form that is used in conjunction with the Bayley test report form, provision is made for recording such observed behaviors as: social orientation (to persons, examiner, mother); cooperativeness; fearfulness; tension; general emotional tone; object orientation; goal directedness; attention span; endurance; activity; reactivity; and sensory areas of interest displayed. The descriptive checklist for recording behavior in each of these areas conveys a vivid image of the baby. To illustrate with "General Emotional Tone," Bayley's descriptive designations include such terms as: cries, fusses, whines, listless, droopy, protests, frowns, unhappy expression, nonexpressive, smiles, coos or babbles with happy intonations, laughs, squeals, crows, animated expression. In a completed record, the baby seems to come alive, and an experienced worker can often see the infant in his mind's eye from the records alone without ever having laid eyes on the child.

References

Bayley, N. 1969. *Bayley Scales of Infant Development: Manual.* New York: The Psychological Corporation.

Bayley, N. 1970. Development of mental abilities. In P. H. Mussen, Ed., *Carmichael's Manual of Child Psychology,* vol. 1. New York: John H. Wiley, and Sons.

Cattell, P. 1940. *The Measurement of Intelligence of Infants and Young Children.* New York: The Psychological Corporation. (Fourth reprinting 1976.)

Gesell, A., and Amatruda, C. S. 1947. *Developmental Diagnosis: Normal and Abnormal Child Development.* New York: Paul B. Hoeber.

McCall, R. B., Hogarty, P. S., and Hurlburt, N. 1972. Transitions in infant sensorimotor development and the prediction of childhood I.Q. *American Psychologist,* 27: 728–48.

12 Examination of Children and Youth

THE PERIOD from childhood through youth covers an extensive range both chronologically and developmentally. Chronologically, it spans the school-age years from preschool through adolescence. Developmentally, it encompasses a broad sequence of continuous change that gradually transforms the child-that-was into the adult-to-be.

The patterns and processes of change that characterize the transformation are masterfully described in the classic writings of Gesell and his co-authors and in the seminal contributions of Piaget, among others. The details are well beyond the scope of this chapter. The focus here is simply on how an examiner fares in the psychological examination of children and youth who are deaf.

Case History

The history of a deaf child begins with its infancy biography and gradually moves into the broadened behavioral sphere that growing up entails. For psychologists to deaf children, a comprehensive history serves the particular purpose of filling information gaps resulting from testing difficulties, interview problems, and observation limitations.

Data of special importance in a case history concern what Muller (1969) calls "the tasks of childhood." For younger children, these include: (1) the growth of self-awareness; (2) the attainment of physiological stability; (3) the formation of simple concepts related to physical and social reality; (4) the appearance of conscience; (5) the learning of social communication and beginning scholastic skills; and (6) acquiring the concepts necessary to everyday life, including appropriate sexual roles. For youth they include: (1) the recognition of limitations; (2) achievement of emotional independence; (3) the choice of a career; and (4) the formation of a personal philosophy.

History items related to Muller's tests are included in Appendix F, the history inventory. The following areas are of special importance in the histories of deaf school-agers.

1. Developmental History

Diagnostic leads to later learning and behavior difficulties can be picked up in the developmental history. For younger children, in particular, such early alerts may provide guides to appropriate interventions at a time when they will do the most good.

2. Health History

Coping with the many pressures and problems of deafness requires considerable physical stamina on the part of a child. Chronic illness in a school-ager means the loss of valuable learning-time that can seldom be made up; physical debility robs a child of the energies needed to master the intricate learnings that lie ahead; and, not infrequently, chronic physical invalidism induces an attitude of psychological invalidism as well. Health history is therefore a continuing consideration in habilitation as well as in rehabilitation, and current health information is an important part of history data.

3. Vision

Vision is a deaf person's major avenue for information from the outside, hence plays a critical role in learning. Given the many documented reports of visual problems among the deaf, including Usher's syndrome (Vernon, 1969), it is of utmost importance that a psychological examiner know the visual status of a deaf school-ager. This would include not only ophthalmological reports but also information concerning visual perception, visual-motor coordination, and visual memory. Visual problems in learning to read must be identified early, so that remedial steps can be taken and this particular reading block overcome where possible.

4. Auditory History

Information concerning the auditory status and history of a school-age child and the auditory status of the child's parents provides an examiner with psychologically important insights. As discussed earlier, the psychological impact of deafness may vary considerably with: (a) age of onset; (b) amount and type of hearing loss; (c) amount and type of usable language preceding deafness; (d) travails leading to diagnosis; (e) age at confirmed diagnosis; (f) family attitudes; and (g) the nature, benefits, and child's acceptance of remedial interventions such as the hearing aid, visual languages, and school placement.

Briefly summarized: The more language the child had preceding deafness and/or the greater the amount of residual hearing, the higher the expectations for linguistic progress. The more disruptive the traumatic impact of acquired deafness, the greater the possibility of serious psychological disturbance. The more frustrating and lengthy the diagnostic search has been, the more likely the presence of family tensions and disturbances in the child's developmental environment. The more helpful the remedial interventions and the sooner they are applied, the better the outlook for adjustment to deafness and for progress in school.

5. *Educational Experiences*

For a deaf child who is cut off from much of the informal, out-of-school learnings acquired by nondeaf children in the course of daily experiences, school represents the principal milieu for developing the skills and attitudes essential for the incorporation and application of knowledge. Among the special considerations in a deaf child's school and learning experiences are the following.

Initial exposures. Whatever the education option a parent initially chooses, permanent negative attitudes to learning may develop even at this beginning stage owing to such factors as: (1) prematurely applied tutorial pressures either by parent or teacher; (2) the forcing of formal instruction before the child is physiologically or emotionally ready; (3) emotional trauma resulting from a child's being sent away from home to board with a tutor or to a residential school; (4) the risks of parent-tutors becoming more tutorial, judgmental, and critical than loving; (5) operating beyond a child's limits of physical endurance; (6) inappropriate school placement; and (7) incompetent teaching.

Equally dangerous is neglect of a child's learning and exploratory "hungers," whether through overprotection, ignorance, or indifference. Such neglect may result in transforming a potentially good learner into a lazy one who may never do full justice to his own potentials. The older the child becomes and the more deeply ingrained the listless learning attitudes, the more difficult they are to correct.

School placement. As previously discussed, deaf pupils attend different kinds of schools and programs, ranging from regular hearing schools to residential special schools. When a school's educational philosophy and the needs of the child are mismatched, the pupil suffers the consequences both scholastically and emotionally. Therefore psychological examiners need to turn to school-placement history to detect whether the school's philosophy coincides with the pupil's best interests, paying special attention to such matters as: (1) whether the methods of instruction and communication are appropriate to a pupil's auditory status, learning abilities, mental capacity, and special learning problems; (2) whether there is adequate provision for a pupil's psychosocial developmental needs; (3) whether there is provision for the treatment of emotional and learning problems; and (4) whether teacher competence is sufficient for dealing with deaf children in general, and the child being examined in particular.

Length of time in school. Serious and permanent scholastic retardations can result from too late a start and too few years in school. Although preschool and infant programs are increasing, there are still numbers of deaf children throughout the country who for one reason or other do not begin school until 8, 10, or more years of age. Such children seldom make up for the delay in beginning school. And there are numerous pupils who leave school before completing the course of study. The less formal education a deaf pupil has had, the more likely the prospect of serious handicaps, and the more difficult they are to alleviate.

Scholastic attainments. Because prelinguistic deafness retards the development of verbal language, it slows the pace of all learning based on verbal-language mastery. To make up for the lag, deaf pupils customarily require an appreciably longer period of schooling than the nondeaf. Even so, the average prelinguistically deaf pupil is about 4 years behind the hearing in scholastic attainment. Where this 4-year retardation extends to 6 and more years, the examiner is alerted to the presence of additional retarding agents such as emotional disturbance, mental incapacity, inadequate instructional practices, special learning disabilities, and language-learning disorders associated with brain damage. Differential diagnostic search is called for.

It must be emphasized that this traditionally accepted 4-year retardation in scholastic attainment should not be viewed as a permanent scholastic "norm" for deaf pupils. It is more likely a "norm" of deficiency in educational management. With improved educational standards, better teaching, a more realistic curriculum, and more appropriate communicative strategies, there is every likelihood that this retardation can be considerably reduced if not eliminated.

6. Family Aspirations and Attitudes

When a deaf child enters the school years, family aspirations begin to evolve and gradually crystallize into plans and goals for the future. A good lead to level of aspiration is history information concerning the educational, occupational, and socioeconomic status of the family. As a rule, the higher the family levels, the higher the aspirations; and the higher the aspirations, the greater the expectations for the child's scholastic success. Both aspirations and expectations can be quite inconsistent with the realities of deaf education or the child's abilities. In many instances, families are not fully informed of these realities by the schools, or if informed feel that their child is bound to prove an exception to the rule. But whatever the situation, when the child does not live up to family hopes, the consequences are registered in his adjustive environment. Where he was once the center of family attention and anticipation, he is now regarded as a lost cause. Not infrequently, emotional problems among deaf school-agers are rooted in such situations. It is therefore essential for a psychological examiner to know whether a child's acceptance by his family is contingent upon attaining the family's aspirations; whether he can attain them; and the extent to which a family will accept modified goals without rejecting the child.

7. Psychosocial Attitudes and Adjustments

With the deaf as with the hearing, the pattern of adult adaptability is fashioned to a considerable extent by the way in which the child was prepared to meet new experiences. When a child is deaf, explanations of the meaning of unfamiliar events are seriously hampered by the problem of communication; and, as a result, many deaf children feel themselves thrown into new experiences rather than prepared for them. Those children whose experiences have happily generated self-confidence and trust in others are able to maintain exploratory drive and emotional equilibrium. But to an insecure child, even everyday events may loom as threats to which he reacts with anxiety, apathy, resistance, and the like. Such a child would rather do without and remain safely protected by a familiar environment than venture out into the unknown. Many of the rigid, inflexible deaf adults of today are nothing more than the frightened, insecure children of the past.

Life is especially hard on a child who becomes deaf during the formative childhood years. Not capable of fully understanding what has happened, the child tends to feel that his parents are somehow responsible for not having prevented it from happening. The parents, on the other hand, in their anxiety to apply the full battery of habilitative compensations, are apt to overlook the critical necessity of reestablishing themselves as symbols of security in the child's new and frighteningly silent world. In such instances, it is not unusual for a child's panic and anger at not hearing to center on the parents for seemingly being more interested in hearing aids and deafness than in the child and his or her emotional needs. Such children often experience disruptive feelings of rejection. Rejection is not generally the case at all; it is simply the child's interpretation of the parents' excessive concern with habilitative aids. Unless special pains are taken to correct this impression, the child's feelings of hostility may become a fixed attitude toward the hearing world.

Another important determinant of social initiative and fraternization with the hearing is the nature of a deaf child's recreational experiences. Many suffer denigrating or at best patronizing treatment at the hands of their hearing peers, and find recreational satisfactions only with the deaf. Some are not permitted by their parents to associate with other deaf children and are in consequence forced to "play" with reluctant hearing children or else go off by themselves; others are recreationally immobilized by strenuous parental overprotection. The ones who fare best are those who are encouraged to develop a wide range of recreational interests with both deaf and hearing peers. They fare best as children, and later as adults.

8. "Preparation-for-life" Knowledge

Traditionally, school age is considered the time when a child is scheduled to be "prepared for life." Referring again to Muller's tasks of childhood (1969), it is a period for acquiring the concepts necessary for everyday living and for the appropriate sex role; a period for achieving emotional independence, choosing a career, and developing a personal philosophy. Considering the obstacles deafness can raise toward accomplishing these crucial tasks, it is essential that a psychological examiner make a special effort to find out how far along the road to independent living a deaf school-ager is for his or her years, and which life areas are in special need of remedial attention. Particularly important is information about a school-ager's sex knowledge and experiences, in view of Kallmann's statement that "sexual delinquency and immaturity, lack of preparation for a successful marriage and a stable family life, and the more extreme forms of deviant sex behavior are by no means less common among the deaf" (1963, p. 245). There are plenty of psychological inventories for such life-adjustment areas as social maturity, values and attitudes, sex knowledge, occupational preferences. Psychological test catalogues and the Buros publications are major reference sources. The trouble in applying the devices to a deaf clientele is that most of the measures are highly verbal and can be extremely difficult to adapt to deaf school-agers both linguistically and conceptually. They can, however, serve as interview guides for examiners who are highly skilled in work with the deaf.

Preparation-for-life information is of value not only in the examination of a particular individual, its importance extends into the whole area of preventive mental health measures for the deaf. To quote Kallmann again, "If we sincerely desire to promote prevention and cure of these delinquency patterns, we shall have to learn to look at them as *deviations* from a normal maturational process that is determined not only by man's biological nature, but also by the family, school, and psychological atmosphere in which he develops" (1965, p. 245, italics added).

9. Focus of Behavior Data

An examiner customarily looks to history data for descriptions of a subject's reported behavior and behavior deviations before conducting his own inquiry. However, a special point must be made concerning the focus of behaviors generally recorded in a case history. This is customarily on the behaving individual. Rarely is there any information about the *elicitor* of the reported behavior, whether teacher, classmate, houseparent, or whoever, or about the situation that evoked or provoked the behavior. But behavior does not take place in a vacuum, nor is it a "normable" constant from person to person or situation to situation. Therefore, in order to evaluate the *relevance* of undesirable behavior and judge whether it was warranted, the focus of the report needs to be broadened to include the behavior of the eliciting figures vis-à-vis the child, the nature of the behavior-evoking situation, and whether certain behaviors are consistently evoked by certain figures. Such history information is particularly important where wide swings and inconsistencies in behavior are reported. The "blame" may lie not so much with the child as with the behavior-evoking figure or situation.

10. Current Communication Patterns

In preparation for meeting a school-ager, the examiner needs to know the child's current preferred modes of and expertise in expressive and receptive communication. While these may be inferred from school history, progress or changes may have taken place in the course of time. Current abilities and preferences need to be described to inform the examiner of which modes to use in interpersonal exchange, what to expect in mutual comprehension, and what alternate approaches or supports may be required.

Psychological Testing

In turning from the infancy to the school-age level, psychologists move from the chronological range of least difference between the deaf and the hearing to that in which differences become increasingly pronounced; from the flexibility characterizing infant evaluation to the rigid rules governing the use of standardized tests; and from the selection of developmental schedules that are equally applicable to deaf and hearing babies to sharp limitations in tests designed and standardized for deaf school-agers.

As a result of this combination of circumstances, most of the tests used with the deaf are measures standardized on nondeaf populations. As previously noted, some support the practice on the grounds that the deaf live in the same world as the hearing and therefore should be tested with the same measures; while others protest the unfairness of testing deaf children with measures and norms based on "hearing" experiences and performance. And finally, there are the "compromisers" who feel a satisfactory solution to the problem is to attach deaf norms to hearing-standardized tests, without realizing that despite deaf norms the tests and test items may still be structurally unsuited to a deaf population.

Psychologists caught in this test-bind are faced with complex problems of test selection. The problem of standardized versus unstandardized is joined by numbers of variations in test format. For example, there are verbal tests which require the use of verbal language for both administration and response. Some deaf persons can take such tests successfully, but most cannot. There are nonverbal tests which use verbal language for directions but not response; nonlanguage tests in which no verbal language is required for either directions or response, performance or manipulative types of tests which can be administered and responded to nonverbally; and there are paper-and-pencil tests in which test items are written, printed, or drawn, and response is made in writing of some kind. Further, there are group tests that can be given simultaneously to upward of 20 subjects and individual tests that are administered to one subject at a time. There are also other kinds of variations among psychological tests that raise provoking questions of choice.

All in all, in attempting to achieve fair test practices with deaf subjects, a conscientious examiner often finds that more time must be spent in searching for appropriate measures than in actual testing. The sections that follow offer guidelines for dealing with this difficult situation.

General Testing Guides

The main focus of this section is on mental and personality testing, since it is in these important examination areas that the testing of deaf subjects poses its most inhibiting problems.

Selecting the Instruments

The "standardization" halo. In selecting psychological tests for deaf subjects, examiners are prone to assume that once a psychological instrument claims to be standardized, it bears a seal of excellence and so warrants consideration for use with deaf individuals. This is of course not so. There are well-standardized tests, poorly standardized ones, and some for which the term "standardized" is simply window-dressing. Whatever modifications need to be made to adapt a test to a deaf subject, the least that can be asked is that the test be well constructed. A good indication of a test's soundness can be found in its standardization details, which are described in the manuals of all responsible tests.

Screening the tests. Once the standardization details of promising tests have been reviewed, a matching process is conducted involving the fit (a) between the content and concepts of test items and a subject's age, experiences, scholastic standing, and concept level; (b) between a test's directions for administration and a subject's ability to comprehend them as they stand; (c) between the manner in which response to test items is to be made (oral, written, manipulative, etc.) and a subject's abilities along these lines; (d) between the demands of unstructured tests, such as projective techniques, and a subject's ability to meet them; and (e) between a subject's ability to take a test after suitable modifications have been made and the feasibility of making modifications without harm to the test. Relevant details about a subject's contributions to these matches are found in the case history, which should be reviewed before test selection. References to test resources and descriptions of tests can be found in psychological test catalogues and in the Buros *Mental Measurement Yearbooks* and other Buros publications and reviews.

Adapting the tests. Where modifications in promising tests are required for deaf subjects, they need to be carefully worked out beforehand, and objective modifications need to be prepared for three eventualities—simplified verbal language, signs, and pantomime—the form to be used depending upon which is most comprehensible to a particular individual. Where such modifications in language are so worked out, it is entirely possible to maintain the intent and objectivity of the original test. The most risky and difficult modifications involve simplifying concepts expressed in test items and questions that are beyond the experiences or grasp of a subject. An example taken from the WISC is: "Why is it generally better to give money to an organized charity than to a street beggar?" (Wechsler, 1949, p. 63). Although items on the WISC Verbal Scale can be tried experimentally with deaf children, this example shows why the Performance Scale of the WISC is preferred for I.Q. purposes. Before using modified tests with deaf subjects, it has been my practice to take the tests myself, with a colleague acting as examiner, in order to assess the conceptual and communicative modifications, their objectivity, and comprehensibility. Whatever improvements seem called for are made, and then the test is tried out with sample deaf subjects with an eye to further improvement, and rechecked with other samples after these improvements have been made.

Pretest Preparations

The test environment. Test rooms should be neutrally cheerful and simply but comfortably furnished. Nothing should suggest a doctor's office, nor should the examiner wear a lab coat. Even with older deaf children, these may arouse unhappy memories of early diagnostic experiences, and inhibit performance. With very young children newly emerging from diagnostic travails, reminders of doctors commonly arouse fear. Room furnishings should include chairs and tables for testing young and older children. For times when parents must be present during testing, a good supply of popular magazines should be available for browsing. Test materials should be neatly arranged, convenient to hand for the examiner but not distractingly visible to the subject; and closed cupboards or files should contain other potentially distracting materials such as office supplies, other tests, and toys. The examiner must keep in mind that deaf children are visual beings; hence visible distractions should be reduced to a minimum. This includes the surface of the test table, which should be free of all materials (test manuals, stop watches, etc.) except those involved in a test task. Stop watches can be particularly distracting to young children and anxiety-provoking to older ones. I have found it convenient to hang the stop watch around my neck on a string that is long enough to center the watch below the tabletop. The child knows it is there, of course, but the watch loses its impact by being less visible and at the same time leaves the examiner's hands free to attend to other matters.

Examiner preparation. Over and above technical competence and the special competencies required of examiners to the deaf, examiners of very young children need to be familiar with the basic facts of child development. Such children are not simplified adults. There are still developmental changes taking place before experiential stability is reached; and children of different developmental levels and experiences may perceive the same test task in quite different ways. Along these lines, research suggests that children even see pictures differently from adults, and that children who have had little experience with pictures perform relatively poorly on tasks involving pictorial representations (Gibson and Olum, 1960, p. 361).

It is highly important, therefore, that examiners of young deaf children be able to see test items through the eyes and experiences of the child. For example, does a given manipulative task fit the child's previous experiences with manipulative play materials or is this a first exposure? "First exposure" children may be seriously penalized in test performance as compared with experienced children of the same age and mental level. Child-examiners must also be able to perceive and interpret minute behavioral clues, and adapt their own behaviors and procedures to what the clues reveal. All these efforts serve to establish empathetic insights and rapport in order to evoke best performance from the child and sound interpretations from the examiner.

Finally, at whatever chronological level is being tested, examiners must enter the test situation fully familiar with the tests and fully skilled in the dextrous manipulation of test materials. Nothing is more boring to a subject of any age, especially a deaf subject, than to have to sit and wait while the examiner is reading up on test instructions, scribbling notes, or fumbling about with test materials. This is the surest way to blunt interest and dull response. Examiners must keep pace with a subject's performance.

Preparing the subject. No subject, even if previously tested, should be plunged into a psychological test without some introductory explanation by a responsible person. With very young children who are not yet test-wise, preparation is smoothly handled where the child is already attending a school in which the examiner is a staff member and makes routine classroom rounds for observation purposes. In such situations, most young children enjoy a break in class routines and happily accompany this familiar, nonthreatening figure to the room where special games are played.

When both examiner and situation are entirely unfamiliar to a young child, special care must be taken on a first encounter not to overpower the child with enthusiastic greetings, especially a timid or mistrustful child. Presumably the intake history which the examiner has read beforehand describes the communicative patterns used by the child, and a smiling "Hello" is addressed to the child in its accustomed communicative mode; or if this is unknown, simply a warm and friendly spoken "Hello." Also, some nontest toys are temptingly displayed to capture the child's interest and convey the message that this is a play situation. If the child shows signs of anxiety unless the mother is present, then she is permitted to stay, but seated off to one side of and slightly behind the child so the child can see her out of the corner of an eye without having to get up and look around to make sure she is still there.

Preschoolers and young school-agers are led into formal testing by way of a brief preliminary period of play with the examiner, using nontest toys. Formal testing begins when the child is ready for more games. In the event a child refuses to respond to these overtures, testing is not forced. The child is smilingly dismissed with a cheerful "Good-bye," and arrangements are made for a return visit which is usually successful. Exceptions to this procedure are certain children with bizarre behaviors who cannot be "prepared" in the usual ways but who can nevertheless be tested, albeit through unorthodox approaches, as illustrated in later discussion.

With older deaf children, who are already test-wise in most instances, preparation can simply take the form of a friendly greeting and an explanation in the subject's preferred communicative mode that the test procedure is a way of finding out about a person's interests and goals as a means of helping to plan for the future and manage current problems. When questions are asked by the subject, they should be answered by the examiner as sincerely but as briefly as possible, since the test session must not be permitted to turn into an interview unless it becomes obvious that the subject's needs so require. In this case, testing is rescheduled for another time.

Influencing Variables

Although many potential variables in testing are controlled through standardization and pretest preparation, examiners must be prepared for others that are still likely to arise, such as test anxiety, motivation, physical or emotional condition at the time of testing, misleading directions, and the subject's previous exposures to the same test. Where such variables threaten test performance, testing should be postponed and special precautions taken to control the offending variables before subsequent testing.

Examiners, too, can be offending variables. Being human, they have personal preferences and competencies which do not necessarily fit every subject, hence influence test performance. It would be too much, for example, to expect every examiner to be equally competent at all chronological levels, with all types of subjects, and all types of tests. Many have their favored pool of tests from which they are unfortunately loath to depart even for a special situation or subject. Most have age-range preferences. And numbers of examiners frankly admit an inability to work with certain types of disablements and certain kinds of subjects. Children are sensitive to such examiner dispositions. and deaf children especially so. Examiners therefore need to face up to their own preferences and limitations and, when they feel ill at ease or out of their depth, to take whatever corrective measures are possible in their particular situation lest they too become a confounding variable.

A Note on Cited Tests

The sampling of tests mentioned in the next sections includes some that are often used by examiners of deaf subjects, some seldom used, and some that warrant further trial. The lists serve an informative rather than a "recommendation" function. Recommendations on the basis of tests alone are almost impossible to make because of the many cautions and criteria involved in conscientious test selection, adaptation, and administration. Whether a test is "good" or not for a deaf subject depends largely on how well these criteria have been established and observed. Even a good test can become a poor instrument when badly matched to a given subject, or poorly adapted, or poorly administered.

Further, in the course of time, test revisions appear. While the changes made are seldom radical, they nevertheless require buying new materials. Where the unrevised version of a test is doing a satisfactory job, examiners must decide for themselves whether this expense is warranted. However, when a test not previously used needs to be ordered, it is wise to consult current test catalogues to see if a revision has been made and what the improvements are in the revised form.

To avoid confusion, the tests cited in the following sections are unrevised versions unless otherwise noted. Examiners may refer to current psychological test catalogues and to the latest Buros *Mental Measurements Yearbook* for detailed test information. To keep abreast of changes in the test market, the reader should ask to be placed on the mailing lists of major test publishers and distributors for their annual catalogues and other announcements.

Finally, Appendices I and J provide publisher and distributor information for easy access to test manuals and materials of those tests and developmental scales cited in the sections on psychological testing.

Mental Testing

Of central importance during the school years are a deaf child's learning potentials. Judgments in this area are often difficult to make, especially when a child's behavior is immature, scholastic attainment is retarded, environmental interplay is limited, and communications are equally so. Therefore, a large share of responsibility falls on mental test information in estimating learning ability.

Mental Tests Used with Deaf School-agers

Table 12.1 rank-lists mental tests used with deaf subjects (preschool through adolescence) as reported by two or more respondents in a survey of psychological practices with the deaf (Levine, 1974). In addition to the hearing-standardized tests cited in Table 12.1, there are several tests standardized on the deaf, namely: the Nebraska Test of Learning Aptitude for Young Deaf Children (Hiskey, 1941); the Ontario School Ability Examination (Amoss, 1936); the Non-Verbal Intelligence Tests for Deaf and Hearing Subjects (Snijders and Snijders-Oomen, 1959); and the Smith Nonverbal Scale, now titled the Smith-Johnson Nonverbal Performance Scale (Smith and Johnson, 1978). Almost half of the respondents reported that their particular test-selections were determined by the triad of ease of administration, ease of scoring, and recommendation by other testers. Advantages and disadvantages were expressed about most of the tests in use, including the popular Wechsler scales.

Descriptive Digests of Selected Mental Tests

The alphabetical listing that follows is an illustrative sampling of tests reported in table 12.1, and annotated by age and test items. All are capable of administration in pantomime or signs.

1. *Chicago Nonverbal Examination.* A paper-and-pencil test for ages 8 years through adult. Tasks include: digit symbol; genus discrimination; block counting in stacked constructions; part/whole discrimination; figure matching; part/whole pictorial relationships; event sequence; progression sequence; pictorial absurdities; pictorial part-to-whole relationships.
2. *Goodenough-Harris Drawing Test.* A paper-and-pencil "one-item" test which is a revision and extension of the Goodenough Draw-a-Man test for ages 3–15 years; involves drawing a man and a woman.
3. *Leiter International Performance Scale.* A performance-type test for ages 2–18 years. Tasks are categorized as: concretistics—matching of specific relationships; symbolic transformation—judging relationships be-

Table 12.1 Mental Tests in Rank Order (*n* =166 Respondents)

Name of Test	Special School			Regular School				Other Agency				Grand Total
	Residential	Day	Total	Special Class	Partially Integrated	Totally Integrated	Total	Diagnostic Unit	Speech & Hearing Center	Rehabilitation Setting	Total	
Wechsler Intelligence Scale for Children (WISC) Performance	32	25	57	47	9	6	62	6	3	1	10	129
Leiter Intelligence Tests	21	19	40	34	5	3	42	7	3	2	12	94
Wechsler Adult Intelligence Scale (WAIS) Performance	31	10	41	18	6	3	27	6	3	2	11	79
Hiskey-Nebraska Learning Aptitude Test	15	10	25	14	7	3	24	1	2	1	4	53
Goodenough-Harris	14	11	25	6	1	1	8	0	2	0	2	35
Wechsler Preschool/ Primary Scale of Intelligence (WPPSI) Performance	10	7	17	7	2	0	9	6	2	0	8	34
Arthur Adaptation Leiter	12	5	17	10	1	0	11	1	1	0	2	30
Columbia Mental Maturity Scale (CMMS)	6	1	7	14	1	2	17	0	0	1	1	25
Merrill-Palmer Scale of Mental Tests	8	5	13	5	1	2	8	0	2	0	2	23
Ravens Progressive Matrices	7	5	12	3	1	1	5	0	0	2	2	19
Ontario School Ability Examination	3	6	9	4	0	0	4	0	0	0	0	13
Stanford-Binet Intelligence	3	4	7	2	3	0	5	0	0	0	0	12
Cattell Intelligence Tests	0	5	5	0	1	0	1	1	1	1	3	9
Chicago Nonverbal Exam.	6	0	6	1	0	0	1	0	0	0	0	7
Wechsler-Bellevue Intelligence Scale II	0	1	1	3	0	0	3	0	0	0	0	4
Snijders-Oomen Nonverbal Intelligence Test	0	1	1	1	1	1	0	2	0	0	0	3
Pintner-Paterson Scale	2	1	3	0	0	0	0	0	0	0	0	3
Denver Developmental	0	3	3	0	0	0	0	0	0	0	0	3
Preschool Attainment (Doll)	1	0	1	1	0	0	1	0	0	0	0	2
Smith Nonverbal Scale	1	0	1	1	0	0	1	0	0	0	0	2
Revised Beta	1	0	1	0	0	0	0	0	0	1	1	2
Calif. Mental Maturity	2	0	2	0	0	0	0	0	0	0	0	2
Porteus Mazes	1	0	1	0	0	0	0	1	0	0	1	2

SOURCE: Drawn from Levine (1974).

tween two events; quantitative discriminations; spatial imagery; genus matching; progression discriminations; immediate recall; speed.

Arthur Adaptation of the Leiter International Performance Scale is a restandardization of the scale on children aged 3–8 years, using portions of the scale appropriate to this age range.

4. *Merrill-Palmer Scale of Mental Tests* (Language Scale omitted). A performance scale for ages 2–5 years. Tasks include such items as: crossing feet; standing on one foot; throwing a ball; paper folding; drawing up a string; cutting with scissors; matching colors; closing fist and moving thumb; copying a circle, a cross, a star; buttons and buttonholes; pyramid buildings; various formboards.

5. *Hiskey-Nebraska Test of Learning Aptitude for Young Deaf Children.* A performance scale standardized on hearing-impaired children for ages 4–10 years. Tasks include: memory for colored objects; bead stringing patterns; pictorial associations; block building; memory for digits; drawing completions; pictorial completions; pictorial identifications; paper folding; visual attention span; puzzle blocks; and pictorial analogies.

6. *Snijders and Snijders-Oomen Nonverbal Intelligence Tests for Deaf and Hearing Subjects.* A performance scale standardized on deaf children for ages 3–15 years. Tasks are grouped according to: form; combination; abstraction; and memory; and include mosaic designs, block design, copying, drawing completion, puzzles, halved pictures, corresponding pictures, picture completion, series continuation, picture analogies, figure analogies, sorting shapes, sorting cards, picture memory, knox cube.

7. *Porteus Mazes.* A "single-item" type of paper-and-pencil test in which mazes of increasing difficulty (Vineland revision, Porteus Maze Extension, and Porteus Maze Supplement) are arranged for ages 3 years through adult.

8. *Raven Progressive Matrices.* A design fill-in test for ages 5 years through adult. The task involves selecting a particular piece, from several exposed pieces, that will complete a given design or "matrix" from which the part had been removed. Design themes are: continuous patterns; analogies between pairs of figures; progressive alteration of patterns; permutations of figures; and resolution of figures into constituent parts. Colored Progressive Matrices sets were constructed in 1947 for children between 5 and 11 years.

9. *Wechsler Preschool and Primary Scale of Intelligence (WPPSI), Performance portion.* Standardized on nondeaf children aged 4–6 years. Test items include: animal house (a color matching/memory task); picture completions; mazes; geometric designs; block designs.

10. *Wechsler Intelligence Scale for Children (WISC), Performance portion.* Standardized on nondeaf children aged 5–15 years. Test items include: digit symbol; picture completions; block designs; picture arrangements; and object assemblies.

11. *Wechsler Adult Intelligence Scale (WAIS), Performance portion.*

Standardized on the nondeaf aged 16 years and over. Test items include: digit symbol; picture completions; block designs; picture arrangements; object assemblies.

Testing Guides and Practices

An underlying imperative in all psychological practice is mutually comprehensible communication between psychologist and subject. The following guides rest on an examiner's ability to engage in such communication with deaf subjects.

1. An important determinant of a subject's test performance lies in his or her clear understanding of test directions. Otherwise poor test performance may be due as much to a misunderstanding of directions as to mental inability. It is therefore essential that an examiner check understanding carefully before proceeding with a test item. In this connection, it is interesting to observe the various ways in which deaf children approach manipulative test items. Some charge right in as soon as the test material is displayed, without waiting for directions. These are generally the test-wise children. Others have difficulty even with suitably adapted directions. In such instances, examiners can devise a few simple practice items if the test lacks sample tasks. It is important, however, that the practice items do not serve as guides to answers. But it is even more important that a subject fully understand what he is expected to do.

2. Testing should be managed so that the subject leaves with a feeling that this has been an interesting, nonjudgmental experience which he would not mind repeating at some future time, as most likely will be the case. Toward this end, testing begins with a task that is within the range of a subject's abilities (as indicated in history information), yet not so simple as to be insulting. Testing should also end on a note of accomplishment, even if a nontest item must be used to achieve this.

3. Where possible, test items should be presented in line with a subject's interests and abilities. Items that have less appeal should be carefully interspersed among those that are more appealing; simpler items among those presenting difficulties. In testing deaf subjects, especially with hearing-standardized tests, it is more judicious to elicit best performance in this way than to rigidly adhere to a prescribed sequence in the face of a subject's resistance or distress.

4. Examiners should guard against taking advantage of a child's wish to please by urging him on beyond the limits of tolerance. When a child is pushed too far, test performance is determined more by adversely influencing variables outside the test frame than by the test itself. Testing should be discontinued when it is apparent that the subject can no longer put forth his best efforts.

5. An examiner's behavior and facial expression should be under wise control when testing deaf subjects. Children, in particular, look to an examiner's face for evidence of appraisal and are extraordinarily sensitive to even minute clues—a raised eyebrow, a slight frown, the twitch of a lip. The examiner's expression should at all times be pleasantly encouraging and nonjudgmental. Also to be avoided is extravagant praise for a good response, because when no praise is forthcoming for a poor one, the child feels let down and discouraged. Instead, the child should be made to feel that it is the effort that counts. Failure is acknowledged by "That was a hard one, but you *tried!* Now let's try another one." Success is quietly enjoyed by both. As the child comes to perceive this nonjudgmental attitude, he will cease to fasten his attention on the examiner's face, and will concentrate instead on the tasks before him and on his own critical faculties.

6. In testing deaf (as well as hearing) children, examiners should not be so eager to record test responses that other equally revelatory behaviors are ignored. These are reviewed later, in the section on Observation.

7. With deviant and disturbed children, unusual flexibility and patience are required to adapt test procedures to the subject's motor compulsions, psychological obsessions, and easy distractibility. Orthodox procedures are replaced by those demanded by the child's behavior and preferences. If, for example, the child insists on sitting on the examiner's lap, testing is conducted in this way. If the child prefers the floor or some other testing locale, then testing is conducted there. Two of my deviant subjects, aged 6 and 7 years, exhibited an autistic pattern that has been likened to a visual agnosia for humans. In one instance, I sat on the floor, completely immobile, for about half an hour, trying to simulate a piece of furniture, before the child approached and permitted sporadic contact. However, no test contact could be established, and testing had to be abandoned. In the other case, a supply of balloons had to be on hand and the child's father had to hover over the child with a demanding expression on his face before the child would perform; and then he would do so only if permitted a break between test items to blow up and play with the balloons. Testing was completed in this case, with an above-average I.Q. In neither instance did the child seem aware of the examiner as a person. Other types of deviant behaviors and obsessions demand relevant adaptations. Completing any test-item under such conditions leaves an examiner possibly exhausted but with a real sense of accomplishment.

8. When an examiner requires the assistance of an interpreter, that person should be carefully selected and coached. Details are reviewed in a later section on Interview.

9. To carry out these practices with deaf subjects, I find that test adminis-

tration is best conducted individually even though the test used is a group test.

Hearing-standardized Mental Tests and the Deaf: Problems and Management

A glance at table 12.1 shows that the intelligence tests most favored for deaf children and youth are performance and nonverbal types of tests, most of which have been standardized on nondeaf populations. Over and above the "fairness" of using hearing-standardized mental tests with deaf subjects, there are other issues worthy of deliberation. A number are briefly summarized here.

Performance scales. There is a general assumption among examiners that the "fairness" issue of using hearing-standardized tests with the deaf is eliminated by using performance or nonverbal types of mental tests. This is a mistaken notion. Even the culture-fair, paper-and-pencil types of mental tests rest on cultural backgrounds and experiential variables, and so do performance tests. For example, Wechsler (1944) found that a test as seemingly culture-fair as Digit-Symbol could not be used with illiterates because they lack experience in the use of pencil and paper. Noted earlier was the poor performance on pictorial tests on the part of children with little or no exposure to pictures. The same principle of background and cultural experiences applies to all tests including performance scales, and may account for the frequent comments from users of the culturally loaded Wechsler children's performance scales that the tests underrate deaf children. Therefore, in using hearing-standardized performance tests as first-tests with very young deaf children, examiners must keep in mind the possibility that they are testing the child's preparatory experiences as much as, or possibly more than, mental ability. In consequence, first I.Q.'s should be regarded as tentative findings subject to verification by later testing.

Another point brought out by the Wechsler performance scales is the practice of using portions of a full scale for arriving at a definitive I.Q. The Wechsler performance scale I.Q.'s are the most widespread example of the practice with deaf subjects. But as Wechsler himself remarked, when an abbreviated form of the Full Scale must be used, "the simplest and safest procedure is to use the Verbal part of the examination alone, and rate the subject on the basis of the I.Q.'s furnished for this part of the scale" (Wechsler, 1944, p. 145). Since this recommendation is not feasible in testing deaf children (or adults), an alternative recommendation is to use a battery of tests and not rely on a single portion of a hearing-standardized full scale as the sole index of mental ability.

Test instructions. Another problem in using hearing-standardized performance scales with deaf children is the lack of standardized directions for deaf subjects. This means that each examiner of a deaf child is free to devise his own. The varying strategies used can lead to considerable variations in response on tests given to the same child at different times by different examiners, as well as to difficulties in securing comparable data from child to child. Steven Ray (1978) sought to counteract these problems by developing a manual of test directions for the administration to deaf children of the revised Wechsler Intelligence Scale for Children (WISC-R).

Assessing validity. The question that haunts all examiners of the deaf is whether hearing-standardized mental tests measure with deaf subjects what they purport to measure with the hearing. One source of information is concurrent validity. This is commonly assessed by estimating the correspondence between a test's scores and those of a dependable established test. And here examiners of the deaf find themselves faced with a further problem: Which of the mental tests used with the deaf can be considered a "dependable established test"? For lack of a definitive answer, the following outside criteria are used as common-sense concurrent validity guides by those who "know" prelinguistically deaf children.

1. An arithmetic achievement level of 4th to 5th grade in older school-agers suggests above-average mental capacity.

2. A reading achievement level of 4th to 5th grade in older school-agers suggests at least average mental capacity.

3. Fairly fluent verbal expressive language suggests better than average mental capacity.

4. A prelinguistically deaf school-ager who is able to compete successfully with hearing peers in full mainstream programs demonstrates at least above-average and generally superior mental capacity.

5. Exceptional alertness on the part of a school-ager or preschooler in grasping thoughts, ideas, and directions, and in creative projects suggests at least above-average mental capacity.

6. Recognized leadership in recreational and other pursuits suggests above-average mental capacity.

These and other real-life criteria can help in assessing the validity for a deaf subject of hearing-standardized mental test scores. Where marked divergence between criteria and scores is found in favor of real-life performance, the fault generally lies with the test or in the manner of testing, and further inquiry is in order. It must be emphasized that the converse of these concurrent validity guides cannot be assumed to indicate mental deficits. There are many deaf children who do not measure up to these outside criteria despite average or better mental endowment. It is the examiner's responsibility to identify the retarding factors.

Interpreting test results. Interpreting scores earned on mental tests requires a clear understanding by the examiner of which *mental behaviors* the test constructor believes to be elicited by which *test items*. Also required is knowledge of the consonance between a subject's experiential background and that of the standardization group of the particular test, and the test-manifested expression of deviations between the two. In the case of deaf subjects, these factors are essential components of the interpreting process.

Test items indicate which components of intelligence are being probed. For example, in the Wechsler Preschool and Primary Scale of Intelligence (WPPSI), the Animal House test item is considered by the test constructor to be essentially a measure of a subject's learning ability involving memory, attention span, goal awareness, and the ability to concentrate (Wechsler, 1963, p. 11); while the Geometric Design task is a measure primarily of perceptual and visual-motor organization (1963, p. 11). At the adult level, Wechsler (1944) considers the Similarities test item to be a measure of logical thinking; Picture Arrangement, a measure of ability to comprehend and size up a total situation; Picture Completion, a measure of ability to differentiate essential from nonessential; and Block Design, a measure of synthetic and analytic abilities. Other mental behaviors evoked by test items include: reasoning; ability to see relationships and make associations; abstractive ability; judgment; learning ability; mental alertness; and comprehension. The kinds of test items commonly used by test constructors to evoke mental response are: analogies; memory for various verbal or nonverbal items; missing parts; symbol matching; similarities and differences; copying directly and from memory; arithmetic problems and reasoning; vocabulary; sentence completion; and problem solving. *It cannot be emphasized strongly enough that interpreting test results is not made by quoting test scores but by evaluating the mental behaviors for which the particular test items and scores stand.*

Where test manuals are not clear about which types of mental activity the various test items are intended to evoke (as is often the case), the examiner must take the time to think this out, possibly with the help of one or another of the many publications on test interpretation which are appearing in the test market. When these publications are used as aids, there is no objection to their use; but when they are used blindly in cookbook fashion, the examiner simply blunts his own professional sensitivities.

Finally, in using hearing-standardized tests with deaf subjects, it is imperative not only that test items be matched to the subject for purposes of examination but that test responses be matched to the subject's background of experiences for purposes of interpretation. The greater the experiential gap between a subject's background and that of the test's standardization group, the greater the likelihood of seemingly off-beat responses which may in actuality be quite in line with the subject's background and experiential viewpoint. It is of course not possible to arrive at exact quantitative estimates of the difference from "hearing" expectations that deafness may impose on test responses. It takes considerable experience even to arrive at a good guesstimate. But after years of psychological practice, perceptive examiners of deaf subjects are able to come up with remarkably astute estimates and interpretations of a deaf subject's mental resources that are often closer to the mark than the test scores themselves.

Special considerations in test selection. In selecting a mental test for a deaf subject of any age, the aim is for as broad a sampling of mental behaviors as possible, and this requires a correspondingly broad variety of test items. It is a rare hearing-standardized test that meets this requirement when used with deaf children. One-item type tests when used alone certainly do not; neither do portions of tests; and even generously itemized hearing-standardized tests become considerably less so when items are omitted that do not "fit" deaf subjects.

One way of getting broader mental coverage is to take advantage of the fact that several mental tests are available that have been standardized on deaf school-agers. Examiners can use these tests or items drawn from them to greater advantage than has been the case thus far. Of special merit is the Snijders–Snijders-Oomen *Non-verbal Intelligence Tests for Deaf and Hearing Subjects,* which covers an age span of 3–15 years and has separate norms for deaf and for hearing populations. There are also the *Hiskey-Nebraska Test of Learning Aptitude for Young Deaf Children* for a narrower chronological range, and the *Smith-Johnson Non-Verbal Performance Scale* for 2–4-year-olds. In each of these tests, the items were selected with deaf subjects in mind, as were the other standardization details.

When, in using such deaf-standardized mental tests, the need arises for obtaining fuller mental or chronological coverage, the test-battery approach is used, that is, a group of tests is administered, of different types (performance, paper-and-pencil, single-item) but all centering on intelligence. The examiner will probably have to dip into the pool of hearing-standardized tests for this purpose, owing to the scarcity of tests standardized on the deaf. There is even a place for verbal items and scales with certain deaf pupils, notably the Verbal as well as the Performance portions of the *Wechsler Adult Intelligence Scale* (WAIS) with deaf youth, as discussed in the next chapter, and the use of verbal tests with deaf pupils being evaluated for ability to succeed in full mainstream programs. When verbal test-items are used, they are administered in the subject's favored communicative mode.

As a rule, the battery approach is used with cases requiring detailed clinical inquiry; and interpreting the results of the mix of mental tests involved demands exceptional clinical judgment and insights on an examiner's part as well as sufficient time for testing, analyzing, and reporting. In ordinary practice, where examiners are under time and productivity pressures, there is an understandable temptation to choose tests for ease of administration and scoring, and to aim for a recordable I.Q. But even in such situations, an item-by-item interpretation needs to be made (and reported) in terms of the mental behaviors for which the scores and items stand; and this not only to supply a realistic picture of a mind at work but also to indicate which areas of mental operation are in special need of remedial attention.

Personality Testing

In the conceptual frame of psychological testing, "personality" is conceived as consisting of traits belonging to the emotional, motivational, attitudinal, and interest make-up of an individual, as distinct from those involved in mental and cognitive abilities; and personality tests, as instruments for exposing and measuring various nonintellectual aspects of behavior (as though this dichotomy were possible, to paraphrase Heim [1970]). Psychological test publishers offer several hundred personality instruments, many of which are controversial in both design and standardization (Buros, 1970).

Personality Tests Used with Deaf School-agers

Table 12.2 rank-lists psychological instruments reported as used in personality testing with deaf subjects by two or more respondents to a survey of psychological practices with the deaf (Levine, 1974). All the cited tests were designed for nondeaf subjects.

They may be classified into several types.

1. *Projective techniques.* Such instruments present a subject with a relatively unstructured and seemingly nonjudgmental task, in order to permit him to structure his response in accordance with the dictates of his own characteristic psychological patterns and reactions. Projective tests included in Table 12.2 are: Machover's Draw-a-Person Test (Machover, 1949); House-Tree-Person Projective Technique (Buck, 1966); Thematic Apperception Test (Murray, 1943); Rorschach Technique (Rorschach, 1942); Rotter Incomplete Sentences Blank (Rotter and Rafferty, 1950); Children's Apperception Test (Bellak, 1954); Make-a-Picture Story (Shneidman, 1947); and Symonds Picture-Story Test (Symonds, 1948).

Although the Bender-Gestalt is often classified and used as a projective personality test, its claim to this classification is questionable. As described by Bender, it "is a paper-and-pencil test in which configurations, originally used by Max Wertheimer for research in visual gestalt psychology, are presented to the individual for copying" (1938, p. 11). Since the test task is one of copying, it permits little if any free personality projection. Bender considers the test a "clinical test" whose value lies in detecting disturbances

Table 12.2 Personality Tests in Rank Order (n = 166 Respondents)

| Name of Test | Special School | | | Regular School | | | | Other Agency | | | | Grand Total |
	Residential	Day	Total	Special Class	Partially Integrated	Totally Integrated	Total	Diagnostic Unit	Speech & Hearing Center	Rehabilitation Setting	Total	
Bender-Gestalt	24	19	43	29	6	2	37	1	3	3	7	87
Draw a Person (Machover)	10	16	26	16	3	2	22	0	1	1	2	50
House-Tree-Person	8	5	13	12	3	2	17	6	2	1	9	39
Thematic Apperception Test (TAT)	7	5	12	2	0	1	3	0	2	2	4	19
Rorschach Test	5	5	10	1	0	0	1	6	2	0	8	19
Vineland Social Maturity Scale	5	3	8	2	0	0	2	0	3	3	6	18
Rotter Incomplete Sentences	5	4	9	3	0	1	4	0	1	0	1	14
Children's Apperception Test (CAT)	2	0	2	1	0	2	3	1	1	0	2	7
Make a Picture Story	4	2	6	0	0	0	0	0	1	0	1	7
Minnesota Multiphasic Inventory (MMPI)	1	1	2	0	0	0	0	0	1	1	2	4
Sixteen Personality Factor Questionnaire	2	0	2	0	0	0	0	0	1	0	1	3
Symonds Picture Story Test	0	1	1	0	0	0	0	0	1	0	1	2

SOURCE: Drawn from Levine (1974).

in the perception of gestalt relationships that are associated with organic brain defects, retardation, regression, and personality defects associated with regression. The great popularity of the Bender-Gestalt as a personality test has been attributed to ease and speed of administration. The test serves its clinical function well; but it was not devised to perform personality description in the usual sense of the "personality" concept and is best used in a battery as a diagnostic instrument.

2. *Personality Inventories.* These instruments present a subject with a list of questions or statements involving personality traits, emotional reactions, interpersonal attitudes and habits, and other behavior styles, to which the subject is expected to give an honest answer on the basis of his own behavioral patterns, preferences, and habits. Two such personality inventories are included in table 12.2: the Minnesota Multiphasic Personality Inventory

(MMPI) (Hathaway and McKinley, 1951), and the Sixteen Personality Factor Questionnaire (16 PF) (Cattell and Eber, 1956–1957).

3. *"Maturity" Inventories.* Such instruments, also of the questionnaire type, are used to assess a subject's level of maturity in various life areas. The Vineland Social Maturity Scale (Doll, 1947), cited in table 12.2, is one such inventory. It is designed to assess an individual's ability to take care of his own practical needs and assume related responsibilities.

There is a clear need for much broader information about deaf schoolagers' preparation for life and level of maturity than has been available thus far. Examiners should acquaint themselves with the contents of such inventories, most of which are cited in psychological test catalogues. Where the inventories cannot be used as they stand with deaf school-agers, they can be used as interview guides and also as guides in the design of school life-adjustment curricula.

Descriptive Digests of Selected Personality Tests

The following digests of selected tests from table 12.2 may assist the reader in gauging the suitability of these tests for deaf subjects (the stated age ranges are for nondeaf subjects) and also to consider which ones lend themselves to administration and response in signs or pantomime.

1. *Machover Draw-a-Person Test (also called Machover Figure Drawing).* Used with ages 2 years and over. Test directions are "to draw a person," and, on completion of the first drawing, to draw a person of the opposite sex. Afterward, inquiry elicits various items of information about the persons drawn.

2. *House-Tree-Person Projective Technique (H-T-P).* Used with ages 3 years and over. Test directions are to draw a "house," and are repeated for "tree" and "person." Then an extensive inquiry is conducted through a series of standardized questions to elicit associations about the subject's home and home life ("house"), life satisfactions and environment ("tree"), and interpersonal relations ("person").

3. *Thematic Apperception Test (TAT).* Used with ages 4 years and over. The TAT material consists of 31 cards containing vaguely provocative pictures in black and white plus one blank card. The subject's task is to tell a story about each picture. For the blank card, the subject is asked to do the same for an imaginary picture. Interpretation is based on the individual's needs as exposed by the stories.

4. *Rorschach Technique.* Used with ages 3 years and over. Test material consists of 10 differently shaped but bilaterally symmetric inkblots, each printed on its own card; 5 are in shades of black and gray, 2 have added touches of red, and 3 are in various pastel colors. The subject is asked to tell what the blots remind him of. Responses are recorded verbatim along with various response-timings, the way the cards are held, and

numerous other behavioral occurrences. Substantial inquiry is conducted after initial responses to the 10 blots are made. Classic interpretation is based on complex scoring procedures and involves ratios and totals rather than single responses; the outcome is an integrated picture of total personality.

5. *The Rotter Incomplete Sentences Blank.* Used with adolescents and adults. The first word or words of a sentence are given, and the subject is asked to complete it in a way that expresses his feelings. An overall adjustment score is derived through the test's scoring procedures. This and other sentence-completion tests are valuable for screening purposes and as interview guides.

6. *Make a Picture Story (MAPS).* Used with ages 6 years and over. Test materials consist of 22 pictorial backgrounds (living room, bedroom, bathroom, schoolroom, etc.) and 67 die-cut figures (male, female, adults, children, minority-group figures, figures with blank faces, nudes, etc.), all held upright by insertion in a wooden base. The examiner places a background before the subject and asks him to choose any figures he wishes to add to the scene and then to make up a story about it. Both scoring and interpretation are complicated procedures, and detailed examples of test interpretation are given in various publications edited by the test constructor.

7. *Minnesota Multiphasic Personality Inventory (MMPI).* Used with ages 16 years and over. The inventory is composed of over 500 statements which the subject is asked to classify as true, false, or cannot say. The range of inquiry is extremely wide, covering numbers of psychopathic conditions as well as other areas of behavior and preference. The inventory statements require a rather high literacy and concept level that cannot easily be transposed to signs. The main value of the Inventory is in differential diagnosis; this is facilitated by computerized scoring and computer printouts of diagnostic and interpretive statements descriptive of the subject's personality.

The *Children's Apperception Test* (CAT) and the *Symonds Picture-Story Test* are adaptations of the *Thematic Apperception Test,* with the CAT using drawings of animals in child-centered human situations; and the Symonds Test, drawings depicting situations of concern to adolescents.

A number of other personality tests used in research with the deaf are described in chapter 7. The *Missouri Children's Picture Series,* the *Hand Test,* and the *Impulse, Ego, Superego (IES) Test,* in particular, warrant broader trials.

Projective Techniques and the Deaf:
Special Considerations

As can be seen in table 12.2, the personality tests most preferred for use with deaf school-agers are the projective techniques. By and large, the basic principles outlined in the section on General Testing Guides also pertain to projective testing. A number of additional considerations are summarized in this section.

Feasible testing age. The "usable age ranges" noted in the projective test digests do not apply to deaf subjects. With the deaf, the rule of thumb for projective testing favors the age range in which response and inquiry are least hampered by lack of expressive language, whether verbal or sign. The safest age-range for such expressive output is in the adolescent years and beyond. There are exceptions, of course. Examiners are therefore advised to language-scan a given subject before proceeding to test, preferably through a preliminary get-acquainted interview rather than a reading achievement test since a reading score will not disclose a subject's expressive facility in the language of signs, which may well suffice for projective test purposes. Certain projective tests are used with very young deaf children, as discussed shortly, but in a less structural manner than required by conventional testing.

"Shortcut" testing. For proper use, projective techniques worth their informational salt require special preparation or training (Anastasi, 1961). This involves a considerable expenditure of an examiner's time and effort. To the time and effort so required are added the time and effort taken up by careful testing, scoring, and interpreting. Projective tests can be major consumers of time. As a result, shortcuts are often used. The most common, especially with deaf subjects, are to play down or omit inquiry in tests where it is required, and to bypass scoring by response-scanning. In the hands of less than expert projective testers, these shortcuts rob a test of its psychological teeth, and leave a tester with little more than biased personality fragments. What emerges is a lopsided personality profile, generally skewed toward deficits. The situation argues against the use of complex projective tests by examiners who, by unskilled shortcutting, shortchange their deaf subjects.

"Matching" projective tests to subjects. After years of exposure to highly structured school environments and routines, numbers of deaf youths, and adults as well, find it hard to handle the loosely structured items of projective tasks. Some are immobilized by Rorschach inkblots. Others are inhibited by sentence completion because they feel their language is not good enough or they experience difficulty in introspective thinking. Some protest a lack of artistic skill when faced with projective drawing tasks; and others find apperceptive story-telling beyond their imaginative faculties. But whatever the situation, in projective testing as in mental testing, an effort should be made to "match" test to subject.

One way of doing this is to include in the pretest get-acquainted interview such questions as: "Have you seen a good movie lately? Can you tell me the story?" (apperceptive story possibilities); "Do you like to look at a cloud in the sky and imagine what it looks like?'' (Rorschach possibilities); ''Do you like to draw?'' (drawing test possibilities). Answers may provide leads, and again they may not. But some such pretest approach should be tried, for it is always possible that inhibited test-response is due as much to the type of projective test used as to the subject's personality.

Another inhibiting factor occasionally arises when the subject is assured that ''there are no wrong or right answers; anything you say is right.'' Deaf subjects know they are being tested; and there must be ''wrongs'' and ''rights,'' or else what's the point in testing? When a deaf subject's facial or other expression protests doubts about the ''no wrong and no right'' formula, an examiner can offer as evidence: ''Many questions have no wrong or right answers. I will tell you some: What color do you like best? Do you like to go to a party? Do you have brothers and sisters?'' and so on. On answering such questions, the subject comes to realize that there are indeed situations in which answers cannot be considered right or wrong, that they simply reflect fact or personal views and feelings. With this realization comes a lessening of constraints as well as a feel for the nature of projective response.

Although an inhibited response pattern (even with a matched test) in itself discloses certain personality traits, it is important to know the rest of the personality picture, the part hiding behind the response-inhibiting defense. Toward this end, I apply generous praise, encouragement, and ''tell me mores'' where it appears safe to chip away at the defense. Since there are no right or wrong answers in projective testing, in contrast to mental testing, this praise procedure is justified by its purpose. However, the need for extra encouragement is noted in recording and reporting.

Childhood projective testing. Projective techniques customarily used with young children take the form of doll-family sets and play-kit tests that include such articles as dolls representing children and adults of both sexes and various age levels, household furnishings, outdoor objects, animals, and other related materials. Some are interpreted through a scoring system, and others inferentially. The assumption in projective play is that a child projects various personality traits and attitudes in its selection and arrangement of the play materials into a kind of mini-story. Interpretation of what the child projects is helped by the child's accompanying remarks or explanations concerning such matters as whom the doll figures represent, what they are doing, to whom and why, and by the child's emotional investments in the scenarios.

When the techniques are used with young deaf children, examiners need to be alert for influencing variables. One is a young deaf child's customary reaction to a display of toys and dolls by an examiner. Often, the child's first thought is that this is a language lesson, and the child begins by *naming* the toys. Even after the examiner has managed to get across the idea that the toys are for playing and not for naming, the child's performance may be affected by his original concept, and he may favor toys that he knows by name or from teaching situations. Hence, examiners must enforce the "play" concept even to participating to a limited extent in play until the child is able to play freely on his own. Other influencing variables include the relatively limited range of a young deaf child's life experiences on which to build stories, the locale in which play is conducted, the examiner's watchful gaze, the child's mood at the time, and affective experiences immediately preceding the play activity. A final problem in using toy and play techniques with young deaf children is the communication difficulty of eliciting their explanatory remarks about the stories they are putting together.

In view of these many influencing factors, I am inclined to use the play technique as a kind of interview situation rather than as a "test," relying on the remarkable pantomimic abilities of most young deaf children to tell their stories for them, as illustrated in the later section on Interview.

Selective versus routine use. Many problems argue against the use of projective techniques for *routine* personality-testing with deaf school-populations. A more feasible procedure would be to conduct routine personality-screening by means of a good behavior-rating instrument such as the *Meadow-Kendall Social-Emotional Inventory for Deaf Students,* devised by Kathryn P. Meadow and standardized on a deaf pupil population. Projective techniques could then be used selectively as diagnostic aids with those pupils rated as emotionally disturbed. The projective instruments so used should be carefully chosen tests of established worth, and should be conscientiously administered, scored, and interpreted.

Personality Self-Report Inventories and the Deaf

With hearing populations, verbal self-report personality inventories are considered great time-savers. They can be self- as well as group-administered, much as achievement tests. Scoring is routinized and often computerized, as in the *Minnesota Multiphasic Personality Inventory,* and interpretation follows well-defined lines. However, these advantages do not hold for a deaf clientele.

Some of the weaknesses of verbal personality inventories were noted in chapter 7. Major deterrents to their use with deaf subjects are the time and effort involved in the exhaustive task of rewording test language, screening and simplifying elusive concepts, and detecting and discarding obviously inappropriate items. A case in point is an item from the *Sixteen Personality Factor Questionnaire:* "Do you think that most of us have so many faults that unless people are charitable to one another life would be intolerable?" Even if such statements could be successfully adapted to an average deaf individual's understanding, we are still left with the question of whether any personality inventory that has undergone such drastic reconditioning could measure with the deaf what it was constructed to measure with the hearing. This is not to say that no deaf people are able to take such inventory tests. Many exceptional deaf persons can do so. But even at this level, how is a deaf individual to answer such questions from the MMPI as: "My hearing is apparently as good as that of most people," or "My speech is the same as always (not faster or slower, or slurring; no hoarseness)"? To answer truthfully would be to risk giving a "maladjusted" response simply because it would not coincide with that expected of an "adjusted" hearing person.

In my opinion, if verbal personality inventories are used with the deaf, they are best used in an exploratory way and should be individually administered and studied. Even the use of manual communication will not override their structural inadequacies as clinical instruments with the deaf-at-large, whether school-age or adult.

Interpreting Personality Test Findings

Problems of interpreting the results of hearing-standardized personality tests when used with deaf subjects are compounded by current issues and problems in personality testing per se. A number have been noted in chapter 7. Detailed discussions can be found in current literature on the subject, including the comprehensive summaries in the *Annual Review of Psychology* publications.

The best an examiner can do in preparation for a formal personality examination of a deaf subject is to know personality tests and testing, to know the deaf, and to know how to communicate with deaf persons. Most importantly, examiners need to bear in mind that all personalities have their share of strengths and weaknesses; there is no such thing as a perfect personality. The presence of deviant test response, though perhaps of diagnostic importance, does not necessarily indicate a malfunctioning personality. Such responses may simply indicate a particular test's diagnostically structured focus which has picked up certain weaknesses in what is nevertheless an effectively functioning personality.

To know whether deviant responses are diagnostically significant requires a *global* rather than a trait-oriented personality picture. But personality tests seldom provide the global view. An examiner must therefore fill in the gaps with information from the case history, observation, and interview. In this way, a picture can be obtained that also includes *personality strengths*. Assessing how well a given personality is likely to function requires balancing the strengths against the weaknesses, with the final assessment the outcome of the ratio between the two. My admiration for the Rorschach technique stems from this system of weighing and balancing in personality scoring and interpretation.

Finally, whatever the test used, identifying positive personality components is generally more important than stressing the negatives, as too often happens. Not only do the positives provide the impetus for managing everyday affairs, they also serve as key supports in counseling and therapy. They must be identified in personality test protocols and interpretation, and included in reporting. In view of the shaky position personality tests occupy in use with the deaf, such identification means that after a test protocol is scored and interpreted according to standardized procedure, it must be reinterpreted in accordance with the examiner's judgment of which responses, while abnormal for hearing subjects, are nevertheless *in line with a deaf subject's background of fashioning* experiences. There are no established guides for this reinterpretation procedure. It is a tricky business and depends almost entirely on an examiner's "knowing" the deaf. But it will indicate roughly the proportion of deviant responses that are more closely related to exogenous factors imposed by the deaf environment than to endogenous deviations in personality.

Achievement Testing

Achievement tests are used in school settings to measure a pupil's level of proficiency in school subjects, generally in terms of a grade score. Tests are available from primary through adult levels but are most heavily used at the intermediate level. The principal measurement targets are language (word knowledge, word discrimination, spelling, reading, language usage, etc.), and arithmetic (computational and problem-solving abilities). Social studies and science are commonly included for upper grade levels, and additional, achievement-like tests or inventories for school-agers are available for such special areas as social insight, health knowledge, and sex knowledge; many more can be found in psychological test catalogues.

Achievement Tests Used with Deaf School-agers

Table 12.3 rank-lists achievement tests reported as used with deaf school-agers by respondents to a survey of psychological practices with the deaf (Levine, 1974). All the tests listed were standardized on hearing populations. They are briefly described in the following digests.

1. *Wide Range Achievement Test (WRAT),* 1976 edition. An easily administered and rapidly scored time-saver that measures level of achievement in the basic scholastic skills of reading, spelling, and arithmetic in the age range from 5 years through adult.

2. *Stanford Achievement Test,* 1973 edition, and *Metropolitan Achieve-*

Table 12.3 Achievement Tests in Rank Order (n = 166 Respondents)

Name of Test	Special School			Regular School				Other Agency				Grand Total
	Residential	Day	Total	Special Class	Partially Integrated	Totally Integrated	Total	Diagnostic Unit	Speech & Hearing Center	Rehabilitation Setting	Total	
Wide Range Achievement Test	3	16	19	30	3	2	35	5	2	1	8	62
Stanford Achievement	27	10	37	8	3	0	11	0	0	2	2	50
Metropolitan Achievement Tests	9	1	10	4	0	1	5	1	0	1	2	17
Gates Reading Achievement	8	1	9	2	0	0	2	0	0	0	0	11
California Achievement	6	2	8	2	0	0	2	0	0	0	0	10
Gray Oral Reading	0	2	2	0	0	0	0	0	1	0	1	3

SOURCE: Drawn from Levine (1974).

ment Tests, 1978 edition. Two of the most comprehensive achievement tests in the psychological market, the former for grades 1.5–9.9, and the latter for grades kindergarten–12.9. They are probably the best formulated and best designed for both subject coverage and flexibility of usage.

3. *California Achievement Tests,* 1957 edition. Concentrate mainly on areas involving language, arithmetic, and reading, for grades 1–14.

4. *Gates Reading Tests* have been replaced by *Gates-MacGinitie Reading Tests,* 1965 edition. They include new items and more timely material for grades 1–12. The test manual provides for conversion of Gates-MacGinitie scores to Gates Reading scores.

5. *Gray Oral Reading Tests,* 1963, 1967 editions. A series of standardized individually administered reading paragraphs for grades 1–12, scored for speed, accuracy, and comprehension.

Special mention should be given to several other tests used with deaf children for achievement and achievement-diagnostic purposes.

6. *Test of Syntactic Abilities* (Quigley et al., 1978). An achievement-analytic test standardized for prelinguistically, profoundly deaf school-agers aged 10–18 years. Its target is syntactic structures, and the 20 subtests evaluate 9 basic structures and pinpoint specific deficiencies in each, thus supplying valuable guides to teachers concerning remedial needs.

7. *Picture Story Language Test* (Myklebust, 1965). Also an achievement-analytic test, but standardized on a representative sample of public-school populations at selected age intervals within the range of 7–17

years. Its target is measurement and analysis of written language ability. Test-samples of written language are secured by having a testee write a story about a standard test-picture.

8. *Stanford Achievement Test for Hearing Impaired Students* (1972). Adapted from the Stanford Achievement Test, this test provides special procedures for testing five scholastic levels of hearing-impaired students, beginning with the primary level.

9. *Peabody Picture Vocabulary Test* (Dunn, 1959). Not an achievement test although it is used as one by various workers with deaf children. It is an untimed, hearing-standardized, individually administered intelligence test in which a subject is given a stimulus word and responds by indicating which in a group of pictures best illustrates the word. With deaf children, the test is generally used in assessing lipreading and/or word knowledge, with the stimulus word signed when necessary.

Using Achievement Tests with Deaf School-agers

The usual practice is for standard-type achievement tests to be group-administered by classroom teachers. When the tests are used with groups of deaf pupils, a great deal of time can be spent in making sure that every pupil clearly understands the instructions for each test. One ingenious teacher devised a strategy that not only saved time but also assured comprehension of instructions. First she screened the language of the test instructions and reduced it to shorter sentences and simpler forms. She then hand-printed the simplified instructions on large sheets of heavy paper, one chart for each set of instructions. Included on the charts were the matching sample tasks. As each test was administered, its corresponding instruction-chart was hung in a position clearly visible to all group members, and then teacher and group read the instructions and performed the sample tasks together. Further clarifications were made as required for certain individuals in the group. Where signing helped to clarify, it was used; and where additional sample tasks were needed, the teacher had on hand a supply of samples she had devised, all of which were simpler than the least difficult of the test's samples, to avoid a too-detailed preliminary practice. The procedure proved exceptionally workable.

But even when test instructions are administered successfully, the examiner must keep a watchful eye on pupils while they are taking the tests. Some of the tricks used by deaf children can be highly amusing. I observed one youngster drawing outlines of one of his hands on sheet after sheet of paper when he should have been working on a computational test-item. When questioned, he replied that this was to give him an extra supply of fingers on which to count when he ran out of his own allotted 10. His face registered wonder and surprise that his inquisitor lacked the wit to appreciate the strategy.

Not infrequently, notoriously poor readers come up with suspiciously ele-
vated reading-achievement scores. When they are individually interview-
checked, it usually turns out that the answers were arrived at through clever
guesswork or through close juxtaposition of key words rather than through
comprehension. The mental agility involved in the operation is to be ad-
mired; but it leaves an examiner wondering what the reading levels of deaf
school-agers would be if the tests were individually administered and the
responses checked through interrogation instead of group-administered and
the responses blind-scored.

Special Clinical Tests

With the steady increase in mentally competent school-agers who are classified as "learning disabled," there is a corresponding emphasis on differential diagnosis. This is so because the label "learning disability" is commonly used as a catchall for a wide variety of learning problems which need
to be sorted out in the service of remedial planning.

Although research has not yet come up with a conclusive picture, definition, or treatment of learning disability (McCarthy and McCarthy, 1969), it
is generally accepted that cerebral dysfunction is an important etiological
factor. Leads to its presence may sometimes be elicited by special clinical
tests designed to probe visual-motor-perceptual manifestations of cerebral
dysfunction. One of the most widely used is the *Bender Visual-Motor Gestalt Test*. Examples of others are:

1. *Benton Revised Visual Retention Test,* 1974 edition. Probes perception of and memory for spatial relations for age 8 years through adult.
Thirty design cards are individually presented to a subject who is required
to reproduce each design immediately on its removal.

2. *Frostig Developmental Test of Visual Perception.* A paper-and-pencil test for assessing five areas of visual perception in the age range 3–9
years: eye–motor coordination; figure–ground; constancy of shape; position in space; and spatial relations.

3. *Lincoln-Oseretsky Motor Development Scale.* Tests unilateral and
bilateral motor abilities at ages 6–14 years. Test items involve a wide variety of motor skills, such as eye–hand coordination, finger dexterity, and
gross activity of hands, arms, legs, and trunk.

When tests such as these are used, two points need special emphasis. The
first is that psychological tests are not invariably successful in detecting cerebral dysfunction; the absence of positive signs does not necessarily indicate the absence of dysfunction. As noted by McCarthy and McCarthy,
"not all frankly neurologically impaired children show impaired performance on these tests" (1969, p. 22). This leads to the second point of emphasis, namely, that clinical tests are used as *part* of a total psychological
examination. Signs of cerebral dysfunction not elicited by such tests or even

in the neurological examination may be picked up in case history data, in regular psychological testing, or in the course of observation and interview.
A very different type of clinical testing is that for color vision. Color vision tests should routinely precede the administration of psychological tests involving color discrimination or projective tests such as the Rorschach, in which reactions to color play an important role. The color vision test that I generally use is the *Dvorine Pseudo Isochromatic Plates,* second edition. The plates allow color-ignorance to be distinguished from color-blindness by means of 22 cards, in 14 of which digits emerge from a multicolor context and 8 of which are designed for children and illiterates.

Vocational Interests

Vocational satisfaction plays an important role in the psychological adjustments of deaf youths after they finish school. It is therefore important to find out what their general vocational interests are while they are still in school, in preparation for later vocational advice and training.

Two of the popular instruments for this purpose are the *Geist Picture Interest Inventory: General Form: Male* (Geist, 1959), of which there is an adaptation for deaf and hard-of-hearing males (Geist, 1962), and the *Wide Range Interest-Opinion Test* (WRIOT) (Jastak and Jastak, 1979). Others are mentioned later in the chapter.

1. *Geist Picture Interest Inventory.* Designed for males in grades 7–16 and male adults. Consists of 44 triads of drawings depicting major vocational and avocational activities. Standard answer sheets provide for recording the 44 choices the subject makes. Eleven interest scores are derived: persuasive, clerical, mechanical, dramatic, musical, scientific, outdoor, literary, computational, artistic, social service. To allow evaluation of the motivations governing the choices, a check list of 68 statements is used on which the subject checks those that apply to his choice.

2. *Wide Range Interest-Opinion Test,* 1979 edition. A pictorial test designed for use with ages 5 years through adult. Consists of 450 pictures arranged in 150 triads. The same pictures are used with males and females but the findings are treated differently. Test results are analyzed in terms of clusters of choices, made by the subject, that have been found to be consistently liked (and disliked) by persons in a given occupation. Attitudes are also included in the scope of examination. The broad occupational categories surveyed include: art, business, services, science, mechanics, farming; job titles, as listed in the Dictionary of Occupational Titles, are provided that correlate positively with interest clusters.

Illustrative Testing Programs

The following programs illustrate the use of tests and test batteries for evaluating hearing-impaired children and youth at two different types of facilities. One, the New York League for the Hard of Hearing in New York

City, is an all-service hearing rehabilitation center; the other is the Whitney
M. Young Magnet High School in Chicago, Illinois. The League's programs
are described by Ruth R. Green, Acting Administrator of the League, and
Frances Santore, Director of Communication Therapies and her associates,
Elizabeth Ying and Nina Hertz. The High School programs are described
by Robert J. Donoghue, Ph.D., School Psychologist for the Hearing-Impaired Program at the school.

Psychological Test Battery:
The New York League for the Hard of Hearing

The New York League for the Hard of Hearing is a nonprofit, multidisciplinary rehabilitation agency providing diagnostic, remedial, and therapeutic assistance to persons of all ages with all degrees of hearing loss, including a sizable deaf clientele. Among the services offered are otological and
audiological services, communications assessment, vocational evaluation
and job placement, public education, and recreation programs. The League's
clients are referred by hospital clinics, physicians, schools, other social
agencies, state and city agencies, and members of the community.

Since the League's services are offered to persons of all ages with widely
different types of hearing impairment and socioeconomic backgrounds,
clearly there can be no "typical" case or test battery. In each instance it is
the psychologist's responsibility to select the instruments that are most suitable for a particular subject and that will best secure the information needed
for optimum understanding and service. Tests most generally used with deaf
children are the following.

1. *Preschool*

Intelligence

Leiter International Performance Scale.
Merrill-Palmer Scale of Mental Tests.
*Wechsler Preschool and Primary Scale of Intelligence, Performance
Scale;* where possible, the Verbal Scale is attempted.

Social maturity

Vineland Social Maturity Scale.

Other

Harris Tests of Laterality. Selected subtests are used to assess eye,
hand, foot dominance.
Peabody Picture Vocabulary Test. To evaluate receptive language
levels, with one form used to evaluate lip-reading reception, and
another form used with deaf children who use sign language to
evaluate signed reception.

2. *Primary/Elementary School-agers*
   Intelligence
      Wechsler Intelligence Scale for Children, revised or unrevised. The Performance and Verbal Scales of the tests are used, but intelligence as indicated by the I.Q. is based on the Performance Scale. The gap, if any, between the scales often shows the extent to which functioning in a mainstream program is feasible.
      Leiter International Performance Scale or the *Columbia Mental Maturity Scale* is substituted for the Wechsler Scale if the child has motor difficulties.

   Visual-perceptual
      The *Bender-Gestalt Test* is used to screen for visual-perceptual dysfunction.

   Maturity/personality
      Vineland Social Maturity Scale.
      House-Tree-Person Test and *Kinetic Family Drawings* are used for information about personality dynamics and adaptations; On the latter test, the child is asked to draw a picture of his or her family.
      Children's Apperception Test is used *only* with children with sufficient verbal skills to express themselves adequately.

   Achievement
      Gates MacGinitie Reading Tests are administered to first-grade children or can be substituted for reading tests on the Stanford Achievement Tests.

      Stanford Achievement Tests are used to measure academic achievement for children who have completed at least first grade. Word meaning, paragraph reading, and arithmetic computation are always administered to see if the child is working up to grade and ability levels and to evaluate whether additional tutoring is required.

Communication Therapies Evaluation:
The New York League for the Hard of Hearing
   The communication evaluation at the League provides a diagnostic summary of a child's comprehension and usage of oral language as well as listening skills. Since the habilitation approach at the League is auditory/oral, primarily a child's oral language skills are evaluated. However, parts of the evaluation can be modified to assess manual sign language skills. The evaluation is 2 hours long (more detailed testing is administered once a child is

enrolled in a therapy program). The procedures of this evaluation are summarized here.

1. *Preschool*

Parent Interview

Parent's perception of child's problems.

Information concerning sounds, words, phrases child uses or responds to.

Parent's response to questions from:

Receptive-Expressive Emergent Language (REEL) Scale. Used to measure language skills in infancy (from birth to 36 months). The test consists of several items which examine normal development of both receptive and expressive language skills at two-month intervals. Information is either supplied by the parent, observed by the examiner, or obtained by direct interaction with the child.

Communication Evaluation Chart. Used to examine language and performance levels of children aged 3 months to 5 years. The language portion of the test evaluates such items as coordination of speech musculature, hearing acuity and auditory perception, acquisition of sounds, and receptive and expressive language skills. The performance skills section is used to evaluate the child's growth and development, motor coordination, and some visual-motor skills

Observation

Parent/child interaction.

Child's play behavior.

Child's spontaneous language while at play.

Receptive language via audition and vision

Tests used in whole or part with children who can be tested

Peabody Picture Vocabulary Test.

Utah Test of Language Development. A checklist of normal language development from ages 1 to 15 years. It is designed to be an objective measurement of expressive and receptive language skills in both normal and handicapped children.

Houston Test for Language Development. This test, which measures the development of language, is divided into two parts. Part I measures aspects of language involving reception, conceptualization, and expression in children aged 6 months to 3 years. Part II examines these same areas of language development in children aged 3–6 years.

Illinois Test of Psycholinguistic Abilities. A norm-referenced test consisting of 10 primary subtests and 2 supplementary subtests which sample some essential skills and functions of both verbal and nonverbal communication. It is designed to be used diagnostically, with children of ages 2–10 years, to identify specific language abilities and disabilities and to serve as a teaching model for developmental or remedial language training. The following individual subtests have been found to be especially useful in assessing the language knowledge and performance of the hearing-impaired population: Auditory Reception, Auditory Association, Auditory Sequential Memory, Grammatic Closure, Visual Reception, Visual Association, and Visual Sequential Memory.

Test for Auditory Comprehension of Language. A detailed screening test that examines linguistic comprehension through picture identification or orally presented lexical, morphological, and syntactical constructs. The basal language age of this test is 3.0.

Procedures used with children who cannot be tested

Toys, pictures, objects are used to assess receptive spoken-language recognition of: body parts, clothing, animals, people, food, common transportation, etc.; own name and family members; familiar commands.

Receptive language via audition alone, using earphones, vibrator, individual hearing aid, or speaking close to child's ear

Ability to imitate vowel sounds, consonant-vowel syllables, changes in pitch, duration, stress, and intonation patterns.

Distance at which the child consistently responds to voice or noisemakers (unaided or with child's aid).

Response to name.

Detection of five sounds according to Daniel Ling (u, a, i, s, /sh/).

If no response to above, try response to drum or bell.

Receptive impression

Examiner's subjective impression of the major receptive modality favored by the child.

Expressive language

Observation

Spontaneous production and imitation of vowels, vowel-consonant or consonant-vowel combinations.

Voice quality.

Motor functioning: grasping and pulling, rings on peg, block stacking.

Like and unlike matching of objects, pictures.

General behavior: attention span, eye contact, response to structured test situation.

Examination of oral-peripheral mechanism, i.e., movement of the articulators and their structural adequacies.

Tests used in whole or part with children who can be tested: as above.

Evaluation results

Discussion with parents of results of evaluation and examiner's recommendations.

2. *School-age*

General communicative information via parent interview and observation, as with preschool child.

Receptive language via audition and vision (objective language tests)

Peabody Picture 'Vocabulary Test.

Illinois Test of Psycholinguistic Abilities.

Detroit Test of Learning Aptitude. Essentially a psychological instrument designed to measure specific cognitive skills underlying the learning process. The examiner is instructed, however, to select from the 19 individual subtests those tasks which are appropriate for the purpose of the testing situation and individual needs of the subject to be tested. In attempting to obtain an overall picture of the hearing-impaired child's verbal and nonverbal response to spoken language, the following subtests have been found to be informative and useful in planning language therapy: Orientations, Verbal Opposites, Oral Commissions, Auditory Attention Span for Related Syllables and Oral Directions.

Houston Test for Language Development. Measures the development of language, divided into two parts. Part I measures aspects of language involving reception, conceptualization, and expression in children aged 6 months to 3 years; Part II examines these same areas in children aged 3–6 years.

Test for Auditory Comprehension of Language.

Also tested are the child's ability to follow familiar questions and one, two, and three-level commands.

Receptive language via audition alone

Distance at which child responds to voice.

Perception of vowels.

Ling's five-sound detection test.

Perception of low, mid, and high consonants and vowel nonsense syllables.

Ability to follow familiar questions and commands.

Ability to imitate changes in pitch, duration, stress, and intonation.

Tonality Test, if applicable. This test, which is presently being standardized, consists of lists of 25 words divided into five sound-frequency groups: low, low-mid, mid, mid-high, and high. A low-frequency word might be "wood," a mid word might be "hat," and a high-frequency word might be "sheet."

Auditory memory for sentence material or a series of clued, isolated words.

Receptive language via vision alone (speechreading)

Costello Speechreading Word Test. Consists of 25 monosyllabic kindergarten-level words, each presented to the child once with voicing for a score of 4 points per word. Forms A or B.

Costello Speechreading Sentence Test. Consists of 50 sentences which are to be presented one time each, with no voice. Comprehension of the sentence is gauged by correct manipulation of props provided or oral repetition of the sentence. One point is given for each sentence that is interpreted correctly.

Also tested is the child's ability to comprehend information in a simple paragraph read with minimal voicing.

Expressive language

Subtests of the *Illinos Test of Psycholinguistic Abilities* and the *Detroit Test of Learning Aptitude.*

Carrow Elicited Language Inventory. Designed to assess a child's mastery of specific grammatical forms based on his ability to imitate progressively larger and more complex sentence constructs. Its use with the hearing-impaired population must take into consideration the child's speech intelligibility and auditory perception/comprehension skills.

Objective articulation test. Routinely the measurement of articulation ability has been considered essential to a thorough understanding of the development of intelligible and fluent oral speech and language skills within the hearing-impaired population. Standardized picture identification tests such as the *Templin-Darley Test of Articulation* and the *Goldman Fristoe Test of Articulation* provide the trained listener with a sample from which to judge the adequacy of the hearing-impaired child's spontaneous or imitative productions of the individual sounds of speech, at the word level and in connected discourse.

Results of the communication therapies evaluation are taken into consideration for determining appropriate educational planning and additional help in speech, language, and hearing development within either a school or a therapy setting.

Psychological Testing Program: Whitney M. Young Magnet High School

The implementation of Public Law 94-142 on September 1, 1978, required, among other things, the creation of an Individualized Education Program (IEP) for each child registered in a special education program. At Chicago's Whitney M. Young Magnet High School, the diagnostic staff of the Hearing Impaired Program (H.I.P.) had anticipated the provisions of PL 94-142 as early as the summer of 1974. This discussion summarizes some of the problems that were foreseen and the solutions ultimately adopted.

The Hearing Impaired Program is a special division of the school, which in itself draws students on a selective basis from the entire city of Chicago. The H.I.P. staff includes about 60 full-time teachers, 25 supportive paraprofessionals, and 12 diagnostic staff personnel. Nearly 300 students, aged 13–21, currently attend the program. Both deaf and hard-of-hearing children are enrolled. Courses of study are tailored to the student's individual needs and include both segregated and mainstreamed class attendance. The philosophy of total communication is an integral factor in the educational process.

Special considerations. Individualized assessment of children in large secondary programs for the hearing-impaired often poses problems not clearly envisaged by legislators. First is the sheer number of students to be evaluated; second is the continuing shortage of qualified examiners; third is the academic structure—no two educational programs are precisely alike in their offerings. Additionally, a time element is involved; students need to be placed academically as soon as possible after entrance. Finally, since the IEP is subject to periodic review and updating, a huge burden is imposed on the diagnostic facility in an educational system.

In planning how to meet these pressures and responsibilities, the diagnostic staff at Whitney M. Young divided the work into two stages. At the professional level, the audiologist, speech therapist, manual sign experts, and psychologists, aided by the school nurse, counselors, and social workers, focused on their specific areas of interest. The needs of each diagnostic area were then assessed carefully in order to develop a structured program of evaluation from which a standard test battery applicable to all students could be drawn. This test battery was intended to relate directly to the H.I.P. school program, be efficient and reliable in terms of the temporal aspect, and provide for the analysis of most if not all of the psychological factors considered relevant to the educational process.

The Center for Evaluation, Diagnosis, and Research (CEDAR), which was responsible for all diagnostic activities within the H.I.P. program, quickly recognizes the difficulty of administering a global diagnostic process to a large number of students, given the time available. Thus, the test battery was modified by each professional area, and only those portions directly involved with current educational placement were administered at any one time.

Tests used in the evaluation program. Given the foregoing situation, the H.I.P. high-school psychologist considered three aspects of the evaluation process: (1) initial screening and placement at entry; (2) on-going academic/vocational placement within the school program; and (3) postsecondary preparation, whether in terms of additional training or of job placement. To meet these needs, his evaluation program contained the following tests.

1. At entry into the secondary-school program (initial screening)

   Intelligence
   Wechsler Adult Intelligence Scales (performance), or
   Wechsler Intelligence Scales for Children (performance), or
   Wechsler Intelligence Scales for Children, Revised (performance)

   Achievement
   Wide Range Achievement Test, and
   California Achievement Test, or
   Stanford Achievement Test

   Personality
   House-Tree-Person, and
   Bender-Gestalt
   Rorschach Psychodiagnostic

2. Second academic year reassessment (vocational decision)

   Achievement
   Stanford Achievement Test, or
   California Achievement Test

   Aptitudes
   Work Sample Evaluation Program (JVS Philadelphia)
   Purdue Pegboard
   Revised Minnesota Paper Form Board (AA)
   Minnesota Clerical Test
   Farnsworth Dichotomous Test for Color Blindness
   Hooper Visual Organization Test
   Maquarrie Test for Mechanical Ability
   Manipulative Aptitude Test

3. Third academic year reassessment (career-counseling stage)

Intelligence
Wechsler tests as at entry

Achievement
Achievement tests as at entry

Career interest exploration
Picture Interest Inventory (Weingarten)
Geist Picture Interest Inventory
Wide Range Interest-Opinion Test (WRIOT)
Kuder Occupational Interest Inventory

Aptitudes
SRA Pictorial Reasoning Test
Computer Program Aptitude Battery
Short Employment Test (Verbal, Numerical, Clerical)
Manipulative Aptitude Test

Test interpretation and staffing. Under the Individualized Education Program, each student is entitled to an individual staffing conference where input is offered by both diagnostic and supportive personnel as well as teachers, parents, and school administrative representatives. In a school setting, the psychologist has two responsibilities each time a student is evaluated. Besides his commitment to the student, the psychologist must also consider the implications of his findings for the educational program itself. Thus he has to familiarize himself with administrative procedures and resources, curricular offerings, teaching philosophies and methodology, facilities and equipment, community resources, diagnostic testing in other areas such as audiology and speech, bicultural and bilingual factors, and social and socioeconomic conditions in the geographical area. All these aspects and more are vital to the provision of adequate services by the psychologist.

The psychologist's role in a staffing conference, therefore, is far from cut-and-dried; he is expected not only to present his test results but also to offer guidance on the question of placement. To do this effectively, he must consider the test findings in terms of the prevailing educational program, pointing out possible placements available, or be in a position to suggest alternative placement. His role is to offer himself as a resource but not to make decisions; he should relate his findings to information provided by other members of the staffing team, thus contributing to a group decision that will benefit the student and also receive administrative and parental support.

Team staffing is most important for test interpretation. It is here that the psychologist obtains the additional background data that is often inadvertently omitted from case reports and test results. Some questions that can be answered here and that can affect the final psychological interpretation are:

1. Is there any current evidence of aural deterioration? Is a hearing aid worn? How effective is it in the presence of ambient noise?
2. Is medication currently prescribed? What is the effect on behavior? What condition does it purport to treat?
3. Is there any evidence of social drug addiction? Type used? Effect?
4. How does the student perform visually? Are glasses worn?
5. What is classroom performance like? Attitude, application, skills, etc.?
6. By what medium are ideas most comfortably exchanged receptively and expressively?

Observation

The observing eye of an experienced examiner is one of his major clinical instruments. With it he can spot soft pathological signs, perceive suggestive lines of inquiry that need following, and gather a wealth of behavior detail. Without it, the psychological examination is simply a mechanical exercise.

The ideal comprehensive examination would include systematic observation of a subject in as wide a variety of real-life situations as possible—in the home, at school, in recreational activities, and above all in group interactions and interpersonal encounters. This ideal is particularly desirable in the examination of prelinguistically deaf children, whose auditory disability produces ramifications that can greatly hamper psychological testing and interview. Observation fills the gaps. It is crucial at preschool levels, where children are under the influence of a variety of authority figures whose management can determine the social and interpersonal patterns that will be the child's for life. Observation here must include the behaviors of these figures vis-à-vis the child.

However, in the real world, observation procedures such as these and as summarized in chapter 10 can rarely be conducted by overtaxed examiners in school settings. Nevertheless a great deal can be perceived through informal observation by a sharp, clinical eye right in the school or in the psychologist's office, as summarized in the following sections.

General Observation

Health and physical condition. Does the child's physical appearance suggest good health, debility, actual illness? Does he seem "over-energized," "under-energized"? Does he appear to have other physical disabilities, such as the wearing of eyeglasses might suggest? Are there any physical abnormalities or disfigurations present to add to the burden of deafness? What are the possible educational and emotional implications? Is medical referral suggested on the basis of observed physical signs?

Motor manifestations. Is there evidence of impaired motor coordination or control? Is motor activity hyperactive or underactive, random or purposeful, listless or positive? Are any bizarre manifestations present, such as posturing, automatic movements or mannerisms, excessive yawning, gulping, catching of breath? Are there tics, twitching, spastic or athetoid movements, postural deviations, poor balance, peculiar gait? What may be the neurologic and psychiatric implications of the observed motor patterns? Is neuropsychiatric referral called for?

Appearance and dress. How does the subject's general appearance strike an observer? Does his clothing conform to the fashion of the day? Are there evidences of compulsive meticulousness, excessive slovenliness, unusual femininity in a male or masculinity in a female, bizarreness? Is there evidence of careless personal hygiene?

Hearing aid management. Does the subject wear a hearing aid? If not, is there evidence that he could profit from one? If he wears an aid, does he carefully adjust the volume controls as required; fuss with it unnecessarily; forget to turn it on; put it on when entering the psychologist's office, and take it off immediately on leaving? Do oral communication skills appear to benefit from the use of an individual aid? What are the audiological implications?

Interpersonal and Group Behavior

General mood. Does the subject give the impression of interest in others, eagerness to be part of the group, self-assurance, attention-seeking, irritability, apathy, indifference? Is he friendly, bored, hostile, a "loner"? Is he actively cooperative, passively accepting, withdrawn? What are his tolerance levels for frustration, conflict, correction, domination?

Ascendance/submission. What does the subject's dependence/independence ratio appear to be with authority figures, in peer groups, in interpersonal confrontations? Is he a "natural leader"; does he insist on the leadership role and refuse to participate otherwise; does he habitually defer to others to do his thinking for him and seem lost without someone to lean on? Is the subject's dependence/independence ratio the same for all situations and with all figures, or does it alter perceptibly in certain situations with certain figures, and if so, how and with whom?

Psychological Test Behavior

During the administration of test instructions. Does the subject concentrate on understanding the test instructions; does he simply look pleasantly at the examiner but make no observable effort to understand; plunge into the test before instructions are completed; habitually stop to ask questions about procedure after having begun the task; appear reluctant to begin unless specifically encouraged by the examiner?

During test performance. Does the child think out his approach before beginning; perform step-by-step planning while working out the test task; proceed entirely on a trial-and-error basis? Does the child continually look to the examiner for hints and clues? What are the child's span of concentration; distractibility; use of systematic procedure; tempo of operations; manual dexterity and visual-motor skills? What of the child's initiative and independence; needs for encouragement and praise; ability to profit from mistakes; meticulousness of operations?

Management of difficulties. When the child is faced with difficulties, does he concentrate on solving them himself; show immediate discouragement and refuse to go on with the task; expect to be helped; accept only sufficient help to get him over a rough spot so that he can proceed on his own; use difficulties as an attention-getting device?

Exercise of critical faculties. Does the subject notice errors as he proceeds with a task and correct them before he continues; is he aware of errors only when he is "stuck"; does he check his work before announcing he is finished or does he claim to be finished and then immediately change his mind? Does he express satisfaction on completion of a task?

Behavior on concluding the test. Is the subject eager to know how he did, indifferent, discouraged? Does he want to know the correct answers to items that have given him difficulty? Does he seem a good candidate for future testing, indifferent, reluctant? Is he eager to leave the test room or does he offer to stay and help the examiner put the test materials in order? Does he appear exhilarated, depressed, fatigued?

Personality rating through mental test behavior. Personality leads are disclosed in all human behaviors, including those observed during mental testing, as illustrated in the following rating form, slightly modified from one devised by Stutsman for preschool children many years ago (Stutsman, 1931, pp. 261–62).

Rating of Personality Traits in
Mental-Test Situations

Name .... *Age* .. *Date* ....
  1. Self-reliance:
     extreme; moderate; average; slightly lacking; markedly lacking
  2. Self-criticism:
     extreme; moderate; average; slightly lacking; markedly lacking

3. Irritability toward failure:
   extreme; moderate; average; very slight; none

4. Degree of praise needed for effective work:
   Type 1—moderate praise helpful
   Type 2—indifferent to approval
   Type 3—praise induces self-consciousness
   Type 4—constant praise expected but harmful
   Type 5—constant praise needed

5. Initiative and independence of action:
   marked; average; very little

6. Self-consciousness:
   not conspicuously present; conspicuously slight; inhibited reactions; show off

7. Spontaneity and repression:
   1. Freedom to work: marked; average; very little
   2. Tendency to ask for what he wants: marked; average; very little
   3. Amount and type of interpersonal communication
   (This category replaces the Stutsman items related to talking and voice quality)

8. Imaginative tendencies:
   marked; average; very little

9. Reaction type to which the child belongs:
   Type 1—slow and deliberate
   Type 2—calm and alert
   Type 3—quick and impetuous

10. Communication skills and exchange
    (This title replaces Stutsman's "Speech Development")

11. Dependence on parent:
    present; not observed; reactions indicate indepedence

12. Other observations

Stutsman stressed that the foregoing outline is "merely offered as a suggestion of the possibilities of using the [mental] test situation for the study of personality" (1931, p. 262).

Classroom Observation: Teacher–Pupil Interactions

The alarming rise in behavior and learning problems among nondeaf pupils has resulted in a vigorous research analysis of teaching styles and practices. The outcome is a sweeping movement in teacher-training programs and evaluation procedures toward demonstrated competence in actual classroom performance (Heath and Neilson, 1974; Hunter, 1977; Rosenshine, 1971).

The movement is not as strong as it deserves to be in the education of deaf children. Yet, next to competent parents, competent teachers represent a deaf child's strongest habilitative lifeline. The extent to which learning disabilities among deaf pupils are simply a reflection of teaching disabilities is a pressing topic for investigation.

In schools for the deaf, psychologists are the traditional referents for problem pupils, and the focus of psychological inquiry has traditionally been the problem child. However, current research findings concerning pupil-behavior correlates of teacher effectiveness means that psychologists must move out of their offices into the classrooms and must be prepared to include educational practices, teacher competence, and teacher–pupil interactions within the frame of diagnosis. To carry out this task requires further competencies on the part of psychologists to the deaf. Not only must they "know" the deaf, they must also know and be able to evaluate the educational influences and teacher practices that go into the fashioning of a deaf pupil.

Formal observational analyses of teacher competence and teacher–pupil interactions pose complex problems of recording, scoring, and interpreting which need not concern us here. But even informal classroom observations can sound important warnings for psychologists trained to interpret them. In my opinion, every psychologist in a school for the deaf should schedule regular class rounds in the form of brief, informal, "sitting-in-for-a-few-minutes" visits for self-instruction on the operational aspects of teaching deaf children at the various chronological levels, and to acquire familiarity with teaching styles and pupil reactions, in particular the reactions of children with deviant behavior. No diagnostic examination of a problem pupil is complete without classroom observation.

Hunter (1977) cites a number of scales devised for evaluating the behavior of teachers and of deviant pupils. Important targets in teacher observations are: (1) the affective climate of the classroom; (2) sensitivity to potential problems and conflicts; (3) skill in structuring and applying corrective comments, measures, and constructive feedback; (4) ability to stimulate creative thinking; (5) organization and clarity in the presentation of lessons; (6) ability to exercise democratic controls; and (7) personal enthusiasm. Several other behaviors can be added for teachers of deaf children; (8) sensitivity to the tolerance limits of a deaf child; (9) ability to head off crisis situations through distracting counteractivities; (10) an understanding acceptance and wise management of frustration outbursts; (11) flexibility and variation in the presentation of daily lessons; and (12) empathy with and respect for the dignity and feelings of deaf children. Excellent preparation for "classroom observation'' is for a psychologist to serve a teaching apprenticeship in a class for deaf children as part of the training required for psychological practice with the deaf.

A milestone in analyzing teacher–deaf-pupil interactions will be attained when a method is devised for simultaneous recording of a pupil's deviant behaviors and a teacher's eliciting and response behaviors. Until that time comes, the observing eye of the well-prepared psychologist will have to gauge the extent to which problem behavior in a given child is related to problem teaching. Where a relationship appears to exist, the wisest possible judgment will have to be exercised in the delicate matter of suggesting remediations in a way that will not antagonize the teacher.

Psychopathic Behaviors

The well-prepared psychologist can also note signs of severe emotional disturbance and psychopathology in the course of informal observation. In themselves, the signs do not ordinarily point to a diagnosis, for similar signs can be associated with various psychopathic conditions, just as the sign "fever" is associated with a wide variety of physical illnesses. In both instances, the signs signify that something is wrong and so alert the observer to the need for differential diagnostic inquiry.

Checklists of signs commonly associated with childhood behavior/ conduct disorders, psychiatric conditions, and antisocial behavior can be found in the case history inventory in Appendix F. Not all the symptoms listed can be seen on inspection. Some are hidden deep in the psyche. But rarely do signs of disturbance exist in isolation. Unseen symptoms are generally accompanied by ones that "show," hence can be observed.

As to the signs themselves, an examiner should expect to find no great difference in manifestations of disturbance between the deaf and the nondeaf. The more experienced the worker is in psychopathology as well as in work with the deaf, the more sensitive he will be to signs of serious deviance in a context of deafness, and the more skilled in distinguishing passing reactive behaviors from pathologically deviant ones.

Interview

To draw out school-agers through interview is far from the easiest of psychological examination techniques (Rich, 1968). School-agers have a self-conscious aversion to intimate self-revelation, especially to strangers. In the case of school-agers who are deaf, the aversion is compounded by difficulties in interpersonal communication. Nevertheless, the interview represents an important means of assessing how well Muller's "tasks of childhood" have been managed, and how well prepared deaf youth is to meet the responsibilities of adulthood. The basic principles of the interview technique have been discussed in chapter 10. The following guides are offered to facilitate interviewing deaf children and youth.

"Interviewing" the Very Young

A conversational interview with deaf preschoolers and very young deaf school-agers is obviously not possible. These children are still in the process of developing language and communication skills, and their attainments are not yet substantial enough for sustained conversation. But many such children have important information to impart. A substitute means for eliciting such leads is through the doll-family kits that are also used in psychological testing. As in that context, the interviewer must make sure there are at least enough dolls available to represent each member of the child's actual family, by age and sex, plus whatever other important figures there may be in the child's immediate life environment. Again, it is helpful to have individual photographs of these persons at hand so that the child can indicate who the actors are in the scenes played out.

This is, of course, an indirect interview approach, but it can prove amazingly informative at times, particularly with disturbed children. One such child in my experience continually grouped together the dolls representing self, mother, and father, while leaving the doll representing the family baby out in the cold, and eventually hurling it to the floor. Another child gave a graphic doll-play of a fight between its mother and father, with brother, sister and self huddled together, and in pantomime indicated intense fear on the part of the children, and a black eye received by the mother. Some children prefer to place the dolls in fixed positions, and themselves act out various incidents while pointing to the doll that is the central figure in the pantomime. Not infrequently, the mini-stories these very young deaf children tell through doll-play and pantomime point straight to the heart of their disturbance and prepare the way for later parent interviews and remedial interventions.

On his part, the examiner resorts to a mix of pantomime, acting, drawing, facial expression, signs, oral communication, or whatever other communicative strategy seems called for to maintain interpersonal exchange with the child being "interviewed." Finally, when the expressive and receptive skills of both child and interviewer are exhausted, there still remain the case history, observation, psychological testing, and parent interviews to tell the rest of the child's story for him.

"Preparation-for-Life" Interview with Deaf Youths

By the time they reach their teens, many deaf school-agers have already been exposed to interview situations, usually for classroom misdemeanors,

poor study habits, and the like. However, broader preparation-for-life interviewing is rarely a routine school practice. In my opinion, it should be.
Teenagers will soon be leaving the protected school environment, and it is
high time that a systematic effort is made to find out how well prepared they
are to meet the demands of independent living, so that appropriate remedial
measures can be taken as required, and hopefully in time.

In such "preparation" interviews, the interviewer looks to see how well
Muller's "tasks" of youth have been managed, namely: the recognition of
limitations, achievement of emotional independence, the choice of a career,
and the formation of a personal philosophy. In the case of deaf youth,
special considerations include: (a) acceptance of deafness; (b) attitudes toward the self, family, and the hearing world; (c) social, conceptual, and sexual maturity; (d) coping mechanisms, including possible use of drugs; (e)
occupational knowledge and aspirations; (f) interpersonal and group adjustments and attitudes; (g) motivations, initiative, and enterprise; and (h)
"other" topics as determined by the individual case.

As I conceive them, preparation-for-life screening interviews take place in
the school setting and are conducted by a communicatively expert staff psychologist or other staff professional, skilled in interviewing and on friendly
terms with the school's pupil population. The purpose of the interview is
frankly explained at the start: "You will be leaving school soon and you will
have a different kind of life. We want you to have a good and happy life. So
we are having this talk together to see how we can help you, and if you have
any questions or problems." As a rule, this friendly introduction is greeted
with a smile and stony silence. The interviewee waits to see what the interviewer comes up with next. Something is needed to break the ice and get the
interview moving.

Among the good ice-breakers in my experience was a teenage discussion
club I had formed as an elective extracurricular activity for open discussion
on any topic of concern to the youthful members. The club proved to be the
most popular of the school's extracurricular activities; and the lively group
discussions and the togetherness engendered by common concerns and problems went far to dispel any self-consciousness that might have hampered
later individual interviews on personal matters.

Other good ice-breakers are sentence completion tests and apperceptive
test stories. Sentence completion tests often provide quick and striking leads
to the feelings and attitudes of deaf youths toward life, family, and self. The
leads can be used as initial "tell me more about that" or "please explain"
strategies to draw out the interviewee. From that point on, the interviewer
can unobtrusively expand the discussion into other areas. I have found the
sentence completion approach generally more applicable and productive than
apperceptive stories because of the more structured nature of the sentence

task and the less taxing demands on narrative language and imagination. When psychological tests are used as interview openers, they need not be given in their entirety—that would eat into interview time and fatigue the interviewee. A few selected items suffice. If the tests have already been administered during psychological testing, the original protocols can, of course, be used for interview purposes.

The items to be included in preparation-for-life interviews should be carefully worked out beforehand by the examiner in collaboration with other school personnel, and a standard form should be devised for interview coverage and recording. Of great help in developing the form are the numerous psychological inventories available on such topics as occupational preference, knowledge, and aspirations; sex knowledge and activities; family living; personal values; marital readiness; and many more related life-adjustment topics. The interview findings are used as the basis for counseling, remedial interventions, and therapy as required.

Interviews with deaf youths follow the general principles of the interview technique. As a rule, deaf youths tend to be open, refreshingly frank, and perfectly willing to discuss any aspect of personal life with someone they know, respect, and trust. In this regard they differ considerably from most hearing youths, with whom interviews are often hampered by hostile resentment of invasion of personal privacy, false modesty, or flippant shock tactics.

Finally, this discussion has been based on situations in which the interview is conducted by communicatively expert examiners who are known to the interviewees. This ideal is not always achievable with deaf youths, and is seldom the case with deaf adults. Suggestions concerning the management of these more difficult interview situations are summarized in chapter 13.

Summary Comment

A glance at the preceding discussion shows that considerable space has been allotted the subject of psychological tests and testing. This may suggest that this branch of psychological information-gathering outranks the others in importance. More likely it outranks the others in complexity and frustration when the slim test-resources available to psychologists to the deaf have to be stretched, modified, adapted, reinterpreted, and otherwise reconditioned to accommodate the needs of a deaf clientele.

In the final analysis, the relative importance of the four basic branches of psychological examining depends upon which provides the clearest information about a given subject. It would be contrary to known fact to accord this distinction to testing per se. The technique is, after all, a shortcut form of objective evaluation in which the operational unit is made up of three interlocking components—the examiner, the test, and the subject. In this unit, the subject "sets the stage"; the test constrains his performance; the examiner controls the action and interplay. Further, in all instances but particularly with deaf subjects, much of a test's "objectivity" rests with the *subjective* judgment of the examiner regarding its use and interpretation. Hence, the old clinical dictum that no test is better than the person giving it; and hence the difficulty of "recommending" tests for deaf subjects without taking into consideration the subject and the examiner as well as the test.

For examiners who know their psychological techniques and who know the deaf, a good case history may be all that is needed for diagnostic evaluation. Or observation may give the story away, or interview, or any combination of these. In other words, tests may not be necessary at all in certain cases except for supplementary data and for mandated records. But where tests are used, "the significance of test scores is greatest when they are combined with a full study of the person by means of interview, case history records, application blanks, and other methods," to quote Cronbach again.

References

Amoss, H. 1936. *Ontario School Ability Examination.* Toronto: Ryerson Press.

Anastasi, A. 1976. *Psychological Testing.* 4th ed. New York: Macmillan.

Bellak, L. 1954. *The Thematic Apperception Test and the Children's Apperception Test in Clinical Use.* New York: Grune & Stratton.

Bender, L. 1938. *A Visual Motor Gestalt Test and Its Clinical Use.* American Orthopsychiatric Association Research Monograph No. 3. New York.

Buck, J. N., 1966. *The House-Tree-Person Technique: Revised Manual.* Los Angeles: Western Psychological Services.

Buros, O. K., Ed. 1974. *Tests in Print, II.* Highland Park, N.J.: Gryphon Press.

Cattell, R. B., and Eber, H. W. 1956–1957. *Sixteen Personality Factor Questionnaire.* Rev. ed. Champaign, Ill.: Institute for Personality and Ability Testing.

Doll, E. A. 1947. *Vineland Social Maturity Scale: Manual of Directions.* Minneapolis: Educational Testing Bureau.

Dunn, L. M. 1959. *Peabody Picture Vocabulary Test.* Circle Pines, Minn.: American Guidance Service.

Geist, H. 1959. *The Geist Picture Interest Inventory: General Form: Male. Psychological Reports,* Monograph Supplement 3.

Geist, H. 1962. Occupational interest profiles of the deaf. *Personnel and Guidance Journal,* September, pp. 50–55.

Gibson, E. J., and Olum, V. 1960. Experimental methods of studying perception in children. In P. H. Mussen, Ed., *Handbook of Research Methods in Child Development.* New York: John Wiley & Sons. Pp. 311–73.

Hathaway, S. R., and McKinley, J. C. 1951. *Minnesota Multiphasic Personality Inventory.* Rev. ed. New York: Psychological Corp.

Heath, R. W., and Neilson, M. A. 1974. The research basis for performance-based teacher education. *Review of Educational Research,* 44: 463–84.

Heim, A. 1970. *Intelligence and Personality: Their Assessment and Relationship.* Baltimore, Md.: Penguin Books.

Hiskey, M. S. 1941. *Nebraska Test of Learning Aptitude for Young Deaf Children.* Lincoln: University of Nebraska.

Hunter, C. P. 1977. Classroom observation instruments and teacher inservice training by school psychologists. *School Psychology Monograph,* 3: 45–88.

Jastak, J. F., and Jastak, S. 1979. *Wide Range Interest-Opinion Test: Manual.* 1979 ed. Wilmington, Del.: Jastak Associates.

Kallmann, F. J. 1963. Main findings and some projections. In J. D. Rainer, K. Z. Altshuler, and F. J. Kallmann, Eds., *Family and Mental Health Problems in a Deaf Population.* New York: New York State Psychiatric Institute, Columbia University. Pp. 243–48.

Levine, E. S. 1974. Psychological tests and practices with the deaf: A survey of the state of the art. *Volta Review,* 76: 298–319.

McCarthy, J. J., and McCarthy, J. F. 1969. *Learning Disabilities.* Boston: Allyn and Bacon.

Machover, K. 1949. *Personality Projection in the Drawing of the Human Figure: A Method of Personality Investigation.* Springfield, Ill.: Charles C. Thomas.

Meadow, K. P. In press. *Meadow-Kendall Social-Emotional Inventory for Deaf Children.* Washington, D.C.: Gallaudet College.

Muller, P. 1969. *The Tasks of Childhood.* Transl. from the French by Anita Mason. New York: World University Library, McGraw-Hill Book Co.

Murray, H. A. 1943. *Thematic Apperception Test.* Cambridge, Mass.: Harvard University Press.

Myklebust, H. R. 1965. *Development and Disorders of Written Language, Vol. 1: Picture Story Language Test.* New York: Grune & Stratton.

Quigley, S. P., Steinkamp, M. W., Power, D. J., and Jones, B. W. 1978. *Test of Syntactic Abilities.* Beaverton, Oregon: Dormac, Inc.

Ray, S. 1979. *An Adaptation of the Wechsler Intelligence Scale for Children: Revised for the Deaf.* Knoxville, Tenn.: Steven Ray.

Rich, J. 1968. *Interviewing Children and Adolescents.* New York: St. Martin's Press.

Rorschach, H. 1942. *Psychodiagnostics: A Diagnostic Test Based on Perception.* Transl. by P. Lemkau and B. Kronenburg. (1st German ed., 1921.) New York: Grune & Stratton; Berne: Huber.

Rosenshine, B. 1971. Teaching behaviors related to pupil achievement: A review of research. In I. Westburg and A. Bellack, Eds., *Research into Classroom Processes: Recent Developments and Next Steps.* New York: Teachers College Press, Columbia University.

Rotter, J. B., and Rafferty, J. E. 1950. *The Rotter Incomplete Sentences Blank.* New York: Psychological Corp.

Shneidman, E. S. 1947. *Make a Picture Story.* New York: Psychological Corp.

Smith, A. J., and Johnson, R. E. 1978. *Smith-Johnson Nonverbal Performance Scale.* Los Angeles: Western Psychological Services.

Snijders, J. Th., and Snijders-Oomen, N. 1959. *Non-Verbal Intelligence Tests for Deaf and Hearing Subjects.* Groningen, Holland: J. B. Wolters.

Stanford Achievement Test for Hearing Impaired Students. 1972. Washington, D.C.: Gallaudet College, Office of Demographic Studies.

Stutsman, R. 1931. *Mental Measurement of Preschool Children*. Yonkers-on-Hudson, N.Y.: World Book Co.

Symonds, P. M. 1948. *Symonds Picture-Story Test*. New York: Bureau of Publications, Teachers College, Columbia University.

Vernon, M. 1969. Usher's syndrome: Deafness and progressive blindness. *Birth Defects Reprint Series*. The National Foundation–March of Dimes.

Wechsler, D. 1944. *The Measurement of Adult Intelligence*. Baltimore: Williams & Wilkins Co.

Wechsler, D. 1949. *Wechsler Intelligence Scale for Children*. New York: Psychological Corp.

Wechsler, D. 1955. *Wechsler Adult Intelligence Scale*. New York: Psychological Corp.

Wechsler, D. 1963. *Wechsler Preschool and Primary Scale of Intelligence*. New York: Psychological Corp.

13 Examination at the Adult Level

MOST DEAF adults whose school days are behind them are reexposed to psychological examining when the need arises for guidance on vocational and related matters. The usual setting is a vocational rehabilitation facility, and the targets of inquiry are contained in the acronym SKAPATI (Pinner, 1970, p. 45), in which the letters represent:

S Skills: the applicant's use of knowledge to execute or perform effectively and readily.

K Knowledge: his background, adequacy of job-related information, "know-how."

A Ability: his proficiency in any kind of work or activity.

P Physical: his physical and emotional capacity to do the job.

A Aptitudes: his potential or undeveloped abilities.

T Traits: his personal characteristics, which primarily include appearance, attitude, manner.

I Interests: choice of vocation, the kind of work he is interested in doing.

The key figure in obtaining and integrating this and related information is the vocational rehabilitation counselor.

The everyday responsibilities of counselors cover an extensive range (McGowan and Porter, 1967), dealing as they do with an extraordinary variety of disablements. Numbers of these specialists are skilled users of many of the information-gathering techniques used in psychological practice. However, it is a rare rehabilitation facility that is staffed with personnel skilled in applying the techniques to a deaf clientele.

The counselors' usual reactions to deaf clients reflect the dilemmas described in chapter 6, added to which is the heterogeneity arising from differences among deaf clients in vocational background, needs, attitudes, and problems.

For example, some deaf clients, generally fresh from school, have no vocational goals, minimal knowledge of the occupational world, unrealistic aspirations, and little motivation to look ahead into a vocational future that spells independence. Others, also fresh from school, have well-founded career targets in the professional world and simply require some financial assistance for college. Sometimes there are family heads who have been laid off from long-held jobs through no fault of their own—the employer faces a financial crisis and needs to cut expenses. There are also chronic vocational failures who lack the flexibility to adjust to the work culture. And there are what DiFrancesca and Hurwitz (1969) call the "hard-core deaf." These are deaf clients who have been failures in school, work, and society, not through lack of intelligence or the ability to work in competitive employment, but because of deficient social and emotional functioning and an inability to see beyond a personal frame of reference and the dictates of personal gratification. Examples in my experience are a woman in New York City who would not take a job on 34th Street because she had arbitrarily decided not to work anywhere below 42nd Street; a man who left a good job because the exit door was several feet farther from his desk than suited his convenience, and another man who left a good job because the employee's restroom was farther away than suited him. And finally, always represented among deaf clients are the severely undereducated and communicatively disabled, some of good mental potential and others with mental deficits, all of whom present a difficult and frustrating challenge to psychologist and rehabilitation counselor alike.

The typical evaluative disposition of this assorted client population is referral to a psychometric consultant. However, it takes considerably more than psychometrics to find the human being behind the facade of disability. The next section provides some guides toward this end.

History Data

Exhaustive history data are not generally required for the average run of nondeaf rehabilitation clients (See chapter 10). A basic minimum is needed to fulfill legal requirements, and over and above this, whatever extra data that enable a counselor to "get to know" the individual client and formulate appropriate rehabilitative measures. However, in the event a particular client is a deaf person, more detailed history information is generally needed for these purposes than is required for the nondeaf. Background and developmental data are useful to help explain how a given deaf client came to be the way he is, as discussed in earlier chapters. Of more immediate concern in most cases is information dealing with the following topics.

1. *Communication Patterns*

    a. The client's preferred modes of expressive communication and his level of expressive abilities.

    b. The client's preferred modes of receptive communication and his facility in receiving information through these modes.

    c. The "fit" between a client's communicative patterns and the communicative requirements of a given job in relation to training, placement, and advancement.

    d. The fit between a client's communicative patterns and the mental ability required to improve the patterns through tutoring; the communicative modes that should be selected for tutoring; the likelihood of significant gains and the length of time required.

    e. The extent to which improved communicative abilities could broaden a client's vocational horizons; the amount of improvement that would be required; the feasibility of achieving such gains.

    f. The feasibility of aural/oral rehabilitative procedures.

2. *Vocational Factors*

    a. The client's vocational preferences, and the fit with his abilities.

    b. The client's level of occupational knowledge and vocational "know-how" in such matters as: applying for a job, employer–employee and co-worker relations; labor unions, taxes, social security, insurance; shop language; the job market.

    c. The client's objectively determined vocational aptitudes and skills.

    d. The pattern of previous work experiences and problems.

    e. The effect on vocational planning of the client's communicative status.

    f. The client's motivations for improving abilities and learning new skills.

3. *Mental Abilities*

    a. The level of the client's functioning intelligence as demonstrated in school history and life activities; the client's level of potential intelligence as disclosed in psychological testing.

    b. The client's learning abilities; observational faculties; the speed, accuracy, and relevance of his mental operations.

    c. The fit between the client's functioning intelligence and his vocational preferences and aspirations.

    d. The client's reasoning and conceptual abilities, and ability to handle numerical, graphic, or other abstract symbol systems.

    e. The kinds of remedial tutoring, counseling, or other remedial measures indicated.

4. *Adjustment Factors*

    a. The client's attitudes toward and interactions with hearing persons; deaf persons; preferred deaf or hearing group settings.

b. The client's adaptability patterns, and levels of tolerance for correction, stress, frustration, sustained effort.

c. The client's principal motivations; self-concept; dependence/independence ratio; reaction to authority figures.

d. Evidences of emotional disturbance and their possible effects on job-holding. Is psychiatric referral called for?

5. *Socioeconomic and Family Situation*

a. Auditory status of family (deaf, hearing, deaf relatives). Is the client the only deaf family member? Is this a foreign-language home?

b. Socioeconomic status of family.

c. The client's marital status; domestic and financial responsibilities; how well managed.

d. The client's dependence/independence ratio in personal decision-making; in family decision-making.

e. The fit between the client's vocational abilities and family aspirations for him; the family influence on the client's acceptance of vocational realities.

f. Family attitudes toward and influences on vocational rehabilitation procedures and recommendations.

6. *Social Participation*

a. The kinds of social outlets the client has; would like to have.

b. The nature and extent of the client's participation in social activities of deaf groups; hearing groups.

c. The client's organizational and club memberships and his levels of participation: leader, active participant, passive observer.

d. The client's participation in community and civic activities, deaf pride movements, etc.

7. *Physical and Health Status*

a. Other physical or health conditions that must be considered in vocational planning and placement.

b. Is there any cerebral dysfunction, neurological disorder, motor disability, or visual condition that must be taken into account in vocational planning; any conditions that tend to aggravate deafness, such as allergies, tendency to respiratory infections, chronic fatigue?

c. The presence of any otological conditions that must be taken into account in vocational preparation and placement, such as impairment of the balance mechanism, or abnormal sensitivity to certain kinds of noise and pressure sensations.

d. The existence of health complaints by the client that are not part of the medical record. Do these appear hypochondriacal? What do the medical consultants have to say about them?

Many nondeaf rehabilitation clients are able to supply a goodly portion of history information by themselves during the course of intake, as are deaf adults in the exceptional and above-average categories. But with the undereducated and severely communicatively limited, most of this information must be obtained from school records and other informants. The reason can be inferred from the following excerpt (literally transcribed from the sign language) of an intake interview conducted in signs with a deaf client-graduate of a school for the deaf.

INTERVIEWER:	"Tell me about when you were little. Could you hear when you were young?"
CLIENT:	"What mean?"
INTERVIEWER:	"Before. Little. Hear can you?"
CLIENT:	"No. Dumb me. Hear nothing little me."
INTERVIEWER:	"Become deaf how?"
CLIENT:	"I deaf since small—still deaf."
INTERVIEWER:	"How deaf? Sick? Accident? What?"
CLIENT:	"Vomited, ear hurt, stomach hurt, was twisted, sick, very hot, hurt, other different things."
INTERVIEWER:	"How old sick?"
CLIENT:	"Not remember."
INTERVIEWER:	"Mother, father, deaf?"
CLIENT:	"No. Father hearing but signs. Mother hearing, not signs, talks."
INTERVIEWER:	"Brothers? Sisters?"
CLIENT:	"Sister nothing. Brother one."
INTERVIEWER:	"How old brother?"
CLIENT:	"Old thirteen."
INTERVIEWER:	"Deaf brother?"
CLIENT:	"Hearing."

The interview continued for a short while following this exchange, until the client said his arms were tired and he wanted to stop.

But even where history is obtained in this way, the case record should include autobiographic input directly from the client, preferably in written form. Such clients should also be encouraged to tell their own stories in their own way. At the initial meeting with the counselor or psychologist, the client is warmly invited to "Tell me about yourself. Write down what you remember about your life and problems. Then I will know how to help you." Some will not be able to respond at all for lack of the verbal language required for writing. But others who have had somewhat more scholastic success will try to oblige. For example, the client in the excerpt above quite willingly wrote: "I teased in the dormitory. I don't like X school. I knew troubling in X school for the deaf. I didn't never tease. I am very quiet." He continued in this vein, with the word "tease" supplied by the interviewer in response to the client's request to tell him how to spell the verbal equivalent of the sign "tease."

Scant and sketchy though such productions generally are, unusual insights are sometimes afforded by what the client does record. In addition, the client's written record displays his verbal expressive ability and concept productions, and so provides another lead to the nature and level of communication required for counseling and the psychological examination.

Psychological Testing

In principles, practices, basic cautions and problems, psychological testing at the adult level generally follows the pattern described for deaf youth in chapter 12; and tests for adults can be selected from the pool of instruments cited there for deaf youth. However, a number of special considerations in adult test situations warrant attention.

Vocational Factors

There is greater emphasis on vocational testing with deaf adults than with school-agers, and special concern with individual adjustment to the work culture. This, in turn, requires added special competencies of psychologists working in rehabilitation settings. These include familiarity with tests and techniques of vocational evaluation, knowledge of the vocational world and the special requirements of various vocations particularly in communication, and familiarity with the job market in terms of deaf applicants.

Communication Factors

A deaf client's communicative resources take on heightened significance and immediacy in vocational rehabilitation not only because of their pivotal role in vocational planning but also because of the federally mandated involvement of rehabilitation clients in their own Individualized Written Rehabilitation Programs (Randolph, 1978; Walton, 1978). Therefore a first prerequisite in the psychological examination is knowledge of a deaf client's communicative patterns and levels.

In theory, this information and other history data should be in the hands of the psychological examiner before the initial test session. But it often happens that the testee arrives first. If this were an interview, the examiner could take more time in exploring the client's communicative habits. But in a test situation, the matter must be handled more expeditiously because of time constraints.

Communicative orientation can be rapidly elicited through brief pretest conversation, followed by language achievement testing. The pretest conversation would involve an exchange of greetings and introductions, an explanation of the proceedings about to take place, and a request for "any questions?" It would begin with oral exchange, and from that point onward would be guided by the client's reaction to spoken language and shifted in accordance with the client's preferred communicative modes. Paper and pencil should be available for any written communication the client or the examiner wishes to make.

From this beginning, the examination moves into formal testing, starting with language and reading achievement tests, still centering on the communication picture—other achievement tests can be given later on. In addition to providing rapid orientation to the communicative situation, beginning a test session with achievement tests has other advantages. First, the relatively impersonal nature of achievement tests is less anxiety-provoking for tense clients than are personality and intelligence tests. Second, it gives examiners who had no advance information some extra time, while the client is working on the tests, to evaluate their own communicative capabilities vis-à-vis the client and plan accordingly.

Donoghue and Bolton (1971) describe a more formal evaluation system conducted in a facility reserved for deaf clients and staffed by experienced workers with the deaf. In this program, an extra session is allocated for communication screening. Each client is rated by qualified personnel on a five-point excellent-to-poor scale in regard to four expressive and six receptive communication skills. The expressive skills include oral speech, writing, manual signs, and fingerspelling. The receptive skills include unaided hearing, aided hearing, speechreading, reading, manual signs, and fingerspelling.

Naturally, the happiest communicative situation for nondeaf examiners is with exceptional deaf clients who can communicate orally. With such persons, psychological tests can generally be used as they stand, provided certain communicative cautions are observed, as summarized in the section on Interview. However, examiners must guard against the misconception that inability to communicate orally reflects adversely on either mental or linguistic resources. There are many deaf persons, who, despite poor oral communicative skills, manifest superior linguistic and mental caliber in their fingerspelled and written communications and in their level of reading ability. On the other hand, there are even more deaf persons whose oral and written output is fractured and minimal, but whose conversation in the language of signs is an informational joy to an inquiring examiner who is fully conversant with the language.

A common misconception of examiners new in the use of sign language is that any level of linguistic discourse, no matter how complex, can be understood by manual deaf clients once it is signed and fingerspelled. This is decidedly not so. In order for the sign language to convey a meaningful message to such persons, it must be couched in the "vocabulary" and syntactic patterns characterizing the language, and in the conceptual patterns characterizing the individual's thinking processes. For examiners, this is another instance of the imperative to "know" the deaf and to be able to "think deaf" and "talk deaf" when required.

Test Selection

A special consideration in selecting tests for deaf adults is the wider communicative heterogeneity found among them than is usually found among deaf youth in school settings. At one extreme are numbers of uneducated deaf adults as well as individuals whose school days are so far behind that they have become set in communicative habits of their own devising. At the other extreme are professional deaf persons, and those preparing for the professions. Examiners in rehabilitation settings must be prepared for these eventualities and all in between.

With deaf persons who are functionally illiterate in every communication system, a commonly used adult intelligence test is the *Revised Beta Examination;* it is a revision of the first nonlanguage group test to be developed, the Army Group Examination Beta used for testing illiterates and non-English-speaking soldiers during World War I. The Revised Beta Examination consists of six subtests: mazes, digit-symbol substitutions, picture absurdities, paper formboard, picture completion, and perceptual speed. Instructions are conveyed through pantomime plus demonstration exercises that precede each subtest. Achievement testing with deaf communicative "illiterates" is generally conducted at the primary level and is limited to reading and computation. Personality testing is carried out through drawing tests, since they can be easily administered in pantomime. Where evidences emerge of greater than expected abilities, which sometimes does happen, testing carefully moves to a higher plane of inquiry. I have found qualified deaf interpreters to be exceptionally expert in the psychological evaluation of communicative "illiterates."

For deaf adults of average and better communicative resources, as well as for nondeaf adults, there had long been a need for individual intelligence tests suited to adult expectations and standardized on adult populations. But until David Wechsler constructed his first adult intelligence test, no such instruments were available (Wechsler, 1944, p. 15). The Wechsler adult scales made it possible to move into the area of adult mental testing with appropriate instrumentation and professional justification. However, testing the deaf adult population with the Wechsler Full Scale raises the debated issue of using verbal mental tests with the deaf.

There has been a long tradition against the use of verbal intelligence tests with deaf subjects. This is entirely understandable in the case of young school-agers whose language, concepts, and experiences are not up to the demands of verbal tests. But with older teenagers and especially with adults, the informational value of appropriately designed and used verbal mental tests based on adult expectations cannot be lightly dismissed. Individuals at these chronological levels are either entering the mainstream of life, or are already there. To succeed requires a goodly measure of coping abilities; not the least of which is mental ability.

As measured by performance tests, the mental ability of the deaf-at-large is of sound average caliber. But this average expectation is not generally manifested in dealing with real-life concepts and problems. To clarify the psychometric aspects of the situation, several workers with the deaf turned to the verbal portion of the Wechsler Adult Intelligence Scales for a closer look at the level of mental functioning behind the Average Performance I.Q. of older teenagers and adults (Falberg, 1974; Levine, 1956; Ross, 1970). The following excerpts from responses to the Bellevue-Wechsler Verbal Scale (Levine, 1956) illustrate the differences found between a school failure (subject A) and a proficient student (subject B), both with Average Performance Scale I.Q. scores. To conserve space, the test questions are abbre-

Test Item	Subject A	Subject B
Information		
Where is London?	Don't know	England
How many pints in a quart?	Don't know	Two
What is a thermometer?	Tell hot and cold	Measures degree cold or heat
How many weeks in a year?	Twelve	Fifty-two
General Comprehension		
Find stamped, addressed envelope. What do you do?	Take stamp off and save it	Mail it
See fire in movies. What do you do?	Run out of the house	Call manager to make alarm for fire engines
Why keep away from bad company?	Easy to spoil me	Learn many bad things from them
Why do people pay taxes?	Don't know	Support public offices
Similarities		
(In what way are the following the same?)		
Orange–banana	Both yellow, good to eat, healthy	Both fruits
Coat–dress	Both pretty	Both are to wear
Wagon–bicycle	Both have wheels, both toys	Both are used to ride
Air–water	Both windy	We cannot live without either air or water

viated here, but they were adapted in language (Levine, 1960) and method of communication to the needs of the subjects.

The problem of understanding why two subjects, both of average Performance Scale I.Q., performed so differently from one another in life was clarified psychometrically by the Bellevue-Wechsler Verbal Scale in the above study. (The WAIS revision had not yet appeared.) The functioning mental ability with which subject A faced real life, as indicated by the Verbal Scale, was 29 I.Q. points below the mental potential with which she was endowed, as measured by the Performance Scale, and 40 I.Q. points below that of Subject B. The findings obtained from the Verbal Scale had closer concurrent validity with the real-life picture than did the average findings obtained from the Performance Scale. This is not an unusual psychometric picture for deaf subjects, with no lack of ready explanations. What needs further exploring is the predictive value of verbal mental tests when used with deaf youth and adults.

I have made it a practice to experiment with the Wechsler Verbal Scale with even severely communicatively limited deaf adults, for the sake of picking up added clinical insight. To illustrate the procedure with the Verbal Scale question "What should you do if, while in the movies, you were the first person to see smoke and fire?" the question in such cases is administered somewhat as follows, in signs, facial expression, pantomime, and body movement:

"You. Movies go?" (Examiner smiles.)

Subject nods "yes."

"Movies like?" (Examiner still smiles while directing a questioning look at subject.)

Subject nods "yes."

"Imagine here movies." (Examiner indicates test room, using sign for "imagines" plus a dreamlike facial expression. It often takes some time for the "imagine" concept to be understood by the subject, and some playacting may be required. When the concept has finally registered, the examiner continues.)

"O.K. Here movies. You sit. Watch." (Examiner demonstrates by staring at an imaginary screen with a rapt facial expression, as if watching a real movie; then slowly looks around with an anxious facial expression—this in preparation for the next statement.)

"Smell smoke!" (Examiner's facial expression is one of alarm.)

"See fire!" (Examiner's facial expression expresses more alarm, and she looks about as if to locate where the fire is, while at the same time conveying the body-movement message to indicate the fire is not part of the movie but in the movie house.)

"You. What do?" (Examiner directs a pointedly questioning look at the subject.)

In response, one communicatively limited subject pantomimed that he would go to the fire alarm box, smash the glass, and pull the alarm. Most other subjects simply indicate they would run away. But in this and in several other surprisingly good answers (in signs and pantomime), this particular subject showed that he had something more to him that warranted closer study and special help even though his total verbal score was well below the Wechsler average.

The diagnostic values of the WAIS Full Scale, as adapted for deaf adults by Falberg (1974), are becoming increasingly recognized in the field of the deaf. The Performance Scale I.Q. indicates the level of endowed mental resources and is used for the records and as a rough guide to expectations. The verbal I.Q. is used to provide clinical insights and as a guide to remedial and counseling needs. It should be kept in the confidential files.

Some "Concurrent Validity" Guides

Among the criteria that can be used in checking adult test results against real-life accomplishments and expectations are the following.

1. A deaf adult is of at least average mental ability if his reading achievement is at a 4th grade level.

2. A deaf adult is probably of above-average mental ability if his arithmetic achievement score is at a 6th grade level.

3. Where scores in reading and arithmetic achievement fall below these levels, the individual may still be of average mental endowment as indicated by other life accomplishments or by insightful drives and motivations, as demonstrated by the earlier story of Roberto.

4. A deaf adult presents a good mental and adjustment picture if he shows good vocational, domestic, and social functioning, regardless of achievement test scores.

5. Inability on the part of nonoral deaf adults to profit significantly from oral remediation is no reflection on mental ability. The time for instituting oral communication is long past.

6. Spectacular remediation gains at the adult level should not be expected when causes for stubborn, long-term learning disabilities involve such factors as adverse school experiences, deeply rooted emotional disorders, or cerebral dysfunction.

In Recapitulation

A number of the special points that have been made about testing deaf adults are summarized in the following excerpts from a workshop report. It was compiled several decades ago but is as timely now as then (Reports of Workshop Committees, 1950, pp. 14–15).

1. The test results based upon tasks involving verbal concepts and language should be interpreted with special care. Individuals who have lost their hearing early in life or for a considerable time before testing may have acquired language habits enough different from the non-handicapped to depress test scores where language tasks are involved.

2. The older the age of the individual when his deafness occurred, the more it can be assumed that his life experiences are common to hearing persons. Therefore, loss of hearing in later life may not be expected to affect test results involving language tasks as much as loss of hearing in childhood.

3. The test results of deaf people on tests involving language or reading are more safely considered as minimal levels of abilities rather than as the upper limits of abilities.

4. When deafness is an accompanying result of a more basic condition, e.g., birth injury involving the nervous system in general, the psychological test results are to be considered primarily in terms of the more basic condition and secondarily in terms of deafness and other accompanying conditions.

5. The I.Q. as a single score is to be regarded with great caution as an index of mental ability. The sub-test scores of the different mental abilities should be examined most carefully and given emphasis in the total case study.

6. The total test score and the separate items should both be studied for clues to abilities, achievements, and personality traits. A study of responses on separate items at times may give clues to a richer and more accurate interpretation of test data. . . .

7. The totally deaf and seriously hard of hearing should be tested individually, and preferably with individualized tests such as the Wechsler.

8. Special precautions should be taken to make certain that good rapport prevails between the examiner and the deaf client. The use of the manual alphabet and sign language is encouraged as a means of giving test instructions. Otherwise, a natural and somewhat restrained form of pantomime is desirable. The counselors have a special responsibility to prepare the client for the testing experience. If the psychologist does not know the manual alphabet or sign language, the client should be told before hand by the counselor about the nature of the tests, the need for full cooperation, the need to make certain that the client fully understands instructions before each test, and that the test results will be discussed later with the counselor. Lack of rapport definitely influences the test results. Moreover, the psychologist has more difficulty in evaluating the effects of poor rapport in the deaf because of difficulties in free and uninhibited communication.

9. When the background of the deaf person shows gaps in formal educa-

tion, the causes for such a fact should be ascertained and be used in interpreting test scores.

10. Conditions of excessive depression, anxiety, idleness, or seclusiveness over long periods of time may be expected to influence test scores. The test scores will indicate the present level of ability-functioning, but interpretations and prognoses must include an evaluation of the underlying conditions and their interaction upon the psychological test scores.

11. The disability of deafness may be overemphasized in the total case study. Other factors may be much more important, and it is always well to be on guard lest such overemphasis obscure other major factors. For example, lack of formal school achievements may be due not to hearing loss but to physical or mental illness, or to neurotic parental concern over the deaf person, or even to poor attitudes of the deaf person himself.

12. Personality traits such as the will to work, adaptability to the hearing world, persistence in solving problems, method of attacking new problems, self-confidence, etc., may be seen in actual operation before, during, and after a testing session. Qualitative observation of the behavior of the deaf client may yield information of considerable significance in the fuller and deeper interpretation of test performance.

In connection with the stress on interpretation expressed in the preceding summary, I wish to emphasize again that the purpose of psychological testing is not to interpret the test, but rather to interpret the individual behaviors and abilities elicited by the test. The test and its scope of possible findings have already been interpreted, as it were, by the test constructor in the process of standardization. But individual responses are psychologically meaningful only in the light of a subject's background of experiences. If the background conforms to that of the standardization population of a given test, interpretation is facilitated. But if it does not, as in the case of the deaf, the examiner must acquire the necessary familiarity with the "unstandardized" life contexts from which the test responses were derived. It is only in the light of the context that responses convey a meaningful message.

Finally, several other recommendations of the Workshop merit reemphasis.

1. The rehabilitation counselor specializing in work with the deaf and the severely hard of hearing should contact one or more qualified psychologists in different sections of the state and seek to interest them in the need for their services in behalf of the hearing-impaired.

2. The counselor should be responsible for sending the psychologist important data in the case history which would be valuable as background for a

psychological evaluation. This information should be sent before the individual meets with the psychologist.

3. The counselor should deem it his responsibility to inform the psychologist in the special problems of rehabilitating the deaf and the severely hard of hearing. This would entail such things as forwarding bibliographies, discussing special case histories with him, and placing him in contact with schools for the deaf.

4. The counselor should discuss the test results and the case data with the psychologist as a means of mutual benefit, and for the greatest welfare of the client. In the initial stages, these contacts with the psychologist should be frequent. Later they will become less necessary as the psychologist becomes experienced in serving the deaf and the severely hard of hearing, and as the counselor becomes more proficient in interpreting the psychological reports.

Psychological Testing of Adults: An Illustrative Testing Program

Among the numerous publications on the evaluation of deaf rehabilitation clients, Watson's guidelines (1977) warrant special mention for comprehensiveness and organization. This section briefly summarizes the psychological tests and procedures used in adult evaluations at the New York League for the Hard of Hearing, as described by Acting Director Ruth R. Green. At the New York League for the Hard of Hearing, psychological evaluations at the adult level are conducted with persons having all degrees and types of hearing loss who require help in vocational and career planning and in vocational retraining.

It is obvious that the needs of the individual clients will vary with such factors as type, onset, and amount of hearing loss as well as with socioeconomic status, communication characteristics, motivation, and adaptability. It is the psychologist's responsibility to select the tests best suited to the individual for ascertaining such pivotal planning factors as the client's intelligence, social maturity, education level, personality patterns, adaptability, aptitudes, interests, and abilities. Test scores are compared with those of the normally hearing population on whom the tests were standardized, but are interpreted in the light of case history information, in particular the effects of hearing loss on the individual's life as well as test performance.

Tests most frequently used with adults at the League include the following:

1. Intelligence

The *Wechsler Adult Intelligence Scale* is used for information about a client's mental abilities. If hearing impairment is the only disability, the Performance I.Q. is considered a valid measure. However, if the client has a visual-motor coordination problem or visual-perceptual dysfunction, the

WAIS Performance Scale is not a generally reliable index of mental ability. Wherever feasible, the WAIS Verbal Scale is also administered using oral language, sign language, or total communication. For a client with adequate reading skills, the questions can also be presented in written form. In most instances, the Verbal I.Q. is used as a rough index of the individual's conceptual, informational, and expressive abilities, as compared with his potential mental resources as indicated by the Performance I.Q. The gap between the two is a valuable guide in vocational planning and in required remediation. The gap is expected to narrow with appropriate treatment.

The *Revised Beta Examination* and the *Non-Language Multi-Mental Test,* both nonlanguage paper-and-pencil tests, are used to measure the mental abilities of clients with severe linguistic and communicative problems. Again, they have limitations for clients with visual-motor or visual-perceptual dysfunctions.

2. *Visual/Perceptual/Motor Coordinations*

The *Bender-Gestalt Test* is used to screen for disturbances in visual/motor/perceptual coordinations and for short-term visual recall.

3. *Achievement*

The *Stanford Achievement Test* is the preferred test. It is used in preference to the Stanford Achievement Test for Hearing Impaired Students because the administration of the latter requires a pretest and the procedures involved generally take too long to be included in a vocational assessment battery.

4. *Vocational Interests and Aptitudes*

The *Kuder Occupational Interest Survey* or the *Strong-Campbell Interest Inventory* is used to ascertain vocational preferences with clients whose reading level is above 6th grade.

The *Wide Range Interest-Opinion Test,* which presents vocational choices pictorially, is used with clients who have less than a 6th grade reading level, provided the client understands the concepts "most" and "least," since choices must be made among activities "most" and "least" liked.

The *Vocational Interest and Sophistication Assessment* (VISA) is used as a vocational preference inventory with clients who have difficulty with "most" and "least" concepts. This inventory presents pictures of people working at manual, entry-level jobs and provides information about a client's preferences in such matters as sedentary versus physical work, indoor versus outdoor work, etc.

The *Revised Minnesota Paper Form-Board Test* is a paper-and-pencil test with a long history of effective prediction in fields that have a mechanical orientation. It has also proved helpful with clients considering an art-related career.

The *Minnesota Clerical Test* is a paper-and-pencil test of speed and accuracy in tasks related to clerical work, and has proved a valuable assessment tool for clients who wish to enter clerical training. The test consists of two parts: number checking and name checking. It is not unusual for clients with poor reading skills to do well on number checking and poorly on name checking.

The *Purdue Pegboard* is an individually administered test of manipulative dexterity, and gives separate scores for the right hand, the left hand, and for both hands together. It measures gross movements of hands, fingers, and arms, and "tip of the finger" dexterity, which is needed in small assembly work, jewelry making, and other areas requiring fine finger skills.

The *Bennett Hand-Tool Dexterity Test* is also an individually administered test, and provides information about a client's proficiency in using ordinary mechanical tools. As a timed test, it provides information about an individual's performance in timed situations, and is useful for clients expressing an interest in mechanical areas.

The *Graves Design Judgment Test* was devised to measure "aptitude for the appreciation or production of art structure." While not the only measure used at the League with clients expressing an interest in the art field, it has the advantage of evaluating the degree to which an individual responds to the basic principles of esthetics. For clients considering an art career, this attribute is an important consideration in art-aptitude evaluation, which also includes the results of the Minnesota Paper Form-Board, an art portfolio, and, where possible, recommendations from art teachers.

5. Personality

In assessing personality, psychological tests are used in addition to information obtained from the case history, interview, and observation. The tests commonly administered are the *House-Tree-Person* and the *Rotter Sentence Completion Test*. The latter test also provides information about the person's communication patterns and linguistic skills. The *Thematic Apperception Test* may also be given, depending on the individual's expressive abilities. The *Vineland Social Maturity Scale* is used for information about outside activities and levels of social maturity and responsibility. However, questions need to be posed so that yes–no answers are avoided.

Interview

The information-targets of an interview vary with its purposes. These may involve intake, counseling, employment, diagnosis, therapy, and more. But whatever the target, the basic principles of interview techniques are as reviewed in chapter 10. The main differences are in the lines of inquiry followed.

The singular advantages of the interview have not been sufficiently exploited with the deaf. On the one hand, examiners unfamiliar with the group feel a natural reluctance to brave the communications obstacles that interviewing the deaf implies. And on the other, the deaf feel an equal reluctance to tell their stories to uneasy strangers. This is one of the reasons that psychological testing is so overemphasized with this population at the expense of interview.

The way out of the impasse lies in the willingness of interviewers to familiarize themselves with the communication patterns found among the deaf. As noted, for psychologists who habitually serve the deaf or who are planning to do so, knowledge of all communication methods used by this population is an essential competence. But this is too much to expect of workers who see only occasional deaf subjects. Nevertheless, the "occasional" subject must also be given a fair hearing.

The suggestions that follow are offered to facilitate the use of the interview technique with deaf persons, some of whom rely heavily on hearing aid support and others of whom do not. The major application of the technique is with adolescents and adults, since sufficient language for interview is generally found at these age levels.

Oral Interviews

Deaf adults who are expert in oral communication usually have good-to-superior verbal attainments and a broad range of communicative experiences with hearing persons. Sometimes their lipreading and language skills are so exceptional that the interviewer is apt to forget his remarks are not heard but are received visually. The strain on persons who have to *see* rather than hear a flow of conversation can be eased in various ways.

Interviewing lipreaders. Lipreaders may or may not wear hearing aids or benefit from amplified hearing. The following guides apply to both groups.

1. The interviewer and the deaf individual should be seated facing one another and not more than about 4 feet apart.

2. Light should come from behind the interviewee and be directed onto the interviewer's face. In this way, light glare into the eyes of the lipreader is avoided, and he is free to concentrate in comfort upon the speaker's face.

3. The interviewer's speech should be natural, simple, and clearly enunciated, using whatever modification in speed is necessary for clearest comprehension. This can be established through brief experimentation. The interviewer will usually find that his natural manner of speaking requires little if any alteration.

4. To be avoided: grimacing, mouthing, shouting, speaking without

voice, and marked slowdown in the delivery of speech. All of these tend to distort mouth movements.

5. Also to be avoided: talking and smoking or chewing at the same time; resting one's cheek on a hand; bending one's head, turning one's face away, and moving about while talking. All of these conceal or impair mouth movements, as do heavily moustached and bearded faces.

6. The interviewer should guard against fatigue on the part of a lipreader. A tired lipreader is not a successful one. When fatigue sets in, either pause for a rest or a coffee break, or suspend the session for another time unless the subject expressly wishes to continue, possibly in written or manual communication.

7. Watch the lipreader's face for signs of difficulty in comprehension. Puzzled expressions should be attended to immediately. Either the subject has not grasped a particular thought, or the vocabulary used has not been lipread successfully.

8. When difficulties in comprehension arise, clarification is made by rephrasing the concept or rewording the language into simpler and/or more visible forms *but never by continued repetition*. Sometimes key words, expressions, and proper names that are particularly difficult to see on the lips have to be written out.

9. When the interviewer is not sure an especially important line of thought has been clearly understood, it should be expressed in several different ways and then discussed with the subject and clarified further if necessary. An understanding of the single words of the vocabulary used does not guarantee that the whole idea has been grasped by the interviewee.

10. Pads and pencils should always be readily available, one set for the subject and another for the interviewer, with spare pencils in easy reach.

Interviewing hearing-aid wearers. Not all hearing-aid wearers are equally proficient hearing-aid users. Some are remarkable decoders of sounds heard through the aid, and synchronize what they hear through the aid with what they see on the lips to form consistently accurate reception. Others remain caught in the throes of trying to synchronize what they see with what they hear; and still others wear their hearing aids more to inform the public that they are hearing-impaired or because of a wish to please some favored individual than for any personal gains. Again, some brief experimentation will indicate the best communicative pattern to follow.

Generally speaking, the interview room for hearing-aid users should be a quiet one, with special precautions against sudden, loud noises such as telephone bells. Muted buzzers or light signals should be substituted wherever possible. To facilitate lipreading, all the suggestions previously noted should be observed. With very few exceptions, expert hearing-aid lipreaders prefer oral communication and writing. Some of their number who know sign language and who are in a tense emotional state sometimes drift into manual communication in the course of interview; it is less demanding. There are others who will have no part of manual communication. Again, brief experimentation is in order.

The interviewer's speech should be clear, distinct, and visible at all times, with the volume of voice maintained at a level of mutual comfort. The interviewee who uses his residual hearing can adjust the aid for optimal audibility; the one who does not will not benefit from shouted conversation.

For the subject who neither lipreads well nor derives much benefit from the hearing aid and who is not familiar with manual communication, writing will have to serve as the major means of communication, with the language geared to the subject's level of comprehension. Finally, for persons who rely heavily on the hearing aid but whose batteries suddenly go dead, a supply of extra batteries should be on hand.

With hearing-aid users as with the "non-amplified" lipreaders, the interviewer should be sensitive to signs of fatigue. Common signs are sudden difficulty in comprehension, excessive manipulation of volume controls, evidences of visual strain, restlessness, tense facial expression, and a general appearance of exhaustion. Interviews should not be prolonged to the point of fatigue. In the end, more time is saved by arranging for another session than by pushing beyond the limit of comfort.

Understanding the speech of deaf adults. In successful oral communication with deaf adults, one side of the coin represents the lipreader's ability to understand what the interviewer is saying; but the other side involves the interviewer's ability to understand what the subject is saying. As previously discussed, the tones and inflections of deaf voices and the manner and rhythm of utterance differ from nondeaf speech. In addition, there are individual variations, some of which are readily understood, but others of which present difficulty.

1. When difficulties are encountered, a helpful procedure is to let the deaf person talk uninterruptedly for a while to give the interviewer's ear a chance to become attuned to the particular tones and rhythms. If the interviewer experiences embarrassment listening to uncomprehended speech, or if the subject has little to say, it is often helpful to request him to read aloud on one pretext or another. Having a known verbal text to which to refer helps the listeners synchronize the sounds he hears with the printed words for which they stand. During this auditory adjustment period, the interviewer should not strain for precise comprehension but should instead open his ears to the general speech patterns until they finally set into recognizable verbal form.

2. If auditory comprehension is still not achieved, the interviewer himself will have to resort to lipreading, and watch the subject's mouth movements as carefully as his own are being watched by the subject. Whether aware of

it or not, most hearing persons use a certain amount of lipreading among themselves, especially city dwellers whose voices are often drowned in the hubbub of city noises.

3. When a deaf subject's speech still cannot be understood despite the use of lipreading combined with hearing, written or manual communication will have to be used, depending upon the wishes of the subject and the manual abilities of the interviewer.

4. Occasional difficulties arise even in the course of successful oral interviews. The interview should not be permitted to bog down on that account. A casual request to write out key words or expressions or to repeat is not taken amiss by deaf persons. Or the interviewer can ask "Tell me more about that," on the chance that comprehension will come in the course of spoken elaboration. It usually does. But on no account should an interviewer correct the speech of a deaf interviewee.

5. What might be considered a variation of the oral interview can be conducted in writing with nonoral subjects who are expert fingerspellers and proficient in linguistic usage. Words and sentences that would ordinarily be spoken are written instead. Of course, conducting an interview in writing can prove a cumbersome procedure, but it has been done. Interviewers in this situation develop a knack of reading upside-down, while the subject is doing the writing; and use a pad and pencil of their own to jot down questions or comments for the interviewee to read. After awhile, the process proceeds quite smoothly. Although this is not a desirable method, interviews conducted in written form have the advantage of providing unusual written records of verbatim conversation.

Manual Interviews

Manual interviews are conducted both with deaf persons who do not communicate readily through speech and lipreading and with many who do. In the latter case, manual conversation eases the strain of lipreading and talking in prolonged sessions. If the interviewer is himself a deaf person, it is the natural thing for an interview to proceed through manual communication. Also, in cases of emotional stress or disturbance, even proficient oralists sometimes prefer manual communication because it is less taxing. With expert deaf fingerspellers and nonexpert manual interviewers, the communicative situation can be managed through writing, as noted above. But whatever the situation, an interviewer specializing in manual deaf clients must possess communicative expertise in nonverbal patterns of communication—in sign language as well as in the "languages" of pantomime, facial expression, gesture, and body movement.

For nondeaf interviewers, the most challenging communicative situation arises where sign language is the interviewee's only expressive and receptive mode. To prepare for such situations, the interviewer must first learn the vocabulary of the sign language. This is the initial phase of preparation. The next phase involves acquiring expertise in ordering the signs according to the syntax of the language as it is habitually used by deaf adults. When the interviewer has achieved some mastery of vocabulary and syntax, the next and most difficult phase of the operation is acquiring expertise in "reading back" messages signed in a variety of ways by a variety of signers. But still the learning task is not completed. The culminating phase of an interviewer's skills lies in the ability to grasp fundamental meanings from the concepts being expressed by deaf signers, no matter how fractured the language or "off-beat" the concepts seem to be. This is another instance of the imperative to "know the deaf," and extends into an interviewer's ability to express himself in the same style as his subject and at the same conceptual level, or else to risk talking over the head of the interviewee.

Where manual expertise is lacking, an interpreter is called to the rescue.

Interpreted Interviews

To conduct an interview through a third person while at the same time striving for rapport with a deaf subject is not easy. It is particularly difficult when, as not infrequently happens, the interviewee comes accompanied by parents or other close relatives who feel it is their responsibility to function as interpreters. If the family members are hearing persons unskilled in manual methods, they usually carry out the role of interpreter by talking *about* rather than *for* the subject. In the end, more history data, personal views, and family anecdotes are obtained than interview information.

Even if the interviewer does succeed in making direct personal contact with the interviewee under these conditions, the latter generally finds it extremely uncomfortable to unburden himself before a family member. Relatives therefore should not be invited to be present during interviews. The major exceptions are relatives of uneducated deaf adults who have no conventional methods of communication and rely on homemade signs and pantomime that are only understood within the family.

It is, of course, entirely possible that a young deaf adult may prefer to have a parent or relative by his side; or there may be no other person available to serve as interpreter. The interviewer will have to manage as best he can until a qualified interpreter can be found; and, until then, count mainly on the testing sessions for more personal contact with the subject.

Where a choice of interpreters is possible, the subject's preferences should be consulted. Often deaf persons are as loath to unburden themselves before deaf interpreters as before members of their own families, or before hearing interpreters who are known to them. The deaf community itself resembles a kind of family, and complete confidentiality is not always possible. It is best, therefore, to ascertain whether the subject prefers a deaf or hearing person to act as interpreter; someone he knows, or a stranger. Finally, the subject should be assured of the confidentiality observed by the examiner and the qualified interpreter in all aspects of the psychological examination, including the interview.

Some further suggestions concerning the conduct of an interpreted interview are as follows:

1. The interviewer should make every reasonable effort to maintain the focus of interest on the subject and not on the interpreter. In interpreted interviews, there is always a danger of the interview becoming a conversation between the interviewer and the interpreter, with the subject left to play a subordinate background role. This must be guarded against, both to respect the subject's integrity as an individual, and to maintain his interest for future examination procedures.

2. Subject, interpreter, and interviewer should be seated within comfortable visual range of each other, but the subject should be seated nearer the interviewer to indicate to him that he is the focus of interest and the interviewer the figure of authority.

3. The interviewer should address himself directly to the subject even though it is the interpreter who is doing the understanding.

4. The interpreter should be given preliminary orientation as to the conduct of the interview, and should be instructed to wait until the interviewer completes his statements before attracting the interviewee's attention. When the interviewer completes his remarks, he turns to the interpreter as a signal to begin.

5. While the interviewer's remarks are being transposed into sign language, the interviewer should observe the facial expression and behavior of the subject to see how his remarks are being received and responded to.

6. If the interviewee's attention remains fixed on the interpreter for longer than necessary, he should be recalled by a light tap on the arm.

7. Both interviewer and interpreter must maintain control over their facial expressions at all times to avoid conveying false or disturbing impressions to the subject.

8. There should be no side conversations about the interviewee between interpreter and interviewer. The subject should be kept informed of whatever passes between them. If it is wiser that he not be informed, the discussion had best take place in his absence.

9. The interviewer must maintain friendly control over the proceedings at all times lest closer rapport develop between the subject and the interpreter than between the subject and the interviewer.

10. In selecting an interpreter, the safest course is to use the roster of

qualified interpreters in the regional offices of the Registry of Interpreters to the Deaf, and preferably to choose an interpreter with some training or experience in serving in psychological settings. Even with such an individual, it is the interviewer's responsibility to provide preliminary orientation to the task in hand. A postinterview discussion with an experienced interpreter can prove highly informative and rewarding to an uninitiated interviewer of deaf persons.

General Conduct of the Interview

Some procedures for the initial meeting between an examiner and a deaf client of unknown communicative habits have already been suggested. Where both are able to communicate satisfactorily, and greetings and introductions have been exchanged, the interviewer continues by asking, "How can I be of help to you?" in a sincerely interested manner. With deaf subjects a direct beginning is better than involved explanations about psychological examinations, for these are apt to be more confusing than enlightening to most deaf clients. In addition, the nature of the response to this direct lead provides clinically valuable information concerning the subject's insight into his own needs and problems. For example, if the presenting problem is chronic vocational failure, the response may be stated as "I need a job"; "I can't hold a job"; or "I am not happy with my work." Each of these tells something about the individual and his perception of his problem.

Whatever the answer, it creates a natural opportunity for the examiner to give some preliminary explanation of the procedures to come. Thus: "In order to give you the best help, I want to find out what kind of job you will be happiest and most successful with. To do this, I must know more about you. So we will talk together and do some tests. We call this 'guidance.' It is done all the time with hearing people as well as with deaf people. This is the way we fit the right person to the right job. Do you understand?"

Such explanations can of course be tailored to suit the subject's language and concept levels, his experiences and problems, and any answer he may have made to the lead question, even an "I don't know how you can help me." In the latter case, the need to "know more about you" is all the more important. It makes sense—and this is an important consideration in work with the deaf. Explanations and procedures that have common-sense appeal inspire confidence. Therefore, practical explanations should be given deaf adults in regard to every phase of the examination process.

At this point, the interviewer presents the client with the next lead opportunity, and that is to tell his story ("Tell me about yourself [or your problem]") in his own way. How the person responds to this invitation also tells a story. Among those who respond, some will present their problems as the result of their own deficiencies while others see their problems as due entirely to outside factors—a hostile world, treacherous friends, demanding relatives, etc. But not too many deaf persons will respond to the open invitation at a first meeting with a stranger. To those who live as highly structured an existence as do most deaf persons, the free field of an unstructured interview presents too wide an expanse and too few guides for comfort. At this early stage, the person is uneasy and shy; he does not know what to say or how to begin. And personal questions before the subject is ready for them may arouse more embarrassment and uneasiness than no interview structure at all.

As with deaf youths, the most practical course in these cases is to use some of the less complex psychological tests as ice-breakers. Achievement tests, figure drawings, and especially sentence completions can be used for the purpose. Once the ice is broken, the interview takes a conversational turn along the path indicated by its purpose and in the communicative/concept manner suited to the interviewee. Where personal problems are the targets of interview, some that are commonly presented by deaf adults involve work and work-related matters, marital adjustments, family management, sex performance and preferences. A helpful aid in interviews involving sexual behavior is Woodward's (1979) compilation of sex-related vocabularly in the American Sign Language. An even greater aid is the artless candor with which most deaf persons, once their confidence is won, discuss their problems and respond to questions involving even the most intimate of details. Some leading interview questions can be culled from the 280 statements in the *Handicap Problems Inventory* of Wright and Remmers, and from the *Bronfenbrenner Hearing Attitude Scale* in Appendix E.

A final note on interviewing deaf persons concerns the interviewer's behavior. As expressed by Betty C. Wright, "The deaf and the hard of hearing are very observant. (They have to be.) The way you stand or sit, the way you shrug your shoulders (perhaps in impatience), the way you walk from your desk to the door tell a great deal to the keen observer. Your manner, your poise, your smile, the expression in your eyes and on your face, the way you use your hands, all tell a story of indifference or understanding" (1956, p.19). In interviewing the deaf, the interviewer must be alert to the fact that he is as closely observed as observing; and because his *behavior* conveys a message on its own, it is essential that he guard against conveying false impressions or revealing through act or facial expression what had best remain concealed.

Observation

Just as an interviewer's behavior tells a story to a deaf client, so does a client's behavior tell a story to an interviewer. All the points noted by

Wright in regard to interviewers apply equally to interviewees; and many other points noted in the discussion of deaf youths apply equally to deaf adults. Behaviors indeed speak more loudly and often more truly than words and are great informers about moods, self-concept, attitudes, feelings, emotional disturbances, and more.

Regarding emotional disturbance, a checklist of observable signs is included in the case history inventory in Appendix F. More detailed listings have been compiled by Vernon (1969). By and large an examiner should expect to find no great differences in observable signs of serious psychopathy between the deaf and nondeaf. Readers with particular interest in mental illness and the deaf are referred to Robinson's excellent publication *Sound Minds in a Soundless World* (1978). Readers with special interest in studies of nonverbal behavior in psychopathological conditions are referred to the works of Ekman and Friesen (1974), Ruesch (1957), and Ostwald (1963, 1977).

Observation is also an increasingly favored technique in the vocational evaluation of deaf persons. Although the usual kit of vocational aptitude tests is still used, Pimentel (1967) complains that several of the tests are highly verbal and can only be used with verbally proficient deaf clients. He states further that none of the customarily used tests "is sufficiently specific to assist the deaf client in narrowing his occupational choices to one or two possibilities with any valid degree of confidence" and that "tests of vocational interest necessarily presuppose a level of occupational information which most young deaf adults do not possess unless they have been exposed to an effective formal guidance program on occupational information" (1967, pp. 26–27).

To bypass most of these difficulties, a more rewarding approach is observation of a client's performance in on-the-job situations. Through this "work-sample" method, an individual tries out a variety of miniature job replications that reproduce the important elements of the job itself, both as to skills and general situation. Among the areas open to observation in this approach are an individual's tolerance level to frustration and correction; enterprise and initiative; capacity for self-direction and assertion; dependence/independence ratio; and potentials for vocational advance. Pimentel (1967) reports that one such work-sample method, the Tower System, has demonstrated exceptional promise with deaf clients.

Although observed vocational aptitudes and abilities are rated by a vocational evaluator rather than a psychological examiner, informal observations of a subject's work behavior add to the findings obtained from the other psychological examination approaches, and whenever feasible should be included in an examiner's scope of inquiry. In general, acquiring a vocational skill presents no particular problems to deaf clients. Most are able to perform as well as or better than their hearing peers. The overriding vocational problems of the deaf are rooted in insufficient preparation for adjusting to the work culture and insufficient knowledge of the routines, practices, and procedures of the occupational world.

References

DiFrancesca, S. J., and Hurwitz, S. N. 1969. Rehabilitation of the hard core deaf: Identification of an affective style. *Journal of Rehabilitation of the Deaf*, 3: 34–41.

Donoghue, R., and Bolton, B. 1971. Psychological evaluation of deaf rehabilitation clients. *Journal of Rehabilitation of the Deaf*, 5: 29–37.

Ekman, P., and Friesen, W. V. 1974. Nonverbal behavior and psychopathology. In R. J. Friedman and M. M. Katz, eds., *The Psychology of Depression: Contemporary Theory and Research*. Washington, D.C.: Winston & Sons.

Falberg, R. M. 1974. Panelist on current developments in the psychological evaluation of deaf individuals. *Journal of Rehabilitation of the Deaf*, 8: 131–41.

Levine, E. S. 1956. *Youth in a Soundless World*. New York: New York University Press.

Levine, E. S. 1960. *The Psychology of Deafness*. New York: Columbia University Press.

McGowan, J. P., and Porter, T. L. 1967. *An Introduction to the Vocational Rehabilitation Process*. Washington, D.C.: U.S. Department of Health, Education, and Welfare.

Ostwald, P. 1963. *Soundmaking: The Acoustic Communication of Emotion*. Springfield, Ill.: Charles C. Thomas.

Ostwald, P., ed. 1977. *Communication and Social Interaction: Clinical and Therapeutic Aspects of Human Behavior*. New York: Grune & Stratton.

Pimentel, A. L. 1967. The Tower System as a vocational test for the deaf client. *Journal of Rehabilitation of the Deaf*, 1: 26–31.

Pinner, J. I. 1970. General employment: The responsibility of an employment interview. *Journal of Rehabilitation of the Deaf, Monograph No. 2*, pp. 43–56.

Randolph, A. H. 1978. The elements of the IWRP and the roles of an SCD. *Journal of Rehabilitation of the Deaf*, 12: 17–21.

Reports of Workshop Committees: First Institute for Special Workers for the Aural Disabled. 1950. Rehabilitation Service Series No. 120. Washington, D.C.: Office of Vocational Rehabilitation.

Robinson, L. 1978. *Sound Minds in a Soundless World*. U.S. Department of Health, Education, and Welfare Publication No. (ADM) 77-560. Washington, D.C.

Ross, D. R. 1970. A technique of verbal ability assessment of deaf people. *Journal of Rehabilitation of the Deaf*, 3: 7–15.

Ruesch, J. 1957. *Disturbed Communication*. New York: W. W. Norton.

Vernon, M. 1969. Techniques of screening for mental illness among deaf clients. *Journal of Rehabilitation of the Deaf*, 2: 23–36.

Walton, P. 1978. Communicating the Individual Written Rehabilitation Program to a deaf client. *Journal of Rehabilitation of the Deaf,* 12: 23–28.

Watson, D. 1977. *Deaf Evaluation and Adjustment Feasibility: Guidelines for the Vocational Evaluation of Deaf Clients.* Silver Spring, Md.: National Association of the Deaf.

Wechsler, D. 1944. *The Measurement of Adult Intelligence.* Baltimore: Williams & Wilkins Co.

Woodward, J. 1979. *Signs of Sexual Behavior: An Introduction to Some Sex-related Vocabulary in American Sign Language.* Silver Spring, Md.: T. J. Publishers.

Wright, B. C. 1956. *Orientation Training for Vocational Rehabilitation Counselors: A Syllabus on Special Problems of the Deaf and the Hard of Hearing for Orientation Institutes.* Washington, D.C.: American Hearing Society.

Wright, G. N., and Remmers, H. H. 1960. *The Handicap Problems Inventory.* Lafayette, Ind.: Purdue Research Foundation.

14 Psychological Reporting

THE FATE of many an individual rests with a psychological report. Striking evidence is surfacing in the wake of PL 94-142; and the importance of psychological reports, or more particularly the *trouble* with psychological reporting, is receiving unprecedented attention. Multidisciplinary polls held on the subject have disclosed a shattering number of deficiencies (Tallent, 1976). The major underlying theme is the failure of psychologists to transform an anonymous "case" into a particular human being. "All too often [psychologists] don't present a comprehensive picture of a unique individual," and "Very frequently, [the reports] are made up of too many stock phrases which do not give any feeling for the individual client" (Tallent, 1976, p. 37). As summarized by what Tallent describes as "one unhappy psychologist,"

> They [the reports] are
> Over-imaginative,
> Over-academic,
> Over-syllabic,
> And not over soon enough! (1976, p. 42)

Tallent also remarks that the term "gobbledygook" appears frequently and prominently in the polls.

Psychological reports fare no better in the judgment of multidisciplinary workers with the deaf. Participants at the Spartanburg Conference voiced sharp dissatisfaction with the manner and language in which reports are put together. To recapitulate: a common complaint was that instead of conveying a meaningful and usable message, many psychological reports do little more than present test results in technical jargon, almost as if psychologists are so preoccupied with testing that they cannot see the individual for the test scores. A strong Conference recommendation was that there should be more concern with the totality of the individual. Toward this end, psychological reports should be expressed in precise, concrete, practical terms; should be prescriptive in nature; and should reflect the psychological, social, medical, and educational background in relation to feasible, relevant recommendations. Or, as previously quoted from the remarks of one Conference participant, they should tell "where the client was; where he is; where he should be; and how to get him there." Equally stressed was the need to gear the language and concepts of the report to the understanding of the particular receiver, even though this might require composing reports in different narrative styles for different receivers.

The validity of the criticisms leveled against psychological reports cannot be denied. Yet a word of explanation is in order in behalf of psychologists to the deaf. It is obvious by now that communication is the major problem of early severe deafness. What is less obvious is that communication is also a major problem of team disciplines specializing in deafness. In fact, communication difficulties in deaf–hearing message exchange are often matched if not exceeded by communication difficulties in multidisciplinary message-exchange. Thus, psychologists on deafness rehabilitation teams are, more often than not, the frustrated receivers of cryptic, abbreviated "trade-language" input from other disciplines. This they are not only expected to decipher but even to interpret in terms of human implications. It is not surprising, therefore, to find gaps in psychological reports that can only be filled by meaningful communications from contributing disciplines. An imperative complement to "the trouble with psychological reporting" would be a poll among psychologists on "the trouble with medical, otological, neurological, audiological, and psychiatric reporting." Ideally such a poll should be followed by a concerted multidisciplinary effort toward meaningful intercommunication, in the service of the deaf victims of team bafflegab. Another handicap to good psychological reporting is the productivity demand under which psychologists to the deaf labor, in particular school psychologists. The need to grind out periodic I.Q.'s for mandated records on hundreds of deaf pupils generally precludes taking the time for painstaking examination, hence for gathering the data for good reports. These few observations should not be taken as an attempt to justify poor psychological reports. They are simply offered in partial explanation of why there are so many of them.

To compose a good psychological report is no simple matter. Among the major requirements are: (a) a sufficient body of psychological data on which to base the report; (b) the time necessary to digest the data and envisage the human counterpart; and (c) a report-writer with technical, organizational, and narrative flexibility as well as the ability to grasp what special information the referring agent needs to have in order to institute appropriate remediation.

Since psychological reports are prepared in many different settings and for many different purposes, there is no standard form to follow. However, the following general headings typify the content and organization customarily found in psychological reports. In regard to deaf subjects, a sample Psychological Report Form is presented in Appendix G.

Psychological Report Categories

1. Identifying Information

Included here is information involving such details as name, address, birth date, which serve to tell who the client is, his setting in time and place, and other related basic information.

2. Reason for Referral

This is a brief statement of the reason or problem that has led to a request for a psychological examination, together with the name and position of the referring agent and the date of referral. In the case of a "problem" referral, the statement should include a description of the presenting problem, and if feasible a quote from the referring individual. Where there is no problem, as in routine I.Q. testing, this should be noted.

3. Background

This section of a report summarizes previous examination findings, significant events in the individual's background, and serves as setting for the interpretation and evaluation of current findings.

4. Psychological Examination

The results of the current psychological examination are reported in this section. Psychological testing is recorded in terms of the category of behavior examined, the tests used (full names) in each category, and the findings obtained.

Each interpretation made for a respective behavior category should refer to the original test findings on which the interpretations are based.

Writing should be descriptive, technical concepts should be expressed in narrative language, and the reader should be given a clear picture of the individual behind the test findings in terms of potentials, abilities, behaviors, strengths, weaknesses, and special problems.

5. Examination Analysis

In this section, current examination findings are related to previous findings, and past and present life events; and a summation is made of the flow of behavior characterizing the individual. Such factors as discrepancies between past and present behaviors, seemingly ingrained traits, sharp behavior changes, pathological signs, signs of cerebral dysfunction, and other diagnostically important facts are specially noted.

6. Psychological Evaluation

This section summarizes the known facts about a client in biography-like narrative, including behavioral manifestations and associated psychological implications. For most report-readers, this is the section that "tells the story"; hence writing should be in an explanatory vein so that the reader can follow the reasoning that has gone into the writer's evaluation.

Except where especially called for, diagnostic labeling is best left out of Psychological Evaluation. Where an evaluation says all that needs to be said, there is no need to add a label, let alone to risk label-stigmatizing children. Generally a Diagnostic Impression suffices.

7. Recommendations

Specific procedural recommendations should only be made where the psychologist possesses special knowledge of or expertise in the area involved, such as education, vocational training, or psychotherapy. Otherwise, recommendations are best made in general, common-sense terms derived from psychological insights, and should leave the relevant procedural steps and strategies to the experts in the particular area.

Report Sample

Examples of various kinds of psychological report-writing can be found in Tallent (1976), and an excellent example of a Devereux Foundation report is in Copel (1967). The following excerpt from a psychological report on a deaf client to a vocational rehabilitation counselor illustrates the manner in which simple language can be used to convey pivotal planning guides:

Test Findings and Implications

While a Full Scale I.Q. rating of 114 on the Wechsler-Bellevue Scale suggests that R—— is a young man with High-Average to Superior intelligence, it would appear that the Performance I.Q. rating of 125 suggesting Superior mental ability is more accurately descriptive of him. R—— demonstrates exceptional skill in handling tasks requiring visual-motor organization and speed, seems readily able to size up and evaluate the motivations of people in different social situations, and also is extremely alert and sensitive to the finest detail in his environment. It is noted further that R—— has a well-developed fund of general information and demonstrates a capacity for good practical judgment. He tends to be somewhat limited in terms of the ability to conceptualize his thinking.

A reading test was given to determine whether R—— had sufficient reading skill for handling the various tests in this battery. The results indicate that he reads at a sixth-grade level and this seems sufficient for purposes of present testing. The chances are that he is capable of an even higher level of reading ability.

An evaluation was made of his arithmetic proficiency. The results indicate that his achievement in this area is at a seventh-grade level. This suggests that he is not strongly equipped for handling material requiring the use of complex numerical processes, although in comparison with his deaf peers he rates above average.

When compared with applicants for mechanic's helper jobs, R—— reveals a rather limited understanding of the mechanical principles involved in everyday situations. He does demonstrate rather well-developed ability to perceive spatial relations when compared with shopwork applicants.

An evaluation was made of his manipulative skills. In using one or both hands and a simple tool in the assembly of small parts, he demonstrates low average manipulative dexterity when compared with unselected male applicants. This also does not appear to be an optimal functioning.

The ACE Examination for College Freshmen was given to evaluate his college potential. While he is apparently limited from a quantitative standpoint, he nevertheless shows promising ability in this area. He seems particularly limited in linguistic skills when compared with college freshmen who are normally hearing.

In summary, the available data reveal that R—— is a seventeen-year-old boy of Superior intelligence. It is possible that he will be able to learn new and complex material quickly and retain such information with effectiveness. R—— seems to have sufficient reading skill for handling most types of paper work in a fairly satisfactory way. He does appear to have a problem with more advanced mathematics. At the same time, however, he is an exceptionally bright young man who is very quick to grasp instruction and who can probably profit enormously from remedial work in the basic skill subjects such as arithmetic and reading. It seems quite probable, particularly in view of his excellent intellectual equipment, that R—— will be able to adapt satisfactorily to Gallaudet College for the deaf, given sufficient preliminary tutoring in preparation.

The preceding illustrates a simple report-approach dealing with a limited line of inquiry. Other types of reports require conceptualization and expression in keeping with their purpose. For example, where reports are used as preparation for a diagnosis in the area of psychopathology, a tightly reasoned presentation is required in which items of evidence are presented step by step as they contribute to a final conclusion. In reports in which the focus is on the nature and significance of a symptom that needs to be analyzed and identified with some dynamic syndrome, a cause-and-effect type of presentation is useful (Tallent, 1976). In short, the manner of conceptualizing a report rests with the expertise of the writer in deciding how best to organize a precise but concise narrative about a center of inquiry while at the same time doing full justice to the human being behind the report.

References

Copel, S. L. 1967. *Psychodiagnostic Study of Children and Adolescents.* Springfield, Ill.: Charles C. Thomas.

Tallent, N. 1976. *Psychological Report Writing.* Englewood Cliffs, N.J.: Prentice-Hall.

A CONCLUDING COMMENT

A LAST GLANCE through the pages of this book as it goes to press shows that a substantial portion has been given over to guides for the psychological examination of deaf subjects. Although there is no question about the urgent need for this kind of information, it must be strongly re-emphasized that quality psychological practices with a deaf clientele are more heavily dependent on understanding the ways in which deaf environments fashion their human occupants than on knowledge of psychological tests and measures. Of course knowing the techniques of psychological examination is important, but such knowledge can be acquired through class instruction, demonstration, and texts on the subject. However, knowledge about inhabitants of a "soundless world" cannot be acquired simply by reading about them or exposing them to psychological examination. It comes with getting to know them as human beings rather than as topics in a book of subjects of research. A major effort of this particular book has been to contrive guides toward this end and to challenge the reader's imagination and judgment.

In trying to accomplish this purpose, I did what I usually do when writing about the deaf, and that is pray for the explanatory force and magic phrases that will hopefully transform the deaf experience into a vicarious equivalent that would fire the understanding of nondeaf readers. In addition, I have placed major emphasis upon a perspective that I believe holds exceptional explanatory promise, namely the environmental perspective. I have placed equal explanatory values upon personal communications from the deaf professional contributors who appear in this book—Robert Donoghue, Max and Frances Friedman, Martin L. A. Sternberg, and the poet Naomi Leeds, who graciously permits me to use her poem on "eyes that hear" (see page 161) whenever I need to inject some beauty into an otherwise tedious narrative; and from the anonymous deaf contributors—rehabilitation clients (among whom Roberto is my special delight), psychological subjects, and deaf pupils, all of whom provide anecdotal illustrations of one kind or other to various points of discussion. To my nondeaf personal-communicants—Ruth R. Green, Frances Santore, Elizabeth Ying, and Nina Hertz—I give special thanks for enriching this book with summaries of their special programs. Finally, I remind my readers of the historic roots of many of the ideas considered to be "new" and of the special genius of their innovative forbears.

The reader may wonder why these acknowledgments come at the end of the book instead of, as is customary, at the beginning. It is because I believe that the readers of this book in particular need to know *what* the contributions are that the author is grateful for, not only the names of a few of the contributors; there are so many who are anonymous. Hence, we read *first*, and then give *insightful* thanks.

The one exception to this order concerns the two distinguished deaf professional persons who have honored me with the Epilogue to this book —Barbara A. Brauer and Allen E. Sussman. It is eminently fitting that this "last word" be said by persons who have themselves lived the deaf experience.

EPILOGUE

A LLEN E. S USSMAN AND B ARBARA A. B RAUER

T HE MESSAGE in Dr. Levine's book comes at a most opportune time. The past decade has witnessed an increasing and overdue protest by physically disabled people regarding their treatment in a denigrating and indifferent human environment. As expressed during several epoch-making legislative events of the decade (such as Public Law 94-142, Section 504 of the Rehabilitation Amendments of 1973, the White House Conference on Handicapped Individuals, and the President's Commission on Mental Health), the insistence, demands, recommendations, and pleadings of physically disabled individuals and groups still await action.

That psychology has begun to use this environmental orientation in studying the relations between environmental deficits and accompanying deficits in deaf persons is evident in the publication of this book. The efforts of the Spartanburg conference of 1975, called by Dr. Levine to set guidelines and standards for the provision of psychological service to deaf persons, are producing hoped-for results. In particular, the establishment of the Task Force on Psychology and the Physically Handicapped, under the auspices of the American Psychological Association's Board of Social and Ethical Responsibility for Psychology, holds great promise for furthering Dr. Levine's pioneering work.

Dr. Levine's earlier benchmark book, *The Psychology of Deafness,* dealt with the psychosocial aspects of deafness through a humanistic approach. The deaf individual was not impersonally presented as a statistic, nor portrayed as a population stereotype, nor viewed through an amalgam of diagnostic classifications and labels. In this book Dr. Levine continues to present the deaf as living, thinking, perceiving, and experiencing individuals with the same capacity to feel as their fellow human beings who hear. Moreover, she emphasizes a crucial concept—that hearing persons would be much like their deaf peers if reared in a similar silent environment.

The underlying message is that environmental conditions can be greater handicapping factors than is the disability of hearing loss per se. Inability to recognize this fact has resulted in continuing denigration for deaf persons, and daily insults, both large and small. They and not the environments in which they are reared are held responsible for their deficiencies. What is more, the biases accompanying this viewpoint continue to hamper realization of the full potential of deaf individuals and to deprive them of opportunities to participate fully in society.

It is time to place the blame where it belongs—on the fashioning forces in the deaf individual's environment that shape the person for better or worse. It is time to analyze these forces objectively and painstaking; for, as Dr. Levine maintains, to truly understand deaf individuals, it is first necessary to know and understand their shaping environments and to perceive how deficits in the environment manifest themselves in the deaf individual.

By shifting from deficits in the individual to deficits in the environment, this book provides a refreshing and daring perspective for workers with the deaf. We see it as a precursor of further written works and research on deafness with an environmental orientation and more specific attention to those sociocultural components that enhance or impair the psychological integrity of deaf persons. Such writings and research should be targeted to family, including parents and siblings, to school, teachers, peers, community; and should focus on the significance of communicative modes and how they affect deaf people, with special attention to educational approaches, communication philosophies, rehabilitation services, preventive and interventive mental health methods, and psychological procedures. If prevention is to be part of a unified and rational psychological approach to problems of the deaf, then measures to improve the life environment of the deaf population are a crucial necessity. This book leads the way by exposing conflicting issues and discordant options in the rearing-environments of deaf children in relation to the human outcomes.

We look forward to research dealing with the identification, assessment, and amelioration if not elimination of environmental forces inimical to the psychosocial integrity of deaf persons. By the same token, we look forward to research and other strategies for disclosing the influences that are *conducive* to the development of psychologically healthy and socially effective deaf individuals. There are many such persons, and yet they are a comparatively unknown group to research. We are in urgent need of models of health, psychological integrity, and social effectiveness from within the highly heterogeneous deaf population, a population that is customarily viewed through the prism of psychopathology. Observers seldom realize that the view is more likely that of the milieu than the person.

We have much to learn about what makes psychologically healthy and socially effective deaf individuals as well as how to assess not only their weaknesses but more particularly their considerable strengths and compensatory skills. We need to study their survival strategies and to pass this body of knowledge and insights on to parents, family members, and professional people, all of whom remain inherently and inextricably a part of the "deaf" environment. Finally we—the writers of this epilogue—as deaf persons ourselves and as psychologists, would like to see the environmental orientation of this book be made a realistic and integral part of all training and professional preparation programs in the field of deafness, the better to understand the needs, problems, and psychological fashioning of people who are deaf.

APPENDIXES

APPENDIX A
The Human Ear and Hearing

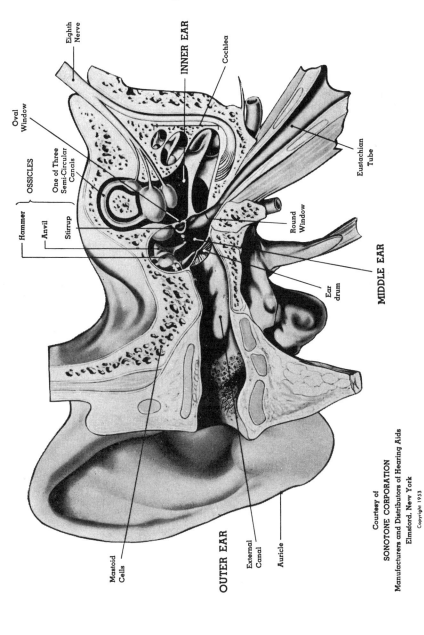

Figure A.1. Sectional diagram of the human ear.

Courtesy of
SONOTONE CORPORATION
Manufacturers and Distributors of Hearing Aids
Elmsford, New York
Copyright 1953

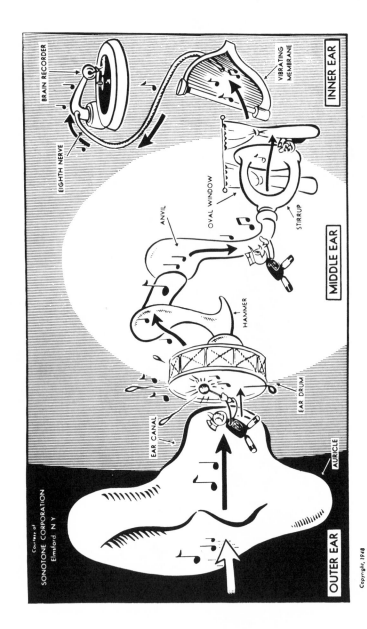

Figure A.2. Diagram of how we hear.

APPENDIX B

Types and Causes of Impaired Hearing

1. Conduction Deafness
   a. Inflammation in the middle ear (otitis media)
   b. Infection and blocking of the Eustachian tubes, commonly caused by adenoid tissue
   c. Damaged (perforated, scarred) ear drum
   d. Obstruction of the outer ear canal, commonly caused by wax
   e. Otosclerosis, which also involves the inner ear in severe cases and is associated with hereditary factors
2. Perception Deafness
   a. Hereditary deafness: genetic factors
   b. Acquired deafness
      (1) Deafness acquired prenatally
         (a) Diseases in the mother during early pregnancy, such as German measles (rubella), mumps, influenza
         (b) Rh blood factor
         (c) Certain drugs taken by the mother during pregnancy, such as quinine
         (d) Pathological condition of the fetus, such as erythroblastosis fetalis
         (e) Developmental anomalies
         (f) Maternal syphilis
      (2) Deafness acquired at birth
         (a) Anoxia
         (b) Traumatic injuries
         (c) Prematurity
      (3) Later acquired deafness
         (a) Infectious diseases, such as meningitis, mumps, measles (morbilli), whooping-cough, scarlet fever

    (b) Hyperpyrexia, especially in childhood
    (c) Various drugs, such as dihydrostreptomycin and quinine
    (d) Noise and blast deafness
    (e) "Dropsy" of some of the tissues of the inner ear, commonly referred to as Ménière's disease
    (f) Avitaminosis, arteriosclerosis, allergy
    (g) Old age

3. Mixed Deafness
    A number of the foregoing conditions, if severe, can cause both perception and conduction deafness.

4. Central Deafness
    a. Acoustic tumors
    b. Certain types of brain damage caused by such conditions as cerebral hemorrhage, multiple sclerosis, syphilis, and abscess, affecting the auditory pathways from the auditory nerve through the brain to the outer temporal lobe
    c. Developmental anomalies affecting these areas

5. Functional and Psychogenic Deafness, and Malingering
    Personality weaknesses and disorders with or without organic impairment of the auditory mechanism, usually associated with neuroses and conscious or unconscious secondary gains phenomena

NOTE: Two types of deafness, *congenital* and *adventitious,* are commonly mentioned in the literature. Neither refers to cause, only to time. A congenital defect is one that is present at birth; an adventitious defect is one that is acquired (or appears) any time after birth. Closely related to congenital deafness in terms of psychosocial, educational, and adjustment problems is prelinguistic deafness (also termed prelingual deafness) which designates a condition of severe hearing loss that is present before the acquisition of speech and language by young children.

APPENDIX C
Manual Methods of
Communication

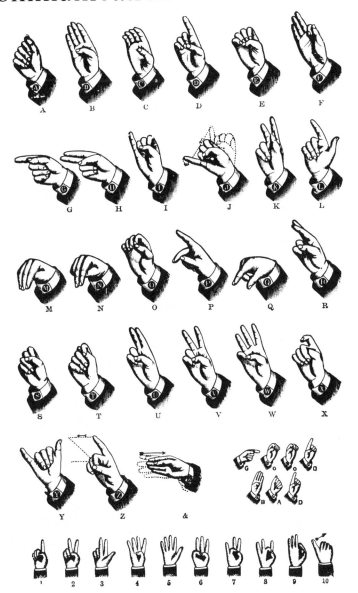

Figure A.3. One-hand manual alphabet.

Photos by Norman W. Crane; posed by Dorothy Kraft, of the Lexington School for the Deaf

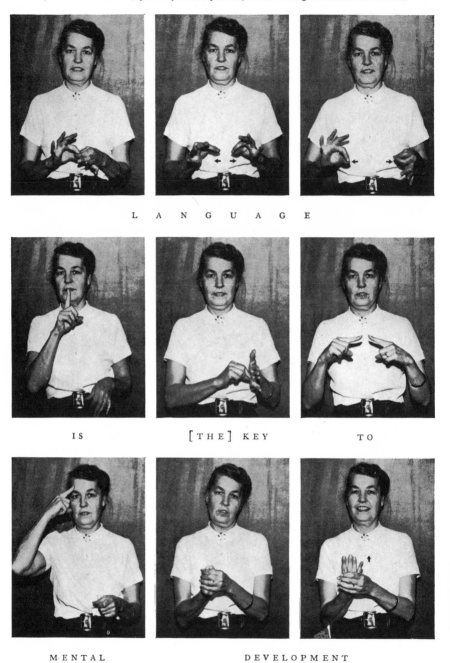

L A N G U A G E

I S   [T H E] K E Y   T O

M E N T A L   D E V E L O P M E N T

Figure A.4. A sentence in Ameslan, "Language is the key to mental development."

APPENDIX D

Experimental Interpreter-Rating Form

This is an experimental evaluation form devised by the writer and associates for the rating of interpreters to the deaf. It is presented here to give the reader an idea of what factors are involved in assessing interpreter competence.

I. FINGERSPELLING
  A. Clarity   ___ 1. Very Good
                      ___ 2. Good
                      ___ 3. Average
                      ___ 4. Fair
                      ___ 5. Poor   ___ stiff fingers
                                       ___ fingers too relaxed
                                       ___ "slurs" words
                                       ___ other (please state)

  B. Hand Position   ___ 1. Very Good
                      ___ 2. Good
                      ___ 3. Average
                      ___ 4. Fair
                      ___ 5. Poor   ___ moves in "typewriter" fashion
                                       ___ too close to face
                                       ___ too far from body
                                       ___ other (please state)

C. Facial Factor
(mouth move-
ments)   ___ 1. Very Good
        ___ 2. Good
        ___ 3. Average
        ___ 4. Fair
        ___ 5. Poor   ___ exaggerated
                  ___ no mouth movements
                  ___ not synonymous with finger-
                      spelling
                  ___ other (please state)

II. SIGNS
  A. Sign Positions   ___ 1. Very Good
            ___ 2. Good
            ___ 3. Average
            ___ 4. Fair
            ___ 5. Poor   ___ too close to body
                      ___ too high
                      ___ too far forward
                      ___ obscures facial movements,
                        especially lips
                      ___ other (please state)

  B. Size of Signs   ___ 1. Very Good
            ___ 2. Good
            ___ 3. Average
            ___ 4. Fair
            ___ 5. Poor   ___ too large
                      ___ too small
                      ___ inconsistent (size of sign var-
                        ies)
                      ___ other (please state)

  C. Clarity of Signs   ___ 1. Very Good
            ___ 2. Good
            ___ 3. Average
            ___ 4. Fair
            ___ 5. Poor   ___ jerky movements, not fluid
                      ___ hesitancy, changing signs
                        halfway through
                      ___ other (please state)

D. Rate of Signing   ___1. Very Good
  ___2. Good
  ___3. Average
  ___4. Fair
  ___5. Poor   ___ too slow
                      ___ fast enough, but skips over
                         material
                      ___ other (please state)

E. Familiarity with
   Sign Vocabulary
                ___1. Very Good (quite familiar & comfortable using
                     signs)
                ___2. Good (somewhat uncomfortable with signs,
                     but communicates adequately)
                ___3. Average
                ___4. Fair
                ___5. Poor (needs more familiarity with signs)

F. Punctuation   ___1. Very Good
  ___2. Good
  ___3. Average
  ___4. Fair
  ___5. Poor   ___ no break in signing for
                       punctuation
                      ___ sporadic punctuation
                       (sometimes punctuates,
                       sometimes not)

III. FACIAL FACTORS
  A. Facial Expression ___1. Very Good
                  ___2. Good
                  ___3. Average
                  ___4. Fair
                  ___5. Poor   ___ expressionless
                                  ___ overly expressive
                                  ___ no eye contact with audience
                                  ___ expressions not synonymous
                                      with speaker's message
                                ___ other (please state)

B. Lip Movements   ___ 1. Very Good
                     ___ 2. Good
                     ___ 3. Average
                     ___ 4. Fair
                     ___ 5. Poor   ___ none
                                         ___ sporadic
                                         ___ exaggerated
                                         ___ not synonymous with signs
                                         ___ other (please state)

IV. BODY FACTORS
    A. Posture   ___ 1. Very Good
                     ___ 2. Good
                     ___ 3. Average
                     ___ 4. Fair
                     ___ 5. Poor   ___ too tense
                                         ___ too relaxed
                                         ___ slouched
                                         ___ unnatural
                                         ___ other (please state)

    B. Body Movements ___ 1. Very Good
                         ___ 2. Good
                         ___ 3. Average
                         ___ 4. Fair
                         ___ 5. Poor   ___ too many (overexaggeration)
                                         ___ too few (stiff)
                                         ___ other (please state)

V. APPEARANCE (dress)
                     ___ 1. Very Good
                     ___ 2. Good
                     ___ 3. Average
                     ___ 4. Fair
                     ___ 5. Poor

Explain: _____

VI. LEVEL OF INTERPRETATION
___ 1. Very Good (appropriate for the audience)
___ 2. Good
___ 3. Average
___ 4. Fair
___ 5. Poor   ___ too intellectual
                     ___ too low-level (low verbal)
                     ___ omission of material consid-
                         ered relevant
                     ___ other (please state)

VII. CONCEPT PRESENTATION
___ 1. Very Good (speaker's concepts are communi-
        cated in excellent fashion)
___ 2. Good (speaker's concepts are adequately
        communicated)
___ 3. Average (not all speaker's concepts are
        communicated, but majority are)
___ 4. Fair (many concepts are not adequately com-
        municated, but speaker is understood)
___ 5. Poor (concepts are not adequately communi-
        cated)

VIII. REVERSE COMMUNICATION SKILLS
A. Ability to read fingerspelling   ___ 1. Very Good
                                           ___ 2. Good
                                           ___ 3. Average
                                           ___ 4. Fair
                                           ___ 5. Poor

B. Ability to comprehend the sign language ___ 1. Very Good
                                            ___ 2. Good
                                            ___ 3. Average
                                            ___ 4. Fair
                                            ___ 5. Poor

C. Ability to interpret the sign language
   verbally for a hearing person   ___ 1. Very Good
                                            ___ 2. Good
                                            ___ 3. Average
                                            ___ 4. Fair
                                            ___ 5. Poor

APPENDIX E

Bronfenbrenner
Hearing Attitude Scale

The following Scale, taken from an unpublished study, "The Psychological Program in the Army Hearing Center at Boston General Hospital," conducted by Urie Bronfenbrenner in the 1940s, was originally devised for the hard of hearing. Scoring and scoring data are not available. However, it is presented here since it is a rare contribution to the study of impaired hearing, and can be selectively adapted to deaf clients as a springboard for interviewing or for an adjustment inventory standardized on the deaf.

1. Being hard of hearing keeps me from doing many of the things I like to do. *Agree Disagree*

2. Since I became hard of hearing, things don't interest me as much as they used to. *Agree Disagree*

3. Other people may become annoyed at being asked to repeat. *Agree Disagree*

4. The strain of trying to hear makes me sweat. *Agree Disagree*

5. The only time I would be willing to wear a hearing aid would be when I am among people who know me well. *Agree Disagree*

6. Being hard of hearing would stop me from taking a job where I have to be the boss. *Agree Disagree*

7. Because of my hearing, people have been unfair to me. *Agree Disagree*

8. When I meet other people I do all the talking so I don't have to listen. *Agree Disagree*

9. Even though I am hard of hearing, I can go to a party and have a good time. *Agree Disagree*

10. Only people who are hard of hearing can help me with my problem. *Agree Disagree*

11. Being hard of hearing is worse than any other handicap. *Agree Disagree*

12. Being hard of hearing gives me the blues. *Agree Disagree*

13. Because I'm hard of hearing some employers may not want to hire me. *Agree Disagree*

14. Because I am hard of hearing, I'm always worried. *Agree Disagree*

15. I don't think I can learn to read lips. *Agree Disagree*

16. Because I am hard of hearing, the only kind of work I can do is common labor. *Agree Disagree*

17. Because I'm hard of hearing, people turn against me. *Agree Disagree*

18. I would rather not know what is going on than admit that I am hard of hearing. *Agree Disagree*

19. Being hard of hearing keeps me from going out in public. *Agree Disagree*

20. Because of my hearing, I have trouble remembering things. *Agree Disagree*

21. I let my hearing trouble get the best of me. *Agree Disagree*

22. Because I am hard of hearing I'm no good to anybody. *Agree Disagree*

23. Being hard of hearing never embarrasses me. *Agree Disagree*

24. Being hard of hearing makes me jumpy. *Agree Disagree*

25. I cannot get along without a hearing aid. *Agree Disagree*

26. If the boss finds out I am hard of hearing I won't be able to hold my job. *Agree Disagree*

27. Because I'm hard of hearing, people stare at me all the time. *Agree Disagree*

28. When I apply for a job, I shall try to hide the fact that I am hard of hearing. *Agree Disagree*

29. Being hard of hearing makes me stay away from my friends. *Agree Disagree*

30. Because I'm hard of hearing, I have a right to feel sorry for myself. *Agree Disagree*

31. Being hard of hearing won't stop me from having a happy family life. *Agree Disagree*

32. If my hearing stays that way life won't be worth living.   *Agree Disagree*

33. A hearing loss is no problem to me.   *Agree Disagree*

34. Being hard of hearing makes me nervous.   *Agree Disagree*

35. I want to learn lip reading.   *Agree Disagree*

36. Because I am hard of hearing, it will be very hard for me to get any kind of a job.   *Agree Disagree*

37. Because I'm hard of hearing, I always get into trouble.   *Agree Disagree*

38. It is hard for me to tell others about my hearing trouble.   *Agree Disagree*

39. As long as I'm hard of hearing, I can't be popular with people.   *Agree Disagree*

40. Nobody has any business telling me how to handle my hearing problem.   *Agree Disagree*

41. If my hearing gets worse I won't be able to take it.   *Agree Disagree*

42. I drink to forget I am hard of hearing.   *Agree Disagree*

43. I think a hard-of-hearing person is bound to make mistakes once in a while.   *Agree Disagree*

44. Being hard of hearing is driving me crazy.   *Agree Disagree*

45. Wearing a hearing aid in public would bother me.   *Agree Disagree*

46. Because I am hard of hearing, I can never get a job that pays good money.   *Agree Disagree*

47. I can't stand having people ask me questions about my hearing.   *Agree Disagree*

48. When people ask me if I am hard of hearing I'd rather not answer.   *Agree Disagree*

49. Because I'm hard of hearing, I stay off by myself.   *Agree Disagree*

50. My hearing gets worse when I am worried.   *Agree Disagree*

51. Being hard of hearing doesn't stop me from living a pretty normal life.   *Agree Disagree*

52. Being hard of hearing makes me feel like crying.   *Agree Disagree*

53. There are some kinds of jobs that a person with good hearing can do better than I can.   *Agree Disagree*

54. Being hard of hearing gets me all tired out.   *Agree Disagree*

55. I don't need anything this hospital can give me.   *Agree Disagree*

56. I may be able to hold my job, but my hearing will keep me from getting ahead.   *Agree Disagree*

57. Being hard of hearing makes me bashful.   *Agree Disagree*

58. I don't think it is fair to have my hearing tested when I apply for a job. *Agree Disagree*

59. Because I'm hard of hearing, I don't go to parties. *Agree Disagree*

60. My hearing changes from day to day. *Agree Disagree*

61. I am hard of hearing, but I still have confidence in myself. *Agree Disagree*

62. Because I am hard of hearing, I don't have any pep. *Agree Disagree*

63. Because other people don't know how loud to talk to me, I may embarrass them once in a while. *Agree Disagree*

64. Because I am hard of hearing, I can't keep my mind on what I'm doing. *Agree Disagree*

65. I won't wear a hearing aid under any conditions. *Agree Disagree*

66. Even though I'm hard of hearing, there is still some kind of work I can do. *Agree Disagree*

67. I can't stand having people kid me about my hearing. *Agree Disagree*

68. When I don't hear what a person is saying I just let it go. *Agree Disagree*

69. Because I'm hard of hearing, I never speak to strangers. *Agree Disagree*

70. Because of my hearing trouble, I don't like people. *Agree Disagree*

71. I have learned how to get along with my hearing trouble. *Agree Disagree*

72. As long as my hearing stays this way I can't be happy. *Agree Disagree*

73. Because I don't always hear what people say, they may lose patience with me once in a while. *Agree Disagree*

74. Being hard of hearing makes me so mad I feel like smashing things. *Agree Disagree*

75. I don't want to go to any hearing classes. *Agree Disagree*

76. Because I am hard of hearing, I won't be able to make a living. *Agree Disagree*

77. Because I'm hard of hearing, I am ashamed to go home to my family. *Agree Disagree*

78. I sometimes make out that my hearing is better than it really is. *Agree Disagree*

79. Because I'm hard of hearing, I don't like to meet new people. *Agree Disagree*

80. I don't care if my hearing does get worse.   *Agree   Disagree*

81. Being hard of hearing has made a completely different person out of me.   *Agree   Disagree*

82. Being hard of hearing makes me feel sad most of the time.   *Agree   Disagree*

83. In applying for most jobs, a person with good hearing has a better chance than I have.   *Agree   Disagree*

84. Because I'm hard of hearing, people get on my nerves.   *Agree   Disagree*

85. If I need a hearing aid, I'll wear it.   *Agree   Disagree*

86. Because I'm hard of hearing, my family will have to support me.   *Agree   Disagree*

87. Everybody makes fun of me because of my hearing.   *Agree   Disagree*

88. When I don't hear what a person has said, I often ask him to say it again.   *Agree   Disagree*

89. Because I'm hard of hearing, I sometimes avoid talking with people.   *Agree   Disagree*

90. I'm glad I'm hard of hearing.   *Agree   Disagree*

91. Being hard of hearing is like having two strikes against you.   *Agree   Disagree*

92. Being hard of hearing makes me feel like giving up sometimes.   *Agree   Disagree*

93. As far as I am concerned none of these questions are worth bothering about.   *Agree   Disagree*

94. I lie awake nights worrying about my hearing trouble.   *Agree   Disagree*

95. I can't stand having doctors look at my ears.   *Agree   Disagree*

96. The only job I can take is one where I can work alone.   *Agree   Disagree*

97. Because of my hearing, nobody wants me around.   *Agree   Disagree*

98. Only my friends should be told that I'm hard of hearing.   *Agree   Disagree*

99. Because I'm hard of hearing, I want to live off by myself.   *Agree   Disagree*

100. I hope my hearing gets better.   *Agree   Disagree*

APPENDIX F

Inventory Guide for Case History Information on Deaf Children and Adults

The outline that follows is not intended for use in routine case-history intake. It is rather an inventory of the kinds of information found useful in the case histories of deaf subjects under diagnostic evaluation. The inventory categories covered in actual history-taking naturally depend upon the age of the subject as well as the information requirements in a given case.

I. INTRODUCTORY DATA

Case no.
Name   Sex
Locating addresses:
   Home   Phone
   School   Phone
   Business   Phone
Birthdate   Birthplace
Ethnic/religious data
Deaf since (age)
Preferred communication method(s)
Deafness in family (specify)

II. PRESENTING PROBLEM

Referred by   Date

Statement of presenting problem

Previous psychologic/psychiatric examinations (date, name of examiner, diagnostic impression, remediations instituted, therapeutic benefits)

III. FAMILY BACKGROUND

A. Direct family line (list information concerning father, mother, full and half siblings, maternal and paternal grandparents under the headings: Name; Age or Birth Date: If Deceased, Cause and Age; Household Member; Education; Occupation; Hearing, Deaf, or Hard of Hearing with Age of Onset; Other Disability)

B. Collateral family line (list foregoing information concerning uncles, aunts, cousins, with close personal relationship to subject and/or with physical or mental disabilities)

C. Parents (See also IIIA.)
   1. Address(es)
   2. Birthplace
   3. In this country since
   4. Date married
   5. Age at birth of subject
   6. Consanguinity
   7. Marital status/compatability

D. Family home and neighborhood
   1. Address(es)
   2. Language(s) spoken in home (including sign language)
   3. Socioeconomic, physical, cultural surroundings

E. Subject's home and neighborhood (if other than D.)
   1. Address
   2. Other occupants (specify)
   3. Socioeconomic, physical, cultural surroundings
Informant(s)

IV. DEVELOPMENTAL HISTORY

A. Prenatal
   1. Parents' attitudes toward pregnancy
   2. Maternal condition during pregnancy: physical   emotional rH factor   injuries/accidents   virus infection (month of pregnancy)   attempts at abortion   other
   3. Attending physician (name, address)
Informant(s)

B. Birth Events
   1. Birthplace
   2. Term   birthweight   labor   delivery   mother's condi-
      tion
   3. Condition of child: normal   resuscitation   jaundice
      cyanosis injuries   prematurity   incubator   malforma-
      tions   congenital abnormalities/anomalies
   4. Attending physician; midwife; other (name, address)
Informant(s)
C. Schedule of infant development (digest of developmental examination)
   1. Motor behavior
   2. Adaptive behavior
   3. Communicative/language behavior
   4. Personal-social behavior
   5. Sensory-perceptual acuities
   6. Orientation to environment
   7. Behavior and physical growth deviations
Examiner   Date
Developmental scale used
Attending physician/pediatrician (name, address)

V. MEDICAL AND HEALTH RECORD

A. General health (date and findings of last physical examination; name
   and address of examining physician)

B. Chronological account of important persistent illnesses, major in-
   juries/accidents, operations, etc., noting especially convulsive disorders, hyperpyrexia, allergies, otological conditions and infections,
   and contagious diseases, noting: Medical Condition; Age of Subject;
   Length of Illness; Treatment; Outcome; Attending physician(s) by
   names and addresses

C. Physical, mental, neurological dysfunctions, and sensory disabilities
   (especially visual) not previously mentioned, noting: Disability; Severity; Age of Onset; Treatment; Outcome; Attending Physician(s) by
   names and addresses

D. List other physical complaints and treatments

VI. AUDITORY HISTORY

A. Discovery of impaired hearing
   1. Age "something wrong" observed
   2. Signs involved
   3. By whom observed

B. Chronological record of diagnostic and treatment experiences and recommendations, noting: Stated Diagnosis; Diagnostician (name, address); Age of Subject; Recommendations Made; Recommendations Carried Out; Outcomes

C. Age of subject when authentic diagnosis was "accepted" by parents

D. Reactions of parents during diagnostic search and to authentic diagnosis

E. Behavioral reactions, patterns, changes in subject during same period

F. Nature of auditory impairment and amount of hearing loss
   1. Otologist's report
   2. Audiologist's report

G. Accompanying involvements: balance impairment   recruitment brain damage   vertigo   tinnitus   psychogenic involvements other

H. Remedial measures
   1. Hearing aid: worn since age   acoustic benefits   subject's acceptance   fitted by (name, address)
   2. Auditory training: since age   benefits conducted by (name(s), addresses)
   3. Special tutoring: speech   lipreading proficiency   conducted by (name, address)
   4. Other:

I. Intrafamily attitudes
Informant(s)

VII. EDUCATIONAL BACKGROUND

A. Infancy and preschool (noting: Name and Address of Facility, i.e., Infant Program, School, Clinic or Hearing Rehabilitation Center, Tutor, Correspondence Course; Type of Instruction; Method of Communication; Day or Residential Placement; If Residential, How Often Home/Visited; Child Adjustments/Problems; Dates Attended; If Changed, Why? General Evaluation of Program)
Informant(s)

B. Schooling (chronology of schools attended, including "outside" tutoring, high school, college, university under the headings used in section VIIA and including degrees earned at college and university levels)

C. Scholastic preferences and class ratings (for achievement test results, see section XIV, Psychological Evaluations)
   1. Best-liked subjects

   2. Least-liked subjects
   3. Highest class grades in
   4. Lowest class grades in
   5. Degrees earned in (specialty)
   6. General school rating: superior   average   poor   failing
D. Scholastic goals
   1. Of subject
   2. Of parents
E. Favored extracurricular activities
Informant(s)

VIII. PSYCHOSOCIAL CHILDHOOD PROFILE

A. Childhood (preschool to puberty) reaction-patterns
   1. Subject's general temperament and emotional pattern
   2. Adjustment to new/unusual events (noting child's age), such as onset of deafness, beginning school, change of schools, change in residence, change in guardianship, broken home, death in family
   3. Parent-subject-sibling relations pre- and post-disability
   4. Recreational interests and activities
   5. Religious training and observances
   6. Sex instruction: by whom   age of subject   reaction
   7. Major "authority" figure(s) in subject's childhood
Informant(s)
B. Summary of habit patterns and problems

	Pattern	If Problem, Since When	Management
General disposition			
Eating			
Motor			
Sensory			
Elimination			
Sleep			
Socialization			
Adaptability			
Learning ability			
Communication			
Independent activity			
General health			
Physical development			
Sex interests			
Other			

Informant(s)

C. Checklist of childhood behavior and conduct disorder-signs
Nail biting
Thumb sucking
Food faddisms
"Psychological" vomiting
Eneuresis
Pronounced disobedience
Persistent night terrors
Habitual temper tantrums
Stealing
Abnormal aggressiveness
Setting fires
Truancy
Other
Informant(s)

IX. VOCATIONAL AND OCCUPATIONAL HISTORY

Note: The categories in sections IX to XIII focus mainly on adult subjects.

A. Vocational training (chronology of vocational training schools attended, courses taken, apprenticeships served, workshops, etc., noting: Training Facility and Address; Dates Attended; Courses Taken; Proficiency; Why Left)

B. Training center reports

C. Special aptitudes

D. Work history
 1. Jobs held while in school (part-time, summer vacation, etc.)
 2. Jobs held since leaving school (Employer Name and Address; Dates Employed; Type of Job; How Obtained; Salary; Why Left)

E. Occupational Preferences and Goals
 1. Of subject
 2. Of family

F. Occupational adjustment problems: inadequate vocational preparation   lack of required skills   insufficient knowledge of occupational world   communication problems   scholastic retardations   unrealistic goals   lack of adaptability   low frustration tolerance   immature attitudes   poor interpersonal relations   health problems   other

G. Reports from employers

H. Economic status

Source of Support	*Occasional*	*Usual*	*Current*	*Weekly Amount*
Salary				
Parents				
Relatives				
Spouse				
Public Assistance				
Other (specify)				

Informant(s)

X. MARITAL ROLE AND PREFERENCES

A. Current marital status: never married   married   separated
widowed   divorced

B. If never married, reason:

C. If marriage contemplated, preferred auditory status of spouse

D. If marriage contemplated, preferred auditory status and sex of children:

E. If currently or previously married
1. Reason for choice
2. Reason if separated or divorced
3. Marital and sexual adjustments and preferences
4. Concept of parent role
5. Economic and family management role
6. Intrafamily relations and attitudes

Informant(s)

XI. SOCIAL INTERESTS AND PARTICIPATION

A. Preferred activities and role
1. Social clubs   member   leader   officeholder   Club names
2. Athletic clubs   member   leader   officeholder   Club names
3. Civic clubs   member   leader   officeholder   Club names
4. Churchgoer
5. Visiting/entertaining friends
6. Movies
7. Card-playing
8. Hobbies (specify)
9. Family events
10. Other
11. No social affiliations

B. Preferred social groups: deaf   hearing   no special preferences

C. Use of telephonic devices (specify)

Informant(s)

XII. SELF-CONCEPT AND ATTITUDES

A. Attitudes toward
1. Deafness
2. Deaf persons
3. Hearing society

B. Concept of self in relation to
1. Others (deaf and hearing)
2. Ambitions, frustrations
3. Assets, liabilities
4. Current problems

C. Insight and judgment in self-evaluation
Informant(s)

XIII. CHECKLISTS OF PSYCHIATRIC SIGNS AND ANTISOCIAL BEHAVIORS

A. Psychiatric signs
Bizarre motor behavior and stances
Thinking and judgment disorders
Mood swings and disturbances
Disorientation: time   place   persons
Phobias, compulsions, obsessions
Ideas of reference   persecution   unreality   sin   guilt
other
Hallucinations: auditory   visual   olfactory   somatic
Memory disorders
Other
Descriptive summary:

B. Antisocial behaviors
Begging
Stealing
Assaultive
Arson
Sex offenses
Addictions
Other
Descriptive summary:

C. Commitment history
1. Psychiatric (note date and place of commitment; by whom; diagnosis; prognosis; date of release; name, address of attending psychiatrist)
2. Prison (note offending act; date of arrest; sentence imposed and

place served; probations; name and address of lawyers and pro-
bation officer; name and address of interpreter)
Informant(s)

XIV. PSYCHOLOGICAL EVALUATIONS

Note: Section XIV includes all subjects of all chronological ages.

A. Intelligence
  1. As indicated by mental test performance (report mental test his-
     tory, where possible under: Date Tested; Test Used; Test Scores;
     Estimated Validity; Method of Administration; Tested by)
  2. As estimated by:

  Learning ability   exceptional   above average   average
                              below average
  Family reports   exceptional   above average   average
                              below average
  Academic level   exceptional   above average   average
                              below average
  Occupation   exceptional   above average   average
                              below average
  Social activities   exceptional   above average   average
                              below average
  Play activities (child)   exceptional   above average   average
                              below average
  Interview   exceptional   above average   average
                              below average
  Observation   exceptional   above average   average
                              below average

  Other
  Remarks
  Informant(s)

B. Personality
  1. As indicated by personality testing (report personality test history
     under: Date Tested; Test Used; Test Results—Diagnostic Impres-
     sion; Estimated Validity; Method of Administration; Tested by)
  2. As indicated by:
     School reports
     Family
     Employer
     Social role
     Marital adjustment
     Antisocial behavior
     Psychiatric history

Interview
Observation
Other
Remarks
Informant(s)

C. Achievement and Special Aptitudes/Abilities
1. As indicated by achievement and aptitude testing (report separately test history under: Date Tested; Test Used; Test Results; Estimated Validity; Method of Administration; Tested by)
2. As indicated by
Classroom performance
Teachers' judgments
Demonstrated aptitudes in job-samples, hobbies, etc.
Other
3. Age/grade achievement ratio   retarded   average   accelerated
Remarks
Informant(s)

D. List other tests administered as for cerebral dysfunction, visual motor/perceptual coordination, color blindness, etc., noting: Date Tested; Test Used; Test Findings; Validity Criterion; Method of Administration; Tested by)
Remarks

XV. SUMMARY OF DATA

XVI. DIAGNOSTIC IMPRESSION

XVII. RECOMMENDATIONS

APPENDIX G

Psychological Report Form

I have found the following form useful in reporting on hearing-impaired subjects.

PSYCHOLOGICAL REPORT

Date of Report:
Date-span of Examination:
Reported by:

Name
Address
Birth date   Sex
(Other identifying data as required by setting)

Audio-communicative Frame of Examination

Hearing Loss
    Age of onset: Cause:
    Current status: Right -   Left -
    Use of hearing aid:
    Deafness in family (specify):

Favored Communication Method(s) (check)
Speech	Examiner-Rating: good	fair	poor
Lipreading	Examiner-Rating: good	fair	poor
Ameslan	Examiner-Rating: good	fair	poor
Fingerspelling	Examiner-Rating: good	fair	poor
Writing	Examiner-Rating: good	fair	poor

Other (specify)
No substantive method

Communication Method(s) Used in Examination
    (including use of interpreter):

Scholastic Status
  Current reading level:
  Current arithmetic level:
  Writing proficiency:

Other Handicapping Conditions (visual, motor, etc.)

Reason for Referral

Statement of reason/description of presenting problem
Referred by: Date:

Previous Psychological Referrals
Note dates, reasons for referral, significant findings, examiner, treatment

---

Present Psychological Examination

I. Psychological Testing   Inclusive Dates:

  Test   Test results/scores   Estimated validity

  A. Intelligence
  B. Personality
  C. Achievement
  D. Interest/Aptitudes
  E. Other (specify)
  Interpretation of test findings by behavior area examined

II. Case History (note significant data)

III. Interview (communication method; general reactions; significant
    data)

IV. Observation (note significant data and general impressions)

Analysis of Total Examination
Narrative summary of integrated findings including a summary of major
psychological strengths, weaknesses, pathological signs, etc. Note also
any special examination problems.

Implications for Habilitation/Rehabilitation
Describe special needs as indicated by psychological examination

---

Recommendations

Examiner(s) _____

APPENDIX H

Questionnaire Used in Survey of Psychological Tests and Practices with the Deaf

EXPLORATIONS IN THE PSYCHOLOGY OF DEAFNESS
Project of the Social and Rehabilitation Service
New York University

Date _____   Agency _____

_____

QUESTIONNAIRE
Psychological Testing
of
Children and Adults with Early Severe Deafness *

I. SETTING
   A. Type (Check which.)
      1. Educational setting
         a. special school for the deaf: residential   _____
            day   _____
         b. regular school, special class for deaf   _____
         c. regular school, hearing-handicapped totally in-
            tegrated   _____
         d. higher education setting (specify type)   _____
         e. other (specify) _____   _____

*Different facilities use different terms to designate this particular population. Two of the terms are used interchangeably in this questionnaire. They are "deaf" and "hearing handicapped." *Both refer to individuals whose hearing loss is so severe and of such early onset as to require special educational techniques or special tutorial services for the acquisition and/or development of speech and language.*

2. Rehabilitation setting
   a. for deaf only   ____
   b. special unit for deaf   ____
   c. generic services, no special unit for deaf   ____
   d. other (specify type) _____ ____
3. Speech and hearing center in:
   a. hospital   ____
   b. university   ____
   c. service agency   ____
   d. other (specify type)   ____
4. Other type of setting (specify type)   ____

B. Number Served
What is the approximate total of hearing handicapped individuals served in your work setting for the past 12 months?

C. Eligibility Requirements
What, if any, are the eligibility criteria used in your work setting for accepting and serving a hearing handicapped individual? ____

II. CLIENTELE
  A. Descriptive Terminology
    1. What criteria does your work setting use in designating a client as "deaf"? _____

    2. If your work setting does not use the term "deaf", what substitute term and criteria are used? _____

  B. Chronological Distribution
What rough percentage breakdown best describes the age range of the hearing handicapped served in your setting in the past 12 months?
    1. below 2 years   ____
    2. 3–5 years   ____
    3. 6–12 years   ____
    4. 13–16 years   ____
    5. 17–25 years   ____
    6. 26–40 years   ____
    7. over 40 years   ____

  C. Predominant Test-Age
In which age range is the greatest proportion of psychological testing done with the hearing handicapped in your work setting?

D. Predominant Communication Methods
What is the predominant form of expressive communication (speech, fingerspelling, sign language) used in daily life by the respective age levels tested in your work setting?

Age level	Form of communication

III. PSYCHOLOGICAL TESTER: GENERAL INFORMATION
A. Staff Position
Which of the following best describes your present activities (check):
1. Full-time psychological worker _____
   a. Exclusively for hearing handicapped _____
   b. Hearing handicapped part of total case load _____
2. Part-time psychological worker (specify time) _____
   a. Exclusively for hearing handicapped _____
   b. Hearing handicapped part of total case load _____
3. Consultant psychological worker (specify time) _____
   a. Exclusively for hearing handicapped _____
   b. Hearing handicapped part of total case load _____
4. Other (specify) _____

B. Responsibilities
1. Check those of the following that are part of your job responsibilities relative to the hearing handicapped:
   a. Individual psychological testing _____
   b. Group psychological testing _____
   c. Psychological counseling _____
   d. Educational advisement _____
   e. Vocational testing _____
   f. Vocational advisement _____
   g. Remedial therapy (tutoring, learning problems, etc) _____
   h. Parent/family counseling _____
   i. Staff inservice training _____
   j. Case follow-up _____
   k. Staff conferences re the hearing handicapped _____
   l. Research _____
   m. Other (specify) _____
2. Which of the above letters (a,b,c, etc.) represent your job responsibilities relative to the non-hearing handicapped? (If "m" to designate "other" is included, please specify.) _____

3. In regard to psychological testing:
   a. About how many hearing handicapped individuals do you test per month? ＿＿＿
   b. About how many *individual* psychological tests do you administer per month to these clients? ＿＿＿
   c. What types of tests are routinely administered to most hearing handicapped clientele (check):
      (1) individual intelligence ＿＿＿
      (2) group intelligence ＿＿＿
      (3) achievement ＿＿＿
      (4) personality ＿＿＿
      (5) vocational ＿＿＿
      (6) other (specify)＿＿＿＿＿＿＿＿＿＿＿＿＿＿＿＿＿＿
   d. What is the average amount of time you allocate for a routine test work-up of a hearing handicapped individual? ＿＿＿
   e. What in your opinion are the major difficulties in testing hearing handicapped subjects?

   _____

   _____

   _____

C. Background
   1. Educational
      a. highest degree ＿＿＿＿＿＿ date earned ＿＿＿＿＿
      b. major and minor subjects ＿＿＿＿＿＿＿＿＿＿＿＿
      c. If a dissertation was written, please give title.

      _____

      d. name of college or university granting degree

      _____

   2. Organization Membership
      Please name professional organizations of which you are a member; also certificates, licenses, boards, etc.

      _____

      _____

   3. Specialty
      In which specialty is your major professional affiliation? (Check)
      a. rehabilitation counseling ＿＿＿
      b. special education (deaf) ＿＿＿
      c. speech therapy ＿＿＿
      d. audiology ＿＿＿
      e. psychology: clinical＿＿ school＿＿ counseling＿＿ educational＿＿
      f. other (specify)＿＿＿＿＿＿＿＿＿＿＿＿＿＿＿＿＿＿

4. Professional Experience
Indicate the number of years of salaried experience in:
a. your major specialty   ____
b. psychological testing of non-hearing handicapped   ____
c. psychological testing of hearing handicapped   ____
d. other work with hearing handicapped (specify work)   ____

5. Personal Experience with Deafness
Indicate personal experiences with deafness preceding professional practice with hearing handicapped (check):
a. personal hearing loss   ____
b. deaf parents   ____
c. deaf children (own)   ____
d. deaf siblings   ____
e. (other) deaf relatives   ____
f. other experiences (specify)_____

g. no previous experience   ____

6. Communication Resources
a. Rate your ability to use the sign language:
excellent___ good ___ fair___ poor ___ none___
b. Rate your ability to read back sign language:
excellent___ good ___ fair___ poor ___ none___
c. Check the main communication resource(s) you use in testing the deaf: speech ___ writing___ fingerspelling___ interpreter___ sign language ___ other _____

7. Special Preparation
Describe briefly the kind of special preparation you had for testing the deaf (on the job; special courses; special program; practicum; etc.); the type of supervision; the setting; and other relevant information and recommendations
_____
_____
_____
_____
_____

IV. SPECIFIC TESTS USED WITH DEAF/HEARING HANDICAPPED CLIENTELE

A. DIRECTIONS

The aim of this section is to find out what tests are being used with the above population, and to get some idea of why the tests being used were selected.

In filling out the following data-collection form, respondents are asked to do the following:

Name of test—Please supply full identifying title of test. For example, if only the performance portion of the WAIS is used, then fill in with WAIS Perf.; or if a test has several forms, identify the one you are reporting.

Used for Age Range—Please supply the age range for which *you* use the test.

Factors Influencing Selection—To get this information within the time/space limits of a questionnaire, we are supplying a numbered list of factors that might possibly influence test selection. The list is by no means comprehensive, but it provides a jumping off function. Here are some of the possible influencing factors:

1. Relative ease of administering the test
2. No particular problems in scoring
3. Takes a relatively short time
4. Recommended by others who test the deaf
5. Recommended in the literature
6. Results of the test closely reflect subject's real life behavior
7. Test results have good predictive value
8. Test manual indicates high validity and reliability coefficients
9. Particular test is requested by work-setting
10. Other—respond in comment form

In answering this section, just put the numeral(s) indicating the factors most important in *your* selection as designated in the above listing. Where other factors are involved that are not in the listing, please write them in.

Comments—all relevant remarks are welcome. (Please use extra sheets as required.) Of particular importance is your evaluative judgment of the test as an instrument for the hearing handicapped, i.e. excellent, good, fair, poor, or other evaluative statement.

B. INSTRUMENTS

1. *Individual Intelligence Tests*

	Used with	Principal Factors	
Name of Test *	Age Range *	Influencing Selection *	Comments

2. Group Intelligence Tests

Name of Test	*	Used with Age Range	*	Principal Factors Influencing Selection	*	Comments

3. Personality Tests and Techniques

Name of Test	*	Used with Age Range	*	Principal Factors Influencing Selection	*	Comments

4. Achievement Tests

Name of Test	*	Used with Age Range	*	Principal Factors Influencing Selection	*	Comments

5. Vocational Aptitudes, Interests, Abilities

Name of Test	*	Used with Age Range	*	Principal Factors Influencing Selection	*	Comments

6. *Other Psychological Tests*

Name of Test	*	Used with Age Range	*	Principal Factors Influencing Selection	*	Comments

C. REPORTING OF TEST RESULTS

How are your test results on the hearing handicapped generally reported? (check all that apply)
1. recorded on cumulative record   ————
2. reported to parents   ————
3. discussed with testee   ————
4. discussed at staff conferences   ————
5. other (specify) ————————————————————

D. USE OF TEST RESULTS

How are the test results used? (check all that apply)
1. in educational planning   ————
2. in vocational training   ————
3. to screen applicants for school admission   ————
4. to establish eligibility for service   ————
5. in differential diagnosis   ————
6. as basis for referral to special workers   ————
   (remedial therapists, psychiatrists, etc.)
7. other (specify) ————————————————————

V. REMARKS, COMMENTS, RECOMMENDATIONS ON ANY ASPECT OF PSYCHOLOGICAL TESTING OF THE DEAF/HEARING IMPAIRED:

TO THE PSYCHOLOGICAL WORKER: THE FOLLOWING IDENTIFYING IN-FORMATION IS OPTIONAL. WHERE PROVIDED, CONFIDENTIALITY IS ASSURED.

Name _____ Address _____ Zip _____

APPENDIX I

A Guide to Test Publishers and Distributors

Tests appearing in this listing are selected from those cited in the sections on psychological and developmental testing. The name of the test is given in the first column of the listing; the source from which it may be ordered, in the second column. For addresses of the publishers/distributors mentioned, see Appendix H. To keep abreast of changes that occur in the test publishing/distributing market, the reader should consult current psychological test catalogues; and for details and reviews of the tests, the Buros *Mental Measurements Yearbooks*.

Title	Publisher/Distributor
INTELLIGENCE TESTS AND DEVELOPMENTAL SCALES	
Standardized on the Deaf	
Drever-Collins Performance Tests of Intelligence: A Series of Non-Linguistic Tests for Deaf and Normal Children	"out of print" (Buros); Originally: A. H. Baird (test materials) Oliver & Boyd (manual)
Hiskey-Nebraska Test of Learning Aptitude for Young Deaf Children	Marshall S. Hiskey
Ontario School Ability Examination	"out of print" (Buros) Originally: Ryerson Press
Snidjers & Snidjers-Comen Non-Verbal Intelligence Tests for Deaf and Hearing Subjects	Swets and Zeitlinger B.V.
Smith-Johnson Nonverbal Performance Scale	Western Psychological Services
Not Standardized on the Deaf	
Arthur Adaptation of the Leiter International Performance Scale	Stoelting
Bayley Scales of Infant Development	Psychological Corporation

Title	Publisher/Distributor
Cattell Infant Intelligence Scale	Psychological Corporation
Chicago Non-Verbal Examination	Out of print
Columbia Mental Maturity Scale	Harcourt Brace Jovanovich
Gesell Developmental Schedules	Examining material: Mr. Nigel Cox; and Albany Medical College
Goodenough-Harris Drawing Test	Harcourt Brace Jovanovich
Leiter International Performance Scale	Stoelting
Merrill-Palmer Scale of Mental Tests	Stoelting
Non-Language Multi-Mental Scale	Teachers College Press
Porteus Maze Tests	Psychological Corporation
Raven Progressive Matrices	Psychological Corporation
Revised Beta Examination, 2nd ed. (Beta II)	Psychological Corporation
Wechsler Adult Intelligence Scale (WAIS)	Psychological Corporation
Wechsler Intelligence Scale for Children, Revised (WISC-R)	Psychological Corporation
Wechsler Preschool and Primary Scale of Intelligence (WPPSI)	Psychological Corporation

PERSONALITY INSTRUMENTS

Personality Inventories

Minnesota Multiphasic Personality Inventory (MMPI)	Psychological Corporation
Sixteen Personality Factor Questionnaire (16 PF)	Institute for Personality and Ability Testing

Social Maturity

Vineland Social Maturity Scale	American Guidance Service

Projective Techniques

Children's Apperception Test (CAT)	CPS, Inc.
Hand Test	Western Psychological Services
House-Tree-Person Projective Technique (H-T-P)	Western Psychological Services
Impulse, Ego, Superego Test (IES)	Psychological Test Specialists
Kinetic Family Drawings	Brunner/Mazel
Machover Draw-a-Person Test	Charles C. Thomas
Make-a-Picture Story (MAPS)	Psychological Corporation
Missouri Children's Picture Series	Jacob O. Sines
Rorschach Technique	Grune & Stratton
Rotter Incomplete Sentences Blank	Psychological Corporation
Symonds Picture-Story Test	Teachers College Press

Title	Publisher/Distributor
Thematic Apperception Test (TAT)	Harvard University Press
Children's Play-Kit Projective Techniques	(Consult test catalogues)

Rating-Assessment Inventory

Meadow-Kendall Social-Emotional Assessment Inventory for Deaf Students	Gallaudet College

ACHIEVEMENT TESTS
General Scholastic

California Achievement Tests	CTB/McGraw-Hill
Metropolitan Achievement Tests	Harcourt Brace Jovanovich
Stanford Achievement Test	Harcourt Brace Jovanovich
Stanford Achievement Test for Hearing Impaired Students	Gallaudet College
Wide Range Achievement Test (WRAT)	Guidance Associates of Delaware

Diagnostic

Picture Story Language Test (Myklebust)	Grune & Stratton
Test of Syntactic Abilities (Quigley et al.)	Dormac, Inc.

Special Areas and Subjects

Carrow Elicited Language Inventory	
Carrow Tests for Auditory Comprehension of Language	Learning Concepts
Costello Speechreading Tests	Doctoral Dissertation by M. R. Costello, "A Study in Speechreading as a Developing Language Process in Deaf and in Hard of Hearing Children," Northwestern University, 1957. Cited in J. Jeffers, and M. Barley, *Speechreading.* Charles C. Thomas, 1971.
Gates-MacGinitie Reading Tests	Teachers College Press
Gray Oral Reading Tests	Bobbs-Merrill
Houston Test for Language Development	Houston Test Co.
Illinois Test of Psycholinguistic Abilities	University of Illinois Press
REEL (Bzoch-League Receptive-Expressive Emergent Language Scale)	Tree of Life Press
Utah Test of Language Development	Communication Research Associates

VOCATIONAL INTERESTS/APTITUDES

Bennett Hand-Tool Dexterity Test	Psychological Corporation
Computer Program Aptitude Battery	Science Research Associates

Title	Publisher/Distributor
Geist Picture Interest Inventory (Hearing and Deaf Forms)	Western Psychological Services
Graves Design Judgment Test	Psychological Corporation
Kuder Occupational Interest Survey	Science Research Associates
MacQuarrie Test for Mechanical Ability	CTB/McGraw-Hill
Manipulative Aptitude Test	Western Psychological Services
Minnesota Clerical Test	Psychological Corporation
Picture Interest Inventory (Weingarten)	CTB/McGraw-Hill
Purdue Pegboard	Science Research Associates
Revised Minnesota Paper Form-Board	Psychological Corporation
Short Employment Tests (The)	Psychological Corporation
SRA Pictorial Reasoning Test	Science Research Associates
Strong-Campbell Interest Inventory	Psychological Corporation
Vocational Interest and Sophistication Assessment (VISA)	Joseph J. Parnicky
Wide Range Interest-Opinion Test (WRIOT)	Jastak Associates
Work Sample Evaluation Program (Jewish Employment and Vocational Service)	Vocational Research Institute, Jewish Employment and Vocational Service

SPECIAL CLINICAL TESTS

Bender Visual-Motor Gestalt Test	Psychological Corporation
Benton Revised Visual Retention Test	Psychological Corporation
Dvorine Color Vision Test	Psychological Corporation
Farnsworth Dichotomous Test for Color Blindness	Psychological Corporation
Frostig Developmental Test of Visual Perception	Consulting Psychologists Press
Harris Tests of Lateral Dominance	Psychological Corporation
Hooper Visual Organization Test	Western Psychological Services
Lincoln-Oseretsky Motor Development Scale	Stoelting

OTHER CITED INSTRUMENTS

(*Note:* where examiners use the following with deaf subjects, they are generally used in part and for purposes other than originally intended)

Peabody Picture Vocabulary Test	American Guidance Service
Detroit Tests of Learning Aptitude	Bobbs-Merrill
Handicap Problems Inventory	University Book Store
Communicative Evaluation Chart from Infancy to Five Years	Educators Publishing Service

APPENDIX J

Publisher and Distributor Directory

Albany Medical College, Albany, New York 12208

American Guidance Service, Inc., Publishers' Building, Circle Pines, Minnesota 55014

A. H. Baird, 33–39 Lothian Street, Edinburgh, Scotland

Bobbs-Merrill Co., Inc. 4300 West 62nd Street, Indianapolis, Indiana 46268

Brunner/Mazel, Inc., 19 Union Square W., New York, N.Y. 10003

CPS, Inc., Box 83, Larchmont, N.Y. 10538

CTB/McGraw-Hill, Del Monte Research Park, Monterey, California 93940

Communication Research Associates, Inc., Box 11012, Salt Lake City, Utah 84111

Consulting Psychologists Press, Inc., 577 College Avenue, Palo Alto, Calif. 94306

Dormac, Inc., Box 752, Beaverton, Oregon 97005

Educators Publishing Service, Inc., 97 Hodge Ave., Buffalo, N.Y. 14222

Gallaudet College, Office of Demographic Studies, Washington, D.C. 20002

Grune & Stratton, Inc., 111 Fifth Avenue, New York, N.Y. 10003

Guidance Associates of Delaware, Inc., 1526 Gilpin Avenue, Wilmington, Delaware 19806

Harcourt Brace Jovanovich, Inc., 757 Third Avenue, New York, N.Y. 10017

Harvard University Press, 79 Garden Street, Cambridge, Massachusetts 02138

Houston Test Company, Box 35152, Houston, Texas 72035

Institute for Personality and Ability Testing, 1602 Coronado Drive, Champaign, Illinois 61820

Jastak Associates, Inc., 1526 Gilpin Avenue, Wilmington, Delaware 19806

Learning Concepts, 2501 N. Lamar, Austin, Texas 78705

Marshall Hiskey, 5640 Baldwin, Lincoln, Nebraska 68508

Nigel Cox, 69 Fawn Drive, Cheshire, Connecticut 06410

Oliver & Boyd, 14 High Street, Edinburgh, Scotland

Parnicky (Joseph J.) Nisonger Center, Ohio State University, 1580 Cannon Drive, Columbus, Ohio 43210

Psychological Corporation, 757 Third Avenue, New York, New York 10017

Psychological Test Specialists, Box 9229, Missoula, Montana 59801

Ryerson Press, 299 Queen Street, West Toronto, Ontario, Canada

Science Research Associates, Inc., 259 E. Erie Street, Chicago, Illinois 60611

Jacob O. Sines, Box 1031, Iowa City, Iowa 52240

Stoelting Company, 1350 S. Kostner Avenue, Chicago, Illinois 60623

Swets and Zeitlinger B.V., Keizersgracht 487, Amsterdam C., The Netherlands

Teachers College Press, 1234 Amsterdam Avenue, New York, N.Y. 10027

Tree of Life Press, 1309 N.E. Second Street, Box 447, Gainesville, Florida 32601

Charles C. Thomas, 327 East Lawrence Avenue, Springfield, Illinois 62703

University of Illinois Press, Urbana, Illinois 61801

University Book Store, 360 State Street, West Lafayette, Indiana 47906

Vocational Research Institute, Jewish Employment and Vocational Service, 1624 Locust Street, Philadelphia, Pennsylvania 19103

Western Psychological Services, 12031 Wilshire Boulevard, Los Angeles, California 90025

APPENDIX K

Information Directories and References

The guides in this Appendix have been selected for their comprehensive yet concise coverage of their respective areas.

Guides to Periodicals and Articles

Ulrich's International Periodicals Directory. This R. R. Bowker annual publication, found in the reference section of most libraries, contains entries for over 60,000 periodicals (as of 1980) from all over the world on some 250 subject areas, including communication, environment, ecology, language, deaf, and other special areas mentioned in this book. Periodicals specifically relevant to "deaf" are included under such headings as: Deaf, Special Education and Rehabilitation, Social Services and Welfare, Medical Sciences. The following information is provided for each periodical in the *Directory.*

1. Name of publication, including translated title, subtitle, title change.
2. Sponsoring organization.
3. Language used in text.
4. Year first published.
5. Frequency.
6. Annual subscription price in country of origin and U.S. rate.
7. Name of editor.
8. Name and address of publishing company.
9. Other details relevant to a particular periodical.

American Annals of the Deaf: April Reference Issue. Founded in 1847, *American Annals of the Deaf* (5034 Wisconsin Ave., N.W., Washington, D.C. 20016) is the official organ of the Conference of Executives of American Schools for the Deaf, and The Convention of American Instructors of the Deaf. The names of selected periodicals relevant to deafness are published annually in the *Annals'* April Reference issue.

dsh ABSTRACTS (Gallaudet College, Washington, D.C. 20002). *dsh ABSTRACTS* is a contribution of Deafness Speech and Hearing Publications, Inc., and prints brief, noncritical summaries of the literature published in all major languages and pertinent to deafness, speech, and hearing. The broad categories covered are: Hearing; Hearing Disorders; Speech; Speech Disorders; and General. The literature summarized in the category Hearing Disorders includes: diagnosis and appraisal; education; etiology and pathology; hearing aids; hearing conservation and noise; medical and surgical treatment; multiple handicaps; psychological factors; social and legal factors; speechreading and manual communication; vestibular system, normal and pathological.

Bibliography on Deafness: A Selected Index. This unique and valuable reference tool was first published in 1966 by the Alexander Graham Bell Association for the Deaf, Inc. (3417 Volta Place, N.W., Washington, D.C. 20007) and has had several supplementary publications since then. Under the editorship of George W. Fellendorf, it marks the first appearance of a cumulative index of significant articles that had appeared in the field's two major periodicals—*The Volta Review* (the Association's official journal), and *The American Annals of the Deaf*—since they began publication, the *Annals* in 1847 and *The Volta Review* in 1899. An invaluable resource for researchers, the *Bibliography,* indexed by subject and author, offers all its users a superb view of developments and perspectives over the course of time to the present.

Guide to Facilities, Services, Programs, Research

American Annals of the Deaf: April Reference Issue. This invaluable *Annals* volume accomplishes the exhaustive feat of providing "who, what, where" information about facilities, services, programs, and research involving the deaf throughout the United States. Its contents are so exquisitely organized that the user is apt to overlook the tremendous quantity of information contained; but there it is when needed.

The *Deaf American* is the official monthly publication of the National Association of the Deaf with its editorial offices at 6374 Kingswood Drive, Indianapolis, Indiana 46256. This journal publishes a wide variety of timely information such as Church and Club directories, in-depth stories and advertisements of special interest to its deaf readers and to professional workers with the deaf.

AUTHOR INDEX

SUBJECT INDEX

Machover Draw-a-Person Test (Machover Figure Drawing), 279, 280, 281
Mainstreaming, 125-30; helping non-deaf children understand the deaf, 45
Make-a-Picture Story (MAPS), 187-88, 279, 280, 282
Maladjustments of the deaf, see Emotional disturbances and maladjustments in the hearing impaired
Mandated planning and accountability, in education of the handicapped, 120-22, 231
Manipulative Aptitude Test, 299, 300
Man-made physical environment, 7, 9-10
Manual Alphabet, 90, 359
Manual communication methods, 131-32, 134, 136, 137, 156; in interviews with adults, 332-33; see also Sign language
Manual English, 102
Manually coded English, 102-4
MAPS, see Make-a-Picture Story
Maquarrie Test for Mechanical Ability, 299
MCPS, see Missouri Children's Picture Series
Meadow, Kathryn P., 285
Meadow-Kendall Social-Emotional Inventory for Deaf Students, 285
Meaning-equivalence of similar concepts in different communication modes, 137
Measurement of Adult Intelligence, The (Wechsler), 231
Media Services, Division of, U.S. Office of Education, see Division of Media Services
Memorizing, in verbal language acquisition by deaf: syntax, 74-81; words and meanings, 71-74
Mental ability: nature-nurture controversy, 5; see also Intelligence; I.Q.
Mental Health Center for the Deaf, New York State Psychiatric Institute, 177, 215
Mental health of the deaf, 31-32, 143; see also Emotional disturbances and maladjustments in the hearing impaired
Mental Measurement Yearbook (Buros), 266, 269
Mental testing, 270-79; see also Intelligence tests
Merrill-Palmer Scale of Mental Tests, 271, 272, 292
Methodical Signs, 100-2
Methods controversy, in education of the deaf, 120, 130-32, 135-38, 140, 144

Metropolitan Achievement Tests, 287-88
Michael Reese Hospital, Chicago, Illinois, Psychosomatic and Psychiatric Institute of, 196
Milieu, in ecological psychology theory, 8
Miller, Mary Beth, 92
Minnesota Clerical Test, 299, 328
Minnesota Multiphasic Personality Inventory (MMPI), 198, 280-81, 282, 285, 286
Missouri Children's Picture Series (MCPS), 189
Mixed deafness, 358
MMPI, see Minnesota Multiphasic Personality Inventory
Monroe Inspection Technique, 186
Motion pictures, captioned, see Captioned films
Motivations of the deaf, 186
Motor development test, Lincoln-Oseretsky, 290
Motor dysfunctions, observation of, 302
Mouth-Hand System of cued lipreading, 88
Muller-Walle method of lipreading instruction, 88
Multidisciplinary message-exchange, communication problems in, 341
Multimodal communication, see Total communication
Multisensory speech-teaching approach, 82-83
Music, psychological effects of, 20

National Association of the Deaf (NAD), 169, 176, 178, 216, 402
National Fraternal Society of the Deaf, 173
National Theatre of the Deaf, 44-45
Natural environment, 7
Nature-nurture controversy, 5
Nebraska Test of Learning Aptitude for Young Deaf Children, 212, 270
Neolithic Revolution, 10
Neurotic traits in the deaf, see Emotional disturbances and maladjustments in the hearing impaired
New England Association of the Deaf, 176
New York League for the Hard of Hearing: selected appraisal programs, 291-98, 326-28
New York State Department of Education, 214
New York State Psychiatric Institute: Department of Medical Genetics, 195, 196; Mental Health Center for the Deaf, 177, 215